Fengli Lan
Metaphor

LIBRI NIGRI

47

Edited by

Hans Rainer Sepp

The *libri nigri* series will be edited at the Central-European Institute of Philosophy, Prague.
www.sif-praha.cz

Fengli Lan

Metaphor
The Weaver of Chinese Medicine

With an Introduction by
Friedrich Wallner

Verlag Traugott Bautz GmbH

Bibliografische Information der Deutschen Nationalbibliothek

Die deutsche Bibliothek verzeichnet diese Publikation
in der Deutschen Nationalbibliografie.
Detaillierte bibliografische Daten sind im Internet abrufbar über
http://dnb.ddb.de

Verlag Traugott Bautz GmbH
D-99734 Nordhausen 2015

Gedruckt auf säurefreiem, alterungsbeständigem Papier

Printed in Germany

ISBN 978-3-95948-020-8

Table of Contents

7 Metaphorizing: A Vital Way to Understand the Human Being

8 Number Metaphors for Constructing the Theoretical System of Chinese Medicine

9 Metaphorizing: A Vital Way to Understand and Modernize Chinese Herbal Medicine

10 Metaphorizing:
A Vital Way to Understand the Concept of Health and Disease

List of Tables

List of Illustrations

Introduction

Metaphor: The Weaver of Chinese Medicine

I am very happy and proud about this book. Because with this book, we execute a radical change in the research on Chinese medicine. But this change inherits dangers of misunderstanding which can be fundamental and destroy the message of this book. Therefore I want to give some hints for correct understanding beforehand. There are two aspects you should consider right from the beginning: The philosophy of Constructive Realism and the role of language in classical China.

The Constructive Realism has shown that Western science is a special case of science. This means other scientific structuralisations are possible and have been already, more or less, realized: The emergence of a specific science is always dependent from a specific culture. Science is always a radicalization of the convictions and implicit presuppositions of a specific culture. The Chinese medicine is a perfect example for such a realization.

The approach of Constructive Realism to compare different sciences is guided by three main ideas: To consider the differences between those sciences, to express their typical way of thinking and to be aware of the peculiarities of these ways of thinking. These three ideas implicate that there are different ways of structuring our knowledge possible and that several already existing besides each other. Those different sciences have emerged out of different ways of thinking, each with their own peculiarities, presuppositions and methods (methodologies). Although incompatible they can coexist next to each other without at least one of them necessarily being wrong. The reason that this is possible can be found in the understanding of science Constructive Realism has developed. Especially in its ontology.

The term "ontology" refers in this context to the relation between science and its object. On the one hand we have scientific theories, which can be seen as proposition-systems. These proposition-systems do not describe their objects; they tell us how to handle the data we get about those objects. The data on the other hand is produced in accordance with the theory (not a specific theory, but the according parts of the theoretical background of the discipline at stake). In order to generate the data it is necessary to focus on certain qualities of the object and exclude others. Which qualities are relevant we are told by the proposition-systems (or theories). With theory and data microworlds – as Constructive Realism calls it – are constructed by reducing the qualities of our world. This leads to the main dichotomy in Constructive Realism: that between "Wirklichkeit" and "Realität". Realität is the dimension of the microworlds – which are constructed by the systematization of certain and the exclusion of other qualities. Wirklichkeit is what is presupposed in this process – the world we live in. The relation between Wirklichkeit and Realität is that of reduction and of reference as well. This understanding of science as a reductive reference is open to the possibility of several ways to refer to the world by selecting different qualities your microworlds are reduced to. This explains how sciences can differ from each other without contradiction.

The main method Constructive Realism has developed to compare these different sciences is strangification. It is based on the idea that scientific theories are systems of propositions which are based on presuppositions. These presuppositions mark the conditions under which the propositions are true. The presuppositions are not always explicit. In fact they rarely are. If we transfer propositions from one system to another the result will get absurd, because the presuppositions needed for these propositions to be true are not given in their new context. With this method we are able to identify the implicit presuppositions that a science is based on.

Only if we know both, these presuppositions, that are the conditions of truth of a scientific theory, and thereby know its epistemic limits, as well as know which qualities are reduced and not part of the microworld, and thereby know its limits of explanation, we can speak of knowledge, that goes beyond simple rule-following within the framework of the microworlds.

If we apply those ideas of Constructive Realism to Chinese medicine, the essential differences between Eastern and Western medicine, that explain their incompatibility, will become clear and possible misleads in researching Chinese medicine will be apparent to us, so we can avoid them. Those mistakes are:

- Looking for similarities. The differences are the key to understanding.
- Giving a scientific legitimation. Although it is possible, it is very destructive to a completely different way of thinking.
- Taking propositions from Chinese medicine out of their original context, without being aware doing so is performing a strangification. The results will very likely be absurd.
- Using terms loaded by Western science.
- Mistaking modern China for classical China.

The differences are:

- The concept of experience. The Western way is to eliminate subjectivity. The Chinese way is to embrace subjectivity. For instance it is common to always refer to the master who offers the experiences.
- The role of generality. In Western science generality is an important quality feature of a theory. The more general, the better. In languages this leads to the idea of universals – the most general concepts that are covering everything. In Chinese language generalizing is unusual. They have something different.
- Intermobiles (if you allow us to introduce this term in lack of fitting vocabulary). They do not abstract terms to more general terms, they connect aspects. It means to connect an object with different qualities and objects in order to achieve a better understanding.
- In China they do not have the body-mind problem.
- The concept of nature. The (historical and intellectual) basis of Western science is that the world has a beginning, that it was constructed, in the sense that it is working according to a construction plan, which means that it has rules. These convictions grew historically. In China they have developed a different concept.
- Holism. We have holism in the Western world, so its mere existence is not enough to pose a difference, but ours is of a different kind. It is the product of our way of reasoning. We are using inductions and go from single experiences to more general experiences. For Chinese medicine holism is the condition of thinking.
- Inductions are unusual in Chinese medicine.

These insights enable us to give you the following useful advices:

- Do not ask for theory, ask for networks.
- Look at the differences.
- Do not generalize.
- Look for examples instead of explanations.
- Try to reduce your position to an observer.

The Chinese medicine is the best historical example for the ideas and convictions of Constructive Realism. In difference to the Western medicine, which follows the concept of analyzing explains the parts. The Western science trusts more the last elements, while classical Chinese thinking is more concentrated to understand the whole. The search for the "last or indivisible elements" seems for the Westerner most important, in Chinese thinking the whole (which must not be identified with system or totality), is represented by a metaphor. Chinese medicine is based on pattern recognition. Looking for the essential the Western science loses the essence.

If you understand the word "metaphor" as we understand it in the Western world, then you have already lost the possibility to understand this book. In our world metaphor can be understood and used in a manifold way: poetical, didactically, indicating what cannot be said or explained (for example pain). In all this cases the use of a metaphor shows the borders of language. In our consciousness there is a contra position between language and reality. Language is somehow arbitrary, can be used like a game, can be easily changed or reformulated. The reality on the other hand we think as unavoidable, serious and solid. Language and reality are strictly divided in our common thinking and unreflected behavior. In classical China language and reality are in a specific way interwoven. They do not contra pone phenomena and reality; The reality does not become the judge for the truth of phenomena, but what is true, what is important and even what is real is decided in the frame of language. Reality appears in language.

The core method in Chinese medicine is *Qu Xiang Bi Lei*, which is completely different from Western thinking. Instead of causal connections the relations it forms can be seen as a type of phenomenology. Just by stating this, before even explaining what *Qu Xiang Bi Lei* is, it becomes evident that Chinese medicine and Western medicine are incommensurable. From what is said above we can add that they are so in four aspects: the methodology, the ontology, the concept of experience and their theoretical structure. As for the methodology *Qu Xiang Bi Lei* is, as we have just said, similar to the position of phenomenology. Instead of induction and deduction it lets the things come for themselves. So on the ontological level, where in the West we have ontological analysis, synthesis and abstraction, Chinese medicine leaves everything as it is. This leads to a different concept of experience. While to Western science it is crucial to keep subjectivity out of your work, traditional Chinese thinking is based on a unification of subjectivity and objectivity. And while the theoretical structure of Western science is that of rules and laws, Chinese science works via pattern recognition and interpretation. It is necessary to keep that in mind in order to understand the following explanation of *Qu Xiang Bi Lei*.

Xiang means image, imagining and elephant. Do not think about elephants, they are not the important point here. This puzzling combination of meanings has historical reasons. The essential point is that image and imagination are the same. In our culture's epistemology the subject is in opposition to the objects and therefore it is necessary to differ between what is really seen in an image and what is just imagination. In Chinese medicine this separation does not exist. Phenomena and Noumena are not divided. What can be seen is already real, not just possible reality. In Western thinking the classic question is about the reality behind what is seen, in classical China there is nothing behind the image. *Xiang* is not representation, it is (an offer of) reality. In Western thinking this would be unthinkable. The picture cannot replace the thing. In Chinese thinking it is the thing.

Let us continue with the explanation: *Qu Xiang* means taking image. It is based on direct experiences gained by observation. An image from the world is taken with the symbols it can bear, to reason from analogy in the way of a metaphor. Relationships between the objects are thereby expressed. *Qu Xiang* means observing *Xiang* and taking *Xiang*. *Bi Lei* means analogizing or reasoning from analogy. It is a process of thought that compares different things and finds the similarities between them, so that it is possible to infer knowledge from one to another.

Chinese thinking does not assume the difference between representation and reality, thus different possibilities of reality are reflected in *Xiang*. The linguistic counterpart of the image (*Xiang*) is the metaphor. At this point then importance of the metaphor in Chinese medicine becomes apparent. It is where reality appears. Like an image and unlike simple propositions a metaphor can offer more than one or two possibilities. If we have a variety of possibilities there must be a way to choose from them. This choice is determined by the intention of acting and the conditions to act out of. *Qu Xiang* is always bound to the possibilities of action. Chinese Medicine is not structured by causality, but by functionality.

Vienna, August 2014 — Friedrich G. Wallner

Author's Foreword

Wide-ranging heated debates between Chinese medicine and Western medicine, the rise of "Integrative Medicine with Chinese at Heart but Western Where Appropriate 医学衷中参西" in the early 20th century, and queries on validity and scienticity of Chinese medicine from some scholars in the world of today, as well as long-term application of Western scientific standards on judging Chinese medicine, all result in that "science" and "Chinese medicine" can not be mentioned in the same breath. Actually whether Chinese medicine is scientific or not depends on how you define "science". Be aware, science originally means "knowledge of any kind". Is Western science the only possible "scientific" approach? Does Chinese medicine have its own claim for truth?

It is not difficult to understand - the possibilities of perceiving the world are manifold, so there are many possible ways of selecting, excluding, and reducing the certain aspects of the analyzed object based on different cultures, and thus many corresponding resolutions. A scientific system can be considered as an artificial and constructed system of data and propositions, a constructed "microworld", a world that selects and reduces qualities of the object in certain aspects. Thus Chinese medicine also has a legitimate claim for truth without getting into contradiction with other different systems like Western medicine. It can also be incompatible with Western medicine for both have different ways of constructing their microworlds.[1]

Chinese medicine can be roughly classified into two parts: one part is the "Dao 道 or Way", i.e. the way of constructing the knowledge system, which needs to be understood based on its culture and philosophy; while the other is the "*Shu* 术 or Skill", i.e. its clinical application, which can be proved in rational ways and by proper methods. As the title goes, this book discusses Dao or Way of Chinese medicine: Metaphor as the weaver of Chinese medicine.

Qu Xiang Bi Lei 取象比类 or Taking Image and Analogizing is the core methodology of Chinese medicine. Its procedure as recorded in *The Book of Changes* – "Observing Object 观物 – Taking Image 取象 – Com-

1 Wallner, Friedrich. How to Research TCM. In Wallner F. G., Kubiena G., Jandl M.J. (eds). 2009: 22-45.

paring and Analogizing 比类 – Understanding Dao 体道" runs through almost all the aspects of Chinese medicine from forming its fundamental concepts, elaborating its theories, to developing its clinical explorations, and thus embodying the three key processes/elements of classical Chinese metaphor studies, i.e., "Imaging/Image 象 – Analogizing/Analogy 比 – Metaphorizing/Metaphor 喻", finally forming metaphors in Chinese medicine, guiding clinical practice, and developing Chinese medicine in both theoretical and clinical explorations. Based on these three key processes/elements, the author advances that *Qu Xiang Bi Lei* is the metaphorizing process and the way of forming metaphors in Chinese medicine, Chinese medicine is a linguistic knowledge system with metaphor as its deep structure, and that metaphor is the weaver of Chinese medicine.

In the recent years, studies on the essence, characteristics, methods, and principles of metaphors in Western scientific discourses have achieved important progress and gratifying outcome[2], but studies on metaphors in discourses of classical Chinese philosophy and science, which originated from *The Book of Changes*, are rarely seen. The significant difference of metaphors in discourses of Western science and Chinese medicine lies in that:

What Western scientific discourse has always been seeking is objective description, Western science takes deduction and induction as its core methodologies, and the functions of metaphors in scientific cognition and exploration has always been in a marginal position in Western science although metaphors can be seen almost everywhere in seemingly objective scientific discourses[3] and metaphors play an absolutely necessary role in scientific exploration and dissemination of scientific thoughts;[4]

While Chinese medicine takes *Qu Xiang Bi Lei* or Taking Image and Analogizing as its core methodology, and is metaphorical from the formation of its concepts, construction of its theoretical framework, to the development of its clinical explorations, and even to the whole system. In other words, the functions of metaphors in scientific cognition and exploration have always been in the core position in Chinese medicine.

---

2 Guo Guichun. Metaphor, Rhetoric, and Scientific Interpretation [M]. Beijing: Science Press, 2007.

3 "Scientific discourses" here refer to "discourses of Western science".

4 Dong Hongle. 2005: Synopsis.

I think that is the fundamental difference in between Western science and Chinese medicine, and that studies on metaphors in Chinese medicine can reveal true values of classical Chinese medicine, bridge the gap between Chinese medicine and Western medicine, promote and realize the integration of the two medical systems.

Along with the formation of a worldwide aging society and the significant variations in disease spectrum, it has become thus clear that Chinese medicine is a real gem worth to cherish and to carry on in the unending quest for human health, well being, and a long life. Then, how to carry on Chinese medicine? *Qu Xiang Bi Lei* 取象比类 or metaphorizing should be one of the most significant approaches to develop and modernize Chinese medicine since it is the core methodology of Chinese medicine.

In publishing this book, I welcome the opportunity of expressing my thanks to Prof. Dr. Friedrich G. Wallner of Faculty of Philosophy, Vienna University, for his invaluable academic collaboration, inspiration, and support in the last years. He developed an interdisciplinary and intercultural philosophy of science (Constructive Realism) during 1985-95, which aims to make the manifold scientific approaches depending on different cultures understandable. As the founding father of Constructive Realism, he has been inspiring me to research Chinese medicine from perspectives of philosophy of science and philosophy of language (Chinese language in particular), which results in the writing of this book.

I am also profoundly grateful to Prof. Dr. Nancy N. Chen of Anthropology Department, University of California at Santa Cruz (UCSC). If without her academic farsightedness, intercultural and interdisciplinary insight as well as her precious support, help, and care, I could not have had the opportunity to continue my study on metaphors in Chinese medicine at UCSC. And her deep-seated attainments in medical anthropology, merticulous scholarship as well as her generous and amiable way of dealing with people will greatly benefit me the whole life time.

Besides, I also thank Lyu Bin of Shanghai University of TCM for his professional technical assistance in type-setting and making the manuscript ready for publication.

Santa Cruz, California

"Language is the outcome of a culture. Language of a nation is the general reflection of the culture of the nation; but we can also say that language is a part of the culture ... and that culture and language have developed together for thousands of years."

- Claude Levi Strauss[5]

We should not content ourselves to the present state of language. We have to trace back to the origins of words if we want to discover the ties which link the words and their references. ... Etymology has thus become not only the heart of linguistics, but also the foundation stone of philosophy of language.

- Ernst Cassirer[6]

Western medicine is an applied medicine based on achievements of modern Western science and technology, while Chinese medicine roots in classical Chinese philosophy and culture, e.g. Daoist School, and thus goes closer to humanities. But both aim to heal the same being, which is composed of body and mind.

- The Author

1 Cultural Differences between Chinese Medicine and Western Medicine

Both transmission of Chinese medicine to the West and dissemination of Western medicine in China started in the Ming dynasty (16th-17th centuries). Some missionaries taught and spread Christian or Catholic religion by practicing Western medicine; meanwhile, they introduced Chinese medicine curiously, esp. their own experiences in Chinese medicine to the West. Over 300 years passed by. At present, Chinese medicine and Western medicine actually coexist no matter in China or in the West. So, Chinese medicine is not only a special medical system with distinctive national features of China, but also a medical system for the humankind of the whole world.

5 Translated from Chinese. Quoted from a secondary source: See He Yumin. 1990: 149.

6 Translated into English from Chinese. Gan Yang, Translator; Ernst Cassirer, Author. 2004: 158. Its Original Version is: *An Essay on Man: An Introduction to a Philosophy of Human Culture* [M]. New Heaven: Yale University Press, 1944.

Chinese medicine and Western medicine share at least 3 common features: 1. the same object - life processes of the human being; 2. the same goal – To prevent and treat diseases; and 3. both are members of "scientific systems", which depends on how you understand "Science". But, Chinese medicine bears strong humane characteristics, and thus goes closer to humanities; while Western medicine, esp. modern Western medicine, is an applied medicine based on achievements of modern Western science and technology, and thus has typical features of modern Western science. What are the cultural differences between the two medical systems? I think that clarifying these differences will be very helpful for you to understand Chinese medicine.

1.1 Chinese Medicine Going Closer to Humanities Rather than Natural Science

There is no breakthrough but only development and enrichment in Chinese medicine since the establishment of its knowledge system about 2,000 years ago; and there is even no real development since the establishment of standardized transmission of Chinese medicine in 1956. Why?

Chinese Medicine has formed a self-contained fruitful paradigm, so can be enriched and developed in the same framework – *Qu Xiang Bi Lei* or Taking Image and Analogizing guided by *Tian Ren He Yi* or The Unity of Heaven and Humankind established about 2,000 years ago, and survives up till today. For example, the theory of Visceral Manifestation embodies the holistic approach of "Four Seasons – Five *Zang* Organs – Yin-Yang – Five Phases" and "The Unity of Heaven and Humankind". While based on reductionism, mechanism and dichotomy, Western medicine takes an analytical approach, and has been continuously refreshing itself because of the application of advanced modern scientific technology and instruments (tools) to develop itself.

In contemporary China, Chinese medicine is classified as a discipline of natural science by the government of China since 1956. For example, there are two major national foundations in China, one is National Natural Science Foundation of China (NNSFC) for sponsoring research projects in the field of natural science, where Chinese medicine is included; the other is National Funds for Social Science for sponsoring research projects in the field of social science, where Chinese medicine is excluded. That is to say, researches on Chinese medicine have to be performed by applying Western scientific methods and evaluated according to Western scientific standards,[7] which inevitably results in that there is even no real development in Chinese medicine no matter in aspect of theoretical or clinical framework. The reason is that Chinese medicine is totally different from and incompatible with Western science and it is not researched in an adequate way, and such approaches to Chinese medicine do not accord with the way of constructing its knowledge system.

1.2 Linguistic Differences

1.2.1 Logographic Writing, Phonetic Writing, and Thinking Modes

Chinese characters or sinograms, the writing forms of Chinese language and one of the most important marks of Chinese civilization, emerged independently around 6,000 years ago, which is identified by the history of Banpo Ruins of Xi'an, Shaanxi Province.[8] The sinogram 家 Jia, which is interpreted as "residence" in *Shuo Wen Jie Zi* or *The Origin of Chinese Characters*[9] 说文解字 and now is Chinese equivalent for English word "home", is composed of two parts 宀 (the image of "the roof of a house" in ancient China for house) and 豕 Shi (the image for swine, pig). Residence or Home should be a living place for human beings, but why there was a pig in the house? You will come to understand this sinogram suddenly if you visit the Banpo Ruin. In the matriarchal clan society, the pig had already been raised and kept in human's residence. It can be seen that the sinogram 家 had been

7 Note: Generally speaking, the researches on Chinese medicine are mainly classified into three major categories: Studies on the History and Literature of Chinese Medicine, Clinical Trials, and Experimental Studies, of which studies on the history and literature are the most difficult to get funds and are usually separated from clinical and experimental studies on Chinese medicine, and almost all clinical and experimental studies are performed in accordance with Western scientific standards.

8 In 1972, Archaeological Institute of China Academy of Science identified the history of Banpo Ruin as around 6,000 years by C14 determination in its labs.

9 *Shuo Wen Jie Zi*《说文解字》literally means "explaining pictographs and analyzing composite sinograms". I prefer to translate the title into *The Origin of Chinese Characters*.

conceived 6,000 years ago; and developed into 家 of the oracle script and bronze script 2,000 years later. See Illus. 1.[10]

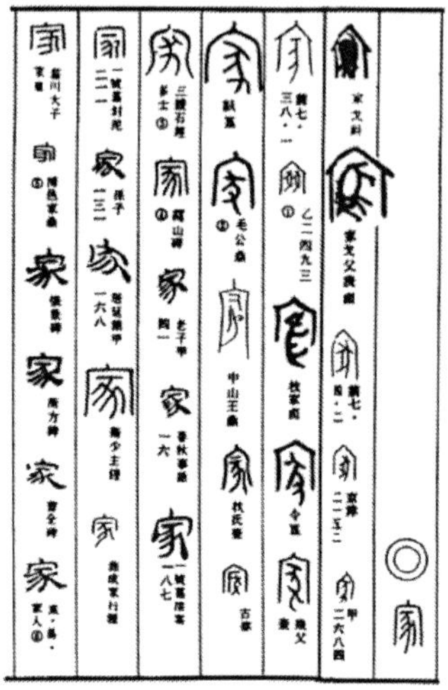

Illus. 1. "Jia 家"(Residence, Home) in *The Great Dictionary of Oracle, Bronze, Seal, and Official Scripts*

Shuo Wen Jie Zi or *The Origin of Chinese Characters* is the first comprehensive systematic dictionary of Chinese characters (or sinograms) arranged by sections with shared components, called radicals (*bùshǒu* 部首, lit. "section headers") and finished in 100 A.D. by Xu Shen 许慎 (A.D. 58? – 147?) of the Eastern Han Dynasty. It is the first dictionary which interprets the original meaning of a sinogram by analyzing its structure and gives the rationale behind it, sometimes the etymology of the sinogram as well. Actually, *Shuo Wen Jie Zi* or *The Origin of Chinese Characters* is far beyond a dictionary, and moreover it can be interpreted from cultural and philosophical perspectives. In this sense it is can be regarded as the earliest monograph on philosophy of Chinese language.

A study on the relationship between *Huang Di Nei Jing* or *Huang Di's Inner Classic* and *Shuo Wen Jie Zi* or *The Origin of Chinese Characters* shows

10 Zuo Min'an. 2005:7.

that "The knowledge of Chinese medicine contained in *The Origin of Chinese Characters* is in direct line of succession with *Huang Di's Inner Classic*; The universal and ecomedical thinking modes of 'Heaven-Earth-Man' in them are cut from the same cloth; The theories of *qi*, yin-yang, and five phases, the theoretical foundation of *The Inner Classic*, can be traced back to their sources through *The Origin of Chinese Characters* which expounds the original meanings of them by analyzing the structures of their sinograms; *The Origin of Chinese Characters* traces back to origins of sinograms and their original meanings through analyzing their structures, therefore, it is important for us to study and read *The Inner Classic*, and to probe into the origin of Chinese medicine as well."[11]

In Chinese logographic writing, the shape of a Chinese character is directly related to its meaning, and both integrate into a unity. The formation of a Chinese character, an organic whole of the shape and the meaning, is one-step made following the rule of nature, reflecting the direct communication between and integration of the subject and the object. The formation also implies an important thinking way, i.e. the imaging thinking.

Integration of the subject and the object is a thread running through classical Chinese culture and science, on the basis of which The Unity of Heaven and Humankind (tian ren he yi, 天人合一) constitutes the foundation of the classical Chinese culture and science.

The imaging thinking is a classical Chinese thinking way, and the process, methods, and rules of which make up "Taking Image and Analogizing" (*Qu Xiang Bi Lei*, 取象比类), the fundamental methodology of classical Chinese culture and science[12]. Chinese characters, which have developed on the basis of the pictographic writing, and their meanings are quite stable and conservative, which promotes the development of imaging and analogizing thinking of Chinese medical experts. Then such thinking modes were set up

---

11 Lan Fengli. 2006, 36（4）: 201-205.

12 The word "traditional" is sometimes disapproving, and means "following older methods and ideas rather than modern or different ones" (*Oxford Advanced Learner's Dictionary*). Chinese culture and science, including Chinese medicine, are based on classical Chinese philosophy, and so I name them "classical Chinese culture and science" and "classical Chinese medicine". They are classical but not old-fashioned or out-of-date because they are still developing in their own framwork.

in the *Huang Di's Inner Classic* and have greatly influenced Chinese medical experts of the later generations.

The logographic writings of yin-yang 阴阳, *wu xing* 五行, and *qi* 气, the extensive imaging and analogizing thinking modes in the *Huang Di's Inner Classic*, and criticism, proofreading, annotations for sinograms from the aspects of the "shape", "pronunciation", and "meaning" in the ancient medical classics made since its appearance, all demonstrate the far-reaching influences of the imaging thinking mode on Chinese medicine. For example, in *Ling Shu* or *Miracullous Pivot* of the *Nei Jing*, the chapter *Xiao Zhen Jie* or *An Explanation of Small Needles* is an interpretation of the part of "Small Needles" of the chapter *Jiu Zhen Shi Er Yuan* or *Nine Needles and Twelve Source Points*. Actually, most of the books on classical Chinese science were composed in this way, i.e. the way of annotating former classics. I think the formation of this common feature results from influences of the logographic writing and the imaging thinking way as well as the writing tradition of Confucian classics.

Phonetic writing, as opposed to logographic writing, is the most common writing form in the world. English, German, French, Spanish, Portuguese, etc. are all phonetic writings, but are different languages composed by the same Latin alphabets. Letrs take English as an example.

English is a kind of phonetic writing. The shapes of English words are directly related to their pronunciations, but have nothing to do with the meanings or the external images of concrete things. That is to say, in the phonetic writing, the shape is separate and independent from the meaning, and the meaning comes from man-made prescripts outside the shape, which indicates that the formation of a word of the phonetic writing is composed of two steps: first, building its shape - spelling of alphabets; second, defining its meaning based on linguistic rules or grammar.

Understanding the meanings of words is based on the sense of hearing, thus jumping out the thinking frame of the visual sense of the concrete images of things, then providing a bigger possibility for logic thinking based on the abstraction, finally forming thinking traditions of abstract inference, conceptual thinking, categorization, and trying to make an objective judgment to the world.

The formation of phonetic writing reflects its two important characteristics: tool – alphabets and abstraction – linguistic rules. Every tool is made to have a certain function according to man's specific aim or intention, thus becoming a medium of connection between man and the nature, and so interrupting the natural direct communication between them. Tool plays a vital role in the Western culture, esp. in the natural sciences, where it is standardized and systematized, and the experimental research approach characterized by the use of various tools is set up.

Actually, the alphabet is the mother of various tools. The thinking way relating to the experimental research approach is abstraction. The rule of abstraction is logic, while linguistic rules or grammar is an embryonic form of logic. The emergence of tool reflects the relationship between the subject and object, i.e., the separation and opposition of them – man remakes the nature. The abstraction pays more attention to being analytical, logical, and restricts imagination.

The tool and abstraction become the foundation of Western culture and science and of the natural science (including Western medicine) in particular. Western natural science manifests in two opposite ways, which have been realized by more and more people as time goes by. The two edges lie in that the environmental pollution and the ecological imbalance, the repay of the nature to the man, always accompany the process of the man conquering and remaking the nature. As regards to Western medicine, the two edges lie in that the severe side effects, drug resistance, and effect being temporary always accompany the notable therapeutic effects.

1.2.2 Chinese Medical Terminology and Western Medical Terminology

Chinese medical terminology is very different from Western medical terminology. For example, a kind of eye disease, which is caused by "pathogenic wind-fire" and marked by acute onset of redness and pain in the eye accompanied by photophobia and lacrimation, is named "wind-fire eye 风火眼" in Chinese medicine. Such a disease is generally diagnosed as "acute conjunctivitis" in Western medicine, which is a kind of "inflammation of the conjunctiva" of the eye. It is interesting that Chinese medicine does not speak of "inflammation"[13] nor does Western medicine speak of "wind-fire", but both can heal the same disease by different methods.

13 It is interesting that the root of the word "Inflammation" is "flame", which means "n. a hot bright stream of burning gas that comes from sth. that is on fire" and "v. to burn with a bright flame" (*Oxford Advanced leaner's Dictionary*).

"Not only the names of diseases, not only the grouping of systems were not the same, but the fundamental perceptual codes that were applied to patients' bodies , the field of objects to which observation addressed itself, the surfaces and depths traversed by the doctor's gaze, the whole system of orientation of his gaze also varied,"[14] What Michael Foucault says about medical perception in different historical periods could apply as well to these different cultural traditions.[15] These different cultural traditions of Chinese medicine and Western medicine are embodied in their specific terminologies.

Undoubtedly, no matter the language of Chinese medicine or the language of Western medicine is a kind of technical language. Modern terminologists define a "technical language" as a form of any given language that is used by people involved in a special field and that has a "terminology", i.e., a set of expressions not used in the common language or, as is often the case, expressions that are used in a different or more specific way than in the common language.

A popular misconception about technical terms is that they are words used *exclusively* by specialists. In actual fact, technical terms in most disciplines largely, if not mostly, come from the common language. Any language only has a certain number of words, and new terms are usually combinations of existing lexical items. Many terms are completely indistinguishable in form from expressions in the common language although they are more specific in meaning. The process whereby common language expressions are given more specific or metaphorical meanings in the technical contexts is called "terminologization". The modern terminological observation that technical terms are largely derived from the common language is reflected clearly both in Chinese medicine and Western medicine. Those acquainted with the language of Chinese medicine are aware that most of the sinograms they come across in Chinese medical texts are used in the common Chinese texts. And most of the Western medical terms are combinations of Latin or Greek morphemes. Actually, about 10,000 Latin or Greek words came into English during the Renaissance Period and finally became a part of English vocabulary.

Actually, both Chinese medical terminology and Western medical terminology can be classified into three categories: 1. words and expressions for

14 Foucault, Michel. 1973: 54.
15 Kaptchuk, Ted J. 2000: 3.

everyday use; 2. specialized terms of their own; and 3. original terms of their own.

1.2.2.1 Three Categories of Chinese Medical Terminology

Both Dr. Nigel Wiseman and Prof. Paul U. Unschuld advocated classifying the basic Chinese medical terminology into two categories:[16] one comprises of words and expressions for everyday use, e.g., 頭 head, 腳 foot, 胸 chest, 腹 abdomen, 心 heart, 肝 liver, 血 blood; the other is composed of specialized Chinese medical terms extended from the common language and formed through metaphor or analogy, e.g., 竅 orifice, 穴 point or hole, 正 upright, 邪 evil, 營 nutrient or camp, 衛 defense or guard, 命門 life gate, 督脈 the governing or supervising vessel.

According to my understanding of Chinese medical terminology, esp. of *Shuo Wen Jie Zi* or *The Origin of Chinese Characters*, I think that Chinese medical terminology can be classified into 3 categories:

The first category is made up of words and expressions from the common language, e.g., some body parts like 心 heart, 肝 liver, 脾 spleen, 肺 lungs, 腎 kidneys, 鼻 nose, 目 eyes, 耳 ears, 頭 head, 腳 foot, 胸 chest, 腹 abdomen, 血 blood; some disease names like 霍亂 cholera, 麻疹 measles, 麻風 leprosy, 瘧疾 malaria, 癲癇 epilepsy; some climatic pathogenic factors like 風 wind, 寒 cold, 濕 dampness, 燥 dryness, 火 fire; some symptoms like 發熱 fever, 頭痛 headache, 痛 pain, 咳嗽 cough, 心悸 palpitation, 健忘 forgetfulness, 頭暈目眩 dizziness, 嘔吐 vomiting, 噁心 nausea, 泄瀉 diarrhea, 便秘（不更衣）constipation.

The second category constitutes specialized Chinese medical terms from daily words and expressions formed through *Qu Xiang Bi Lei* or Taking Image and Analogizing, i.e. the metaphorizing process, e.g., 藏 depots or viscera, 府 palaces or bowels, 經 meridian, 絡 network vessel, 竅 orifice, 穴 point or hole, 正 upright, 邪 evil, 營 camp, 衛 guard, 督脈 governing vessel, 任脈 controlling vessel, 三焦 *san jiao*, 命門 life gate, etc. which usually bear historical, cultural, and medical values at the same time.

16 Wiseman, Nigel. 2001, 22(7): 51-54.

The third category comprises of original Chinese medical terms, e.g., some pictophonetic characters such as 疝, 疸, 癰, 瘍, 痔, 痿, 痹, etc. in *Shuo Wen Jie Zi* or *The Origin of Chinese Characters, Disease Section.*

1.2.2.2 Three Categoriess of Western Medical Terminology

Dr. Nigel Wiseman[17] roughly classified the Western medical terminology into 3 categories and distinguished them as well.

The first category constitutes borrowings from the common language, e.g., fever, chill, cough, cold, hiccough, headache, pain, tenderness, soreness, palpitations, bleeding, hot flushes, forgetfulness, dizziness, vomiting, blindness, jaundice, deafness, nausea, emaciation, diarrhea, constipation, goiter, sores, corn, sty, boil, measles, mumps, and fracture. These words, commonly used by doctors, are known to all speakers and denote conditions that can be identified by most normal adults.

The second category comprises terms devised by modern medicine to describe certain technical concepts: conjunctivitis, anemia, hypertension, paranasal sinusitis, trichomoniasis, arteriosclerosis, optic atrophy, hyperchlorhydria, coronary thrombosis, glomerulonephritis hematoma, cerebrovascular ischemia. Although some of these words (such as anemia, hypertension and conjunctivitis) may be familiar to and even used by non-experts, the conditions they denote cannot be diagnosed by the non-experts with the medical precision. These terms reflect knowledge that lies at a long distance from the lay understanding.

Between these two categories is the third comprising terms of medical origin that do not require any specialist knowledge or instrumentation to understand or identify, e.g., enuresis, lochia, pharynx, larynx, dysphagia, strangury, scrofula, tumor, fistula, miliaria, macule, papule, and diphtheria.

I think that the terms of the first category are actually from words and expressions for everyday use, that of the second category are specialized terms of Western medicine, and that of the third category are original terms of Western medicine.

17 Wiseman, Nigel. The Translation of Chinese Medical Terminology. 1996: 67.

1.2.2.3 Drawing Lessons from English-Chinese Translation of Western Medicine in China

In the course of transmission and exchange of medical cultures, linguistic contact is a forerunner of the contact of different medical cultures. Language, an essential medium, is the carrier of the medical knowledge. The transmission and exchange between different medical cultures will first manifest in the terminology. The foreign terminology comes to be the "envoy" of the different medical cultures. Generally speaking, a foreign medical culture is introduced and disseminated by translating the foreign medical terminology in a proper way. The translated terminology gradually integrates into the native language, finally becomes an organic part of the mainstream medical culture of the nation proper.

The history of translation and dissemination of Western medicine in China shows that Western medical terminology and culture are very closely associated with each other, just like the shadow following the person. It also took a very long time for the formation of standard Chinese translation of Western medical terminology in China. In the early stage of translation and dissemination of Western medicine in China, for example, translation of the term "scarlet fever" had been very confusing, which had many different translations such as "紅熱症，紅疹，疹子熱病，痧病，花紅熱症，猩紅熱", etc.

It can be seen from the history and reality of translating Western medicine into Chinese that the first and third categories of Chinese medical terms have been successfully used to translate the first and third categories of Western medical terms and thus to express Western medical knowledge, and that using the second category of Chinese medical terms, which are specialized terms carring the most distinctive Chinese medical knowledge, to translate specialized terms of Western medicine, has produced serious confusions or even mistakes. Here are two examples:

1. Translating "typhoid" into "傷寒" Typhoid refers to "infection of the intestine caused by *Salmonella typhi* in food and water,"[18] manifesting in fever, diarrhea, even bloody stool; while "傷寒" is a specialized Chinese medical term, bears two meanings in Chinese medicine: in a broad sense, "傷

18 Collin, P.H. 2001: 613.

寒", cold-induced disease, is a general term for various externally contracted febrile diseases, as stated in the *Basic Questions · Discourse on Febrile Diseases* (*Su Wen·Re Lun*) – 《素問 · 熱論》: "今夫熱病者，皆傷寒之類也"; in a narrow sense, "傷寒", cold affection, refers to a condition caused by cold, manifesting in chills and fevers, absence of sweating, headache, floating and tense pulse, as stated in *The Classic of Difficult Issues* (*Nan Jing*) – 《難經·五十八難》: 傷寒有五：有中風，有傷寒，有濕溫，有熱病，有溫病，其所苦各不同." Later on, some translators rendered "傷寒" in Chinese medicine back into "typhoid". Such a translation has confused the differences between "typhoid" in Western medicine and "傷寒" in Chinese medicine, thus causing misunderstanding the both terms or even misleading the readers.

2. Translating "surgery" into "外科學" Surgery refers to "treatment of a disease or disorder which requires an operation to cut into or to remove or to manipulate tissue or organs or parts;"[19] while "外科學" in Chinese medicine refers to a specialty which studies the causes, pathogenesis, and treatments of the diseases on the body surface.[20] Many majors of Chinese medicine, including undergraduates and even doctorate candidates, and some translators as well, translate "外科學" in Chinese medicine into "Surgery". Actually, "外科學" in Chinese medicine should be translated into "external medicine" for the real "surgery" in Chinese medicine declined long ago since Hua Tuo 华佗 died in 208 A.D. So "中医外科学" should be "Chinese External Medicine" not "TCM Surgery" or "Surgery in Chinese Medicine".

We should draw some lessons from the above mentioned translation examples that the second category of Western medical terms should not be used to translate and express the specialized Chinese medical terms. For example, although "風火眼 wind-fire eye" in Chinese medicine and "acute conjunctivitis" in Western medicine actually refer to the same disease, it is ill-advised to translate "風火眼" into "acute conjunctivitis" for such a translation must confuse cultural differences between the two medical systems, and fail to produce such an association of the cause (pathogenic wind-fire) and therapeutic method (coursing wind and clearing fire) with the translation "acute conjunctivitis", thus destroying the independency, wholeness and systematicness of the theoretical system of Chinese medicine.

19 Collin, P.H. 2001: 571.
20 Li Jingwei, Ou Yongxin, Yu Ying'ao, et al. 2001:301.

1.2.2.4 Learning Successful Experiences of Dissemination of Western Medicine in China

Why has Western medicine been successfully transmitted to China? The key lies in that Western medical terminology has been translated into Chinese in a complete, independent and systematic way through literal or word-for-word translation approach, e.g., "Conjunctivitis" is rendered as "結膜炎" not "風火眼"; "Acute contagious conjunctivitis" as "急性觸染性結膜炎" not "天行赤眼"; "Globus" as "球;球(狀)感", and "Globus abdominalis" as "腹(部)球(狀)感" not "癟瘕", "Globus hystericus" as "癔症球, 癔病性窒息(感)" not "梅核氣".

The Chinese terms of Western medicine are so strange to the terminology of Chinese medicine and to the Chinese fraternity as well, but why do translators not adopt the terms of Chinese medicine to translate Western medical terms? Because the translator intends to preserve the systematicness, independence, and completeness (or integrity) of Western medicine, and don't want to make Western medicine in China become a Non-Chinese Non-Western Medicine or Non-Donkey Non-Horse medicine.

1.2.2.5 Etymology-Based Literal Translation Approach: Key to Eliminate Confusions and Ambiguities

Actually, "Translations of Chinese Medical Concepts Being Confusing" is the major problem in translating Chinese medical texts.

It is well known that Chinese medicine is the product of systematizing the knowledge contained in the ancient Chinese medical classics, esp. "the Four Great Medical Classics". Most of the specialized Chinese medical concepts formed for the first time in ancient Chinese medical classics by means of metaphorizing and analogizing, thus embodying the cultural presupposition *Tian Ren He Yi* or The Unity of Heaven and Humankind and the specific core methodology *Qu Xiang Bi Lei* or taking image and analogizing, thus bearing historical, cultural and medical values at the same time.

But when translating a Chinese medical concept, most of translators no matter of China or other countries lay stress only on its medical value and ignoring its cultural and historical values, and thus making the English translation lose the central methodology of Chinese medicine – *Qu Xiang Bi Lei* or taking image and analogizing.

I hold that specialized terms of both Chinese and Western medicine reflect that they are based on specific and different cultural presuppositions and thinking ways; and that Chinese medicine is a systematic, complete, and unique medical system incompatible with Western medicine; and therefore, English translation of concepts of Chinese medical classics, esp. those formed by means of metaphorizing and analogizing, should apply the translation strategy which can reflect their metaphorical connotations and the specific Chinese methodology of *Qu Xiang Bi Lei*, i.e. *Literal Translation Approach Based on Etymology Investigation*, thus observing the only one standard.

As Newmark points out that "However, in communicative as in semantic translation, provided that equivalent-effect is secured, the literal word-for-word translation is not only the best, it is the only valid method of translation. There is no excuse for unnecessary 'synonyms', let alone paraphrase, in any type of translation."[21]

The core knowledge of Chinese medicine is from classical Chinese medical texts, which are written in self-interpreting sinograms. Compared to phonetic writing forms, Chinese language (logographic writing) is more stable and accumulative. In Chinese language, giving the original sinogram new meanings by the way of metaphorizing instead of creating new sinograms is the major way to reflect the changes and developments of the world and the means and process of Chinese people cognizing, understanding and stating the world. After tracing back to the original meanings of sinograms, concepts and statements are not difficult to understand in their contexts in a broad sense, which also provide us extensive but close links among different disciplines of Chinese culture and science. Therefore, etymology investigation is of vital significance for etymology of a sinogram can unify all the migrating meanings of concepts based on the one sinogram with the same etymology. The theoretical system of Chinese medicine is stated and expressed in a natural language with the two major characteristics: being polysemous and ambiguous, which can also be clarified and unified by etymology investigation and metaphor understanding.

21 Newmark, Peter. 1981: 39.

1.2.3 Classical Medical Chinese, Medical English and Epistemology

Ferid Murad (1936–), a Nobel Prize winner in medicine (1998), set up Murad Research Institute for Modernized Chinese Medicine, a modern research centre on Chinese pharmacology named after his name with the collaboration with Shanghai University of Traditional Chinese Medicine in 2003. At that time, he said he was seeking for a language which is able to give a scientific interpretation for pharmacological and molecule mechanisms of the therapeutic effects of Chinese herbal remedies. Chinese medicine has its own discourse, and so why do we need to look for another language to interpret it? Is it possible to find such a kind of language?

Ludwig Wittgenstein (1889-1951) believed that language is a kind of picture, which cannot be proved with facts of the real world. That is to say, we do not need to prove or interpret the logic contained in the discourse of Chinese medicine with the so-called scientific methods, what we should do is to regard it as a picture in which the discourse of Chinese medicine describes man's lifestyle – a harmonious state among man, the nature and the society, how man behaves in the daily life to preserve health, to prevent and treat illnesses, and which is like a picture of the life world.

According to Wittgenstein's idea of philosophy of language - "language games", Chinese medicine is definitely a kind of language, a language game in respect to man, its healthy state, and its connection with the nature; Western medicine is another language game in respect to the body and its diseases; and differences between them is that Chinese medicine does not reduce its language but it enriches it by metaphors. Therefore it makes sense to say: Chinese medicine is a natural language and Western medicine is a formal descriptive technical language. Here is an importance difference for the theoretical understanding of both: Formal languages must be interpreted for getting sense; Natural languages are interpreting themselves.

It's true that the textual criticism, exegetical studies and annotations of ancient medical classics have always been an important academic field of study in Chinese medicine up till now since the era of the *Huang Di's Inner Classic*,[22] which helps practitioners of Chinese medicine of the past dynas-

22 Note: For example, the chapter of *Zhen Jie* or *An Explanation of Needles* of *Basic Questions* 《素問 · 針解》 and the chapter of *Xiao Zhen Jie* or *An Explanation of Small*

ties understand and develop Chinese medicine in both theoretical and clinical explorations.

Now, let's look at the two paragraphs about the origin of man both from the angle of genetics in Chinese medicine and Western medicine respectively:

> 1. "人生於地，懸命於天，天地合气，命之曰人。人能應四時者，天地為之父母（《素問 · 寶命全形論》）。"
> Translation: Man is born on the earth, hanging his life to the heaven. The union of *Qi* of Heaven and Earth makes up a man. Man can adapt himself to the seasons for Heaven and Earth are his parents. (*Basic Questions · Discourse on Protecting Life and Preserving Physical Appearance*)
>
> 2. "Man is metazoon, triploblastic, chordale, vertebrate, pentadactyle, mammalian, eutherian, primate... The outlines of each of his principal system of organs may be traced back, like those of other mammals, to the fishes." (L.A.B.-orradaile)
> 譯文：人屬於後生動物，系五趾，三胚層高級動物，屬脊索動物門，脊椎動物亞門，哺乳綱，靈長目......象其他哺乳動物一樣，他的每一個器官系統的輪廓可以追溯到魚類。[23]

It is clear that the latter is a kind of formal technical language, a typical language of modern Western science, which is only used as a tool to convey information, to identify its reference, and to express points of view. And it has become so boring and dry by the so-called theoretical, objective, and scientific formulations. While discourse of Chinese medicine is a kind of hermeneutic language full of metaphors, and it is closely related to the context of the life world - an inseparable organic whole of man, the nature and the society. It can inspire, hint, and enlighten you to know how Chinese medicine understands man in a direct and original way.

According to Wittgenstein's idea of philosophy of language, the discourse of Chinese medicine and that of Western medicine are different "language games", showing different lifestyles, and describing different "pictures" of life, and so one cannot be interpreted or proved by the other. For example, mixing the discourse of Western medicine with that of Chinese

---

Needles of *Miraculous Pivot*《靈樞 · 小針解》both interpret the chapter of *Jiu Zhen Shi Er Yuan* or *Nine Needles and Twelve Source Points* of the *Spirit Pivot* 《靈樞 · 九針十二原》.

23 Hou Weirui. 1988: 278.

medicine will disturb the cognizing way of Chinese medicine, which is just like to coat or cover the transparent life world with the scientific formal language. Therefore, we should reconsider the current progress of researching, modernizing, or even westernizing Chinese medicine, and what we need to do is to understand the rationality of Chinese medicine from its own discourse, from the "picture" of the lifestyle in the life world its discourse describes. That is to interpret Chinese medicine with itself. I do not deny the approach to apply modern science and technology to study Chinese medicine, but such researches must be in accordance with philosophy of Chinese medicine.

1.3 Differences in Their Philosophical Foundations

Philosophy, the core of culture and the theoretical thinking of the top level, has been guiding the development of medicine and other subjects of science. Western thinking mode is known as analytical thinking, causal thinking, or conceptual thinking, on the basis of which the mechanism, reductionism, dichotomy formed and greatly promoted the development of Western medicine.

Surgery and organ transplantation medicine have developed on the basis of the mechanism which views the human body as a "machine".

On the basis of reductionist ideology or reductionism – that is, seeking to understand a system by breaking it down into its constituent parts, experimental physiology and cellular biology were founded in the 19th century and molecular biology was founded in the 20th century; influenced by such a thinking, Western medicine has studied various systems and organs of the body down to cells, to molecules, and to genes in the recent 2 centuries, and constructed a series branches of learning of basic medicine, thus forming the so-called "scientific" Western medicine.

Dichotomy, philosophy of a division into two opposite parts – A and Non-A, indicates the separation of the subject and object, of the nature and man, of the time and space, of the body and mind, of the ontology and epistemology, ect., and guides the treating principle of Western medicine which treats a condition using drugs which produce opposite symptoms to those of the condition.

Classical Chinese thinking mode is known as correlative thinking, which originated in *The Book of Changes* and is mainly characterized by explaining dynamic life processes by opposing and complementing as the

Yin-Yang Diaphragm suggests. The correlative thinking sees everything in the world as interdependent and interactive. In Chinese medicine, the correlative thinking manifests itself concretely in the yin-yang theory, the five-phase theory, and the visceral manifestation theory, the vessel theory, etc., which evolved in the way of following the features of the heaven and earth (the nature) to the human being from concrete to abstract, from structure to function. In Chinese medicine, disease is regarded as the result of imbalance or disharmony of yin and yang, and the goal of Chinese medical treatment is to restore the balance for each individual under his or her own unique environment.

Actually, correlative thinking mode of Eastern tradition and causal thinking mode of Western tradition depend on each other and complement to each other, to some extent oppose to each other. Both together will surely make a better world for the humankind. More and more scholars of the West and the East have acknowledged this point.

Compared to the Western philosophical thinking mode, classical Chinese philosophical thinking mode is not inferior at all, but can be a perfect complement to the Western philosophical thinking. The two traditions should understand each other, respect each other. Only in this way, each tradition can understand its own culture more thoroughly; the two traditions can promote each other and develop together.

That is to say, there are no ranking cultures. Actually, both correlative thinking mode of Eastern tradition and causal thinking mode of Western tradition have their advantages and disadvantages, thus can complement to each other in an almost perfect way. Intercultural activities such as translation and intercultural philosophy can make them understand each other, promote each other and develop together.

I would like to reformulate Confucius's statement "Men with honor can be harmonious but different" in this way: Medicine of East and West are different but together can make a harmonious world.

In the remote antiquity when Fu Xi 伏羲 ruled the country, he raised his head to observe images on the heaven, bowed his head to observe phenomena on the earth, observed images of birds and beasts and those of the earth, took near images from man and far images of other things from the nature, on the basis of which he then started to make the Eight Trigrams to illustrate the phenomena. Until Shen Nong's 神农 time, tying knots was used to keep records of things; And then things became complicated and numerous, and cheating things started to happen. [Until Huang Di's time,] the historian official Cang Jie 仓颉 created sinograms[24] enlightened by differentiable footprints of birds and beasts.

古者庖犧氏之王天下也，仰則觀象於天，俯則觀法於地，觀鳥獸之文與地之宜，近取諸身，遠取諸物；於是始作易八卦，以垂憲象。及神農氏，結繩為治，而統其事。庶業其繁，飾偽萌生。黃帝史官倉頡，見鳥獸蹄迒之跡，知分理可相別異也，初造書契。

- Xu Shen 许慎[25]

2 *Tian Ren He Yi*[26]: The Ontological Presupposition of Chinese Medicine

The theme of Chinese philosophy is to probe into the relationship between the "heaven and man", or the relationship between "the Way of heaven and the Way of man", regarding the heaven as man's heaven and the man as the heaven's man.

24 For translation of Chinese 汉字 I prefer "sinogram" instead of "Chinese character", which was originally proposed by Prof. Pan Wenguo 潘文国 (1944–) in his monograph entitled "*Sinogram as the Basic Unit and Chinese Language Study*" 《字本位与汉语研究》 published in 2002. The author advanced that Chinese language study should take *Zi* or sinogram instead of *Ci* or word as the basic unit for Chinese language study.

25 See the *Preface* of *Shuo Wen Jie Zi* or *The Origin of Chinese Characters* by Xu Shen 许慎 (?58-147? A.D.).

26 *Tian* 天 in *Tian* Dao 天道 and *Ren* Dao 人道 or *Tian Ren He Yi* 天人合一 is usually translated into Heaven, but actually not the same as in the West. Actually, "*Tian Ren He Yi* 天人合一" is the abbreviation of "*Tian Di Ren He Yi* 天地人合一", i.e. the Unity of Heaven, Earth, and Humankind". "*Tian Ren He Yi* 天人合一" can be literally translated as "the Unity of Heaven and Humankind".

2.1 Etymology-based Understanding of *Tian Ren He Yi*

The writing form keeps the old [thinking] ways 斯文存古道. That is to say, Chinese characters reflect classical Chinese thinking ways and the way of Chinese people understanding the world. *Tian Ren He Yi* 天人合一, the ontological and cultural presupposition of Chinese medicine, also resides in sinograms.

Classical Chinese thinking is empirical and synthetical, tends to seize the holistic feature of things based on experiences. Man is vivid and complicated, while the nature is vast and boundless. How did the ancient Chinese people understand the complicated man and the vast nature? The answer is to relate the man and the nature to each other, guided by the idea of *Tian Ren He Yi* 天人合一 or the Unity of Heaven and Humankind. Such ideas actually imply in Chinese characters.

Man is a small nature, and the nature is a big man. On one hand, sinograms referring to human body's parts, behaviors and characteristics can also denote things in the nature, i.e. one relates to man, while the other relates to the nature. For example, *Shou* 首 originally means head, but also refers to the thing at the top of the handle of a weapon; *Er* 耳 originally means ear, but also refers to any ear-like thing such as the ears of a tripod (鼎); *Xing* 性 originally means man's nature, but also refers to the nature and characteristics of things; *Tian* 天 originally means man's vertex, but also refers to the sky, the heaven, the God, which reflects a subject-centered nature.

On the other hand, sinograms referring to things in the nature can also denote parts, behaviours and characteristics of man, i.e. one relates to the nature, while the other relates to man. For example, *Qi* 气 originally refers to thin, floating clouds in the nature, but later refers to the invisible basic ingredient constituting the man which can be transformed into blood, essence, and body fluid, etc., and the normal functional activities of life which is governed by "*qi*" is known as *Shen* 神; *Shen* 神 originally refers to lightening in the nature, but later on refers to the spirit or mind of the man; *Jing* 经 originally denotes the longitudinal lines of the textiles or the warps, but later on refers to the running routes of the main stems of the man's vessel system 经络系统; etc.

Tian Ren He Yi leads to frequent introspection, self-examination and observation of the nature, therefore it is a kind of circular reasoning: from the man to the nature and from the nature to the man, based on the subject, reflecting the direct communication between and unification of the subject and the object. The subject is the center of the nature, is the one to understand self and the outside world, and so is the norm to understand the myriad of beings. Well-understanding of the subject and the nature means knowing the ways, principles of all the things in the world.

2.1.1 Pan Gu 盤古, the Creator of the World in Chinese Mythology

How is the world created? How is the man created? Why does the man come to this world? Mythology, philosophy and science have always been trying to answer the above questions. Actually, mythology, philosophy and science of a particular culture share some common cultural presuppositions.

"The source of civilization is hidden in the Chaos[27]. ... In order to reveal the source, people not only need to carefully study the unearthed teeth, skulls, and pieces of porcelain, but also need to seek clues from myths and legends of the remote antiquity. Myths are the soul of a nationality. If a nationality does not have myths, its history is just like to originate from a puppet without thinking. It is because of moving myths that it is possible for us to track down our ancestors' footmarks to see their behaviors and their ways of thinking." [28]

Pan Gu 盤古 first appeared in Xu Zheng's *San Wu Li Ji* 《三五历纪》 and *Wu Yun Li Nian Ji* 《五运历年纪》, both of which are lost. But the related contents are preserved in later works such as *Tai Ping Yu Lan*《太平御览》(977-983) and *Yi Shi* 《绎史》.[29]

Pan 盤, a signific-phonetic, is a household utensil, and its shape is usually round.[30] In ancients' eyes, the heaven was also round, as recorded by Xu Zheng 徐整 of the Three-Kingdom Period (220-280) that "The chaotic world is just like an egg."[31] Pan 盤 follows 般, written as I in oracle script

---

27 Chaos refers to the primeval state of the nature according to folklore.

28 Xiao Jiansheng. 2009: 13.

29 The author is Ma Xiao 马骕 (1621-1673) of the early Qing Dynasty. *Yi Shi* 《绎史》 has altogether 160 volumes and 5 sections, namely Remote Antiquity, Three Eras, Spring-Autumn Period, Warring States Period, and External Records.

30 He Jiuying, Hu Shuangbao, Zhang Meng. 1995: 195-196.

31 See *Tai Ping Yu Lan*《太平御览》 (977-983), which quotes *San Wu Li Ji* 《三五

and  in lesser seal script, which indicates both meaning and pronunciation, and means "rotate", as stated in *Shuo Wen Jie Zi* or *The Origin of Chinese Characters* "Resembling the image of rotating a boat. Following 舟 boat and 殳. 殳 refers to what make it rotate. 象舟之旋，从舟。从殳，殳，所以旋也." Gu 古 means ancient, remote antiquity, which was formerly hu 瓠, the bottle gourd.

Pan Gu is not a historical figure but a god created by ancient Chinese people for "Pan Gu grew 1 Zhang (about 3.3 meters) per day as the heaven ascended 1 Zhang per day and the earth thickened 1 Zhang per day for 18,000 years (*San Wu Li Ji,* 《三五历纪》)." And how did Pan Gu separate the heaven from the earth? He separated the heaven from the earth by rotating the chaotic *qi* into lucid yang and turbid yin, which is just like the *Tai Ji* Diagram (or the Yin-Yang Diagram). That was the beginning of the world. Then he died, and all parts of his dead body transformed into various beings in the nature, such as "his breathing into wind & cloud, his voice into thunders, the left eye into the Sun, the right eye into the moon, his head, feet, upper limbs and trunk into the Five Mountains, the blood in the vessels into water in the rivers, the tendons into roads, his flesh into soil, his hair of the head into stars, the body hair into grasses and trees, his bones and teeth into metals in the soil, his essence and marrow into pearls and jades, his sweat into rain, and his spirit into birds, beasts, fishes, and insects, etc." according to the records in *San Wu Li Ji* 《三五历纪》.

Two important ideas can be inferred although there are some contradictory parts about this myth:

1. *Tian Ren He Yi* 天人合一 or the Unity of Heaven and Humankind (Pan Gu, God[32]), the world view of Chinese culture, indicates that the heaven, earth, and man constitute with the same ingredient - *Qi* in the same way, thus uniting and resembling each other, abbreviated as "*Tian Ren He Yi* or the Unity of Heaven and Humankind";

2. *Qu Xiang Bi Lei* 取象比类 or Taking Image and Analogizing is a vital methodology of Chinese culture and science.

历纪》.

32 God or *Shen* is the metaphor of creating. See Lan Fengli. Understanding *SHEN* in Classical Chinese Texts. In Lan Fengli, Wallner F. G.., Wobovnik C (eds.). 2011: 11-27 .

2.1.2 One (一 and 壹): The Origin of All Things

> "One (*yi* 一) is the original great beginning. Dao is based on one (*yi* 一), and then is to separate the heaven from the earth and to create all the things".
> 惟初太始，道立于一，造分天地，化成萬物。
>
> \- *Shuo Wen Jie Zi* or *The Origin of Chinese Characters*

> "The movements under the heaven start from one (*yi* 一)."
> 天下之動貞夫一。
>
> \- *The Book of Changes*

> "At the great beginning there was Non-being, [but] no Being nor Name. That was where one (*yi* 一) started, but still no physical appearance."
> 泰初有无,无有无名；一之所起,有一而未形。
>
> \- *Chuang Tzu. Chapter of Heaven and Earth*

> "Where do the rules start to be established? They start to be established at the great oneness. The great oneness is the root of all the beings and the bottom of all the phenomena."
> 法于何立？立于一画。一画者，众有之本，万象之根。
>
> \- *Arts of Painting. The Great Oneness of Visual Arts*[33]

One is far beyond the number one. In philosophers' eyes, one is the origin of all the things. *Shuo Wen Jie Zi* or *The Origin of Chinese Characters* starts from "*yi* 一", ends with "*hai* 亥", the last of the twelve earthly branches[34]. The interpretation of "*yi* 一" in *Shuo Wen Jie Zi* or *The Origin of Chinese Characters* completely carries on the concepts in the myth of creating the world, thus conceiving the system of the concepts of the genesis of the world in Chinese philosophy. "*Yi* 一" is far beyond the number one, and is the opposite of the multiple as the myriad of beings in the world, and is the exact mysterious being or state before the beginning of the world.[35]

---

33 The author of *Hua Yu Lu* or *Arts of Painting* 《画语录》 is Shi Dao 石涛 (1630-1724), a great artist in Chinese painting. As Kaptchuk said that "The arts in China were nourished by the same naturalist and Daoist sensibility that fed Chinese philosophy and medicine." See Kaptchuk, Ted J. 2000: 17.

34 The twelve earthly branches refer to *Zi* 子, *Chou* 丑, *Yin* 寅, *Mao* 卯, *Chen* 辰, *Si* 巳, *Wu* 午, *Wei* 未, *Shen* 申, *You* 酉, *Xu* 戌, *Hai* 亥.

35 Ye Shuxian, Tian Daxian. 1998: 3.

In Chinese, both 一 and 壹 means one. Actually, 壹 is derived from 一. Yi 壹, written as 壹 in lesser seal script, resembles the image of a pot with a lid. *The Origin of Chinese Characters* interprets it as "undivided. Following 壶 (Pot)." *The Book of Songs · July* reads that "To pick up bottle gourds in August 八月断壶", where Mao's interpretation reads that "*Hu* 壶 refers to the bottle gourd." The bottle gourd stands for the creation myth of the nature: the upper became the heaven and the lower became the earth. See the Illus. 2 for the bottle gourd.

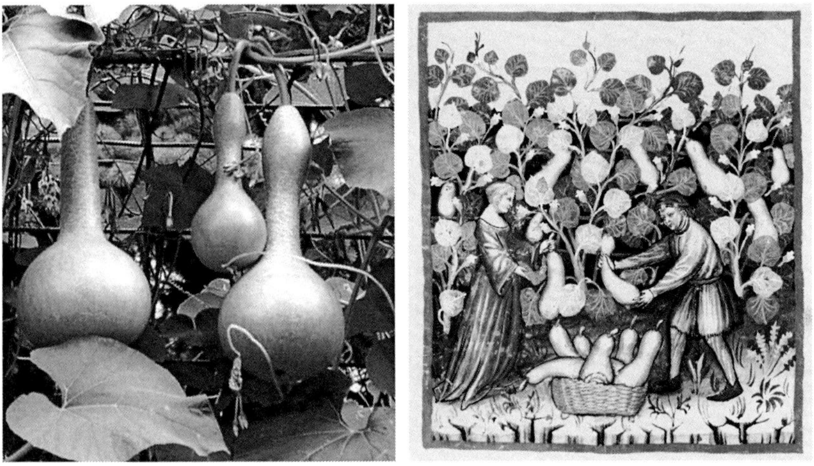

Illus. 2. The Bottle Gourd.
Right: Tacuinum Sanitatis (c1390, Cod. Vindob. p. n. 2644) fol. 22 verso

In Chinese legends, the bottle gourd functioned as a vessel to save people from flooding like Noah's ark. There are unearthed bottle gourds and bottle gourd-shaped potteries from some early ruins of 7,000 years ago in China. Besides, in ancient Chinese people's eyes, the bottle gourd was a symbol for uterus, and so for the female as well. The bottle gourd can be divided into two, which has been an essential utensil for a family, functioning as a spoon or a container. It has long been an original mascot for Chinese people, a symbol of good fortune, happiness, and official salary.

Giradort, Norman J., an American sinologist, believed that the bottle gourd was the sub-type of cosmological egg. He said that the bottle gourd and egg, chaos and nothing, hermaphroditic giant, and incestuous primordial couple can all be understood as the mythological symbol of "the fullness of being", which stresses the primordial unity of the sexes.[36]

The Fu Xi & Nü Wa Coupling Figure has many different versions, from stone figures of the Han Dynasty (206 B.C. – 220 A.D.) to paintings on silk, or paper of later dynasties until the Northern Dynasties (386-581). Paintings on silk or paper tend to be easily destroyed or decomposed, so are difficult to be found. But a large number of them are available in Turpan[37], Xinjiang. The Illus. 3 is one of those paintings. Fu Xi 伏羲 and Nü Wa 女娲 in this painting have high noses and deep eyes, just like persons of mixed blood. Wen Yiduo 闻一多 (1899-1946), a Chinese poet and scholar, did a textual research on Fu Xi. He believed that Fu Xi and Nü Wa, two names but one person, were personified bottle gourds, among which the only difference was the gender.[38]

This figure shows the image of the earliest ancestors in Chinese mythology. In this figure, Nü Wa holds a pair of compasses, which a witch in the remote antiquity used to study celestial phenomena and to communicate the heaven with earth. Fu Xi holds a carpenter's square, which was used to measure the land. The compasses and the square also imply that the heaven was round-shaped and the earth squared-shaped. They hug each other face to face and with their snake-shaped tails twining together. There is a sun above their heads and a moon below their tails. There are many stars and constellations around them.

It is amazing that the shape of their twining tails is the same as that of DNA with double helix, which contains the genetic instructions used in the development and functioning of all known living organisms.

---

36 Translated from Chinese. See the original reference *Myth and Meaning in Early Taoism*. Berkeley and Los Angeles: University of California Press, 1983.

37 Turpan has long been the centre of a fertile oasis and an important trade centre. It was historically located along the northern route of the Silk Road, thus being international and intercultural. It was originally one kingdom called Gushi 故師 which the Chinese conquered in 107 B.C. During the Han era the city changed hands several times between the Xiongnu or Hun 匈奴 and the Han, interspersed with short periods of independence.

38 See the first volume of *The Complete Works of Wen Yiduo*.

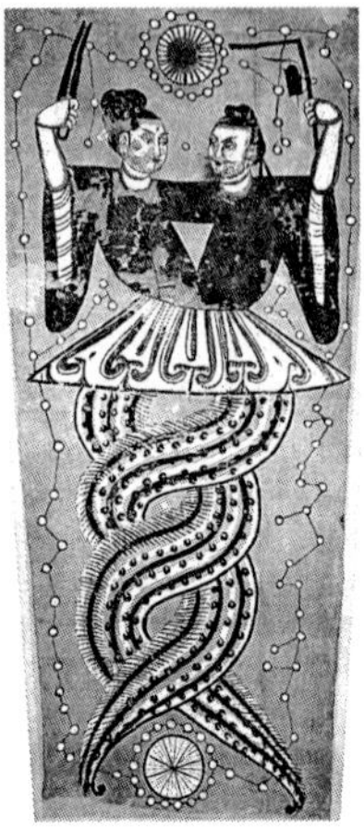

Illus. 3. Fu Xi & Nü Wa Coupling Figure. Unearthed in Xinjiang

Pan Gu 盘古 separated the heaven from the earth. "The chaotic world is just like an egg." And one was the chaotic world and the egg as well. *The Book of Changes* reads that "Therefore there is in the Changes the Great Primal Beginning. This generates the two primary forces (Yin and Yang). The two primary forces generate the four images (the four seasons). The four images generate the eight trigrams. 是故易有太极，是生两仪，两仪生四象，四象生八卦." Here in this quotation one is the *Tai Ji*, the Great Primal Beginning.

Actually, Dao 道 and One 一 can be mutually interpretive. In fact, Dao bears two qualities, i.e., nothing and being. Nothing means without shape or image, i.e., the chaotic world; Being means with shape and image, i.e. the one. So *Lao Tzu* reads that "Dao gives birth to one 道生一", which means that which has physical appearance is generated by that which has no physical appearance.

Qian Zuo Du of *The Book of Changes* reads that "Confucius states that 'Changes start from *Tai Ji*. *Tai Ji* gives birth to two, i.e. yin and yang, so to generate the heaven and earth. In between the heaven and earth there are the seasons of Spring, Summer, Autumn, and Winter, i.e. the four seasons. Each of the four seasons has the qualities of yin and yang, hardness and softness; therefore, the eight trigrams are generated. The eight trigrams establish the Dao of the Heaven and Earth, so the images of thunder, wind, water, fire, mountain and swamp are determined'."

《易·乾凿度》："孔子曰：易始于太极。太极分而为二，故生天地。天地有春、秋、冬、夏之节，故生四时。四时各有阴阳刚柔之分，故生八卦。八卦成列，天地之道立，雷风水火山泽之象定矣."

To sum up, "*yi* 一"is the first beginning of the numbers; "*yi* 壹" represents the image of the bottle gourd, means "undivided". One is far beyond the number one. Philosophers' interpretation of One is the origin of all things. All in all, One is *Tai Ji* or the Great Primal Beginning, the foundation of Dao, and the mystical state before the Genesis of the world.

Shuo Wen Jie Zi or *The Origin of Chinese Characters* starts with "*yi* 一" and ends with "*hai* 亥" for "*yi* 一" refers to *Tai Ji* or the Great Primal Beginning, the foundation of Dao, and the mystical state before the Genesis of the world; while "*hai* 亥" is interpreted as "the image of a pregnant woman, delivering a baby, then starting again from *yi* 一", then transforming again into everything in the world. Such an arrangement also suggests the circular reasoning of Chinese philosophy.

2.1.3 Heaven: Tian 天

Tian is usually translated into Heaven, but actually not the same. *Shuo Wen Jie Zi* or *The Origin of Chinese Characters* interprets "Tian 天" as "Vertex, Supreme; following 一 and 大. 顛也。至高無上，从一大." "Yi 一" is usually translated into one, but as we know it is far beyond the number one, referring to *Tai Ji* or the Great Primal Beginning, the foundation of Dao, and the mystical state before the Genesis of the world". "Da 大" is usually translated into big or great, being composed of "yi 一" and "Ren 人 or Man". See Illus. 4.

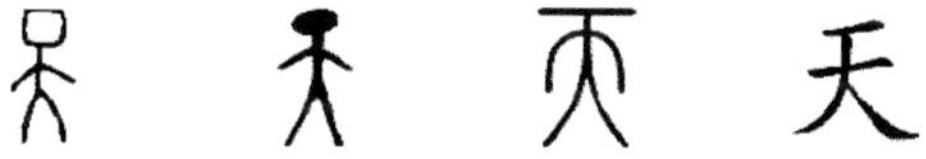

Illus. 4. "Tian 天" from Oracle, Bronze, Lesser Seal to Regular Script

Tian 天 refers to man's vertex, Sky, Heaven, and God. According to the interpretations of "tian 天" and "yi 一" in *Shuo Wen Jie Zi* or *The Origin of Chinese Characters*, *Tian* 天 bears 3 cultural connotations in the ancient China: 1) the mystical *tian*, the master of the world, like God; 2) the natural *tian*, including all of the natural phenomena, opposed to man-made; 3) the existing Heaven or sky, opposed to the earth.

2.1.4 Man: Ren 人

Shuo Wen Jie Zi or *The Origin of Chinese Characters* explains "Ren 人 or Man" as "the most valuable being in between the heaven and earth. 天地之性最貴者也."

Huang Di's Inner Classic. Basic Questions. Discourse on Treasuring Life and Preserving Physical Appearance 《黄帝内经素问·寶命全形論》 states that "Covered by the heaven and carried by the earth, all the myriad beings have come to existence. [But] None is more precious than man. Man comes to life through the *qi* of the heaven and earth; he matures in accordance with the laws of the four seasons. 天覆地載，萬物悉備，莫貴於人。人以天地之气生，四時之法成"; and that "Man is born on the earth, hanging his life to the heaven. The union of the heaven qi and the earth *qi* gives birth to man. Man can adapt himself to the seasons for the heaven and earth are his father and mother. 人生於地，懸命於天，天地合气，命之曰人。人能應四時者，天地爲之父母."

That is to say, the man shares the common constituent – *Qi* with the heaven, and earth. That is to say, the heaven, earth, and man constitute with the same ingredient - *Qi* in the same way, thus uniting and resembling each other, abbreviated as "*Tian Ren He Yi* or the Unity of Heaven and humankind".

2.1.5 Earth: Di 地

As for *Di* 地, *Shuo Wen Jie Zi* or *The Origin of Chinese Characters* explains that "Primordial *Qi* (Yuan Qi, 元气) is essential for separating the Heaven from the Earth; the Heaven is light and lucid, and the Earth is heavy and turbid; the Earth functions to carry all the things. 元气初分，輕清陽爲天，重濁陰爲地。萬物所陳列也."

This interpretation tells us three pieces of information: the essential factor to separate the heaven and earth - Primordial *Qi*; the qualities of the heaven and earth – the heaven being light and lucid and the earth being heavy and turbid; and the function of the earth – to carry all the things.

2.1.6 Three: San, 三

2.1.6.1 The original meaning of "San 三": Three and Many

The kids in the kindergarten all know the truth of 1+2=3. But actually, "San 三" can be three, or multiple, even ad infinitum, and uncountable. The story of Confucius studying *The Book of Changes* is cited in *Shi Ji* or *The Historical Records* by Sima Qian[39] that Confucius read *The Book of Changes* in his old age so frequently that the leather ropes fixing the pages (actually the bamboo slips) were fractured three (three=many) times 韦编三绝, which indicated he studied *The Book of Changes* very diligently.

In the remote antiquity, three was the largest number. For example, sinograms composed by three same parts means many:

淼：(of wide expanse of water) vast;
森：full of trees;
晶：many stars;
磊：many stones;
众：many people;
首：written as in lesser seal script, a lot of hair on the head.

Three in European Languages has the similar connotation[40]:

Thrice (English), Ter (Latin): three; many.
Tres (three, Latin) relates to Tran (beyond).
Très (very, extreme, French) relates to Trois (three).

Actually, using three or times of three for many are very common in Chinese language. For example,

---

39 Sima Qian 司马迁 (145 or 135? – ca. 86 B.C.), was a prefect historian of the Han Dynasty. He is regarded as the father of Chinese historiography because of his highly praised work, *The Historical Records* (Shi Ji, 史记), a general history of China covering more than two thousand years from Huang Di, the Yellow Emperor, to Emperor Han Wu Di. His definitive work laid the foundation for later Chinese historiography.
40 Translated from Chinese. The original reference is *NUMBER: The Language of Science (A Critical Survey Written for the Cultured non Mathematician)* by Tobias Dantzig (1884-1956).

三人成虎：Three (many) people spreading reports of a tiger make you believe there is one around. That is to say, a lie, if repeated often enough, will be accepted as truth.

三折肱而为良医：After having broken his upper arms for three (many) times, he becomes a good surgeon. That is to say, experience is a good teacher.

后宫佳丽三千人：Three thousand concubines of a monarch, which indicates that a monarch could have as many concubines as he liked.

The poem hereafter uses "three thousand feet" as an artistic exaggeration to describe the magnificent sight of the cataract on Mount Lu.

望庐山瀑布	Cataract on Mount Lu
日照香炉生紫烟，	The sunlit Censer perk exhales a wreath of cloud;
遥望瀑布挂前川。	Like an upended stream the cataract sounds loud.
飞流直下三千尺，	Its torrent dashes down three thousand feet from high;
疑是银河落九天。	As if the Silver River fell from azure sky.

(Originally composed by Li Bai[41], Translated by Xu Yuanchong)

2.1.6.2 Three Gives Birth to All Things

Lao Tzu reads that "Dao begets the one, the one begets the two, the two begets the three, and the three gives birth to all things (in the world). 道生一，一生二，二生三，三生万物." Dao and One can be mutually interpretive. In fact, Dao bears two qualities, i.e., nothing and being. Nothing means without shape or image, i.e., the chaotic world; Being means with shape and image, i.e. the one. So "Dao gives birth to one" means that which has physical appearance is generated by that which has no physical appearance. Two refers to the heaven and earth, and yin and yang; "the two begets the three" can be understood as the union of the heaven *qi* and the earth *qi* makes man.

41 Li Bai 李白 (701-762), also known in the West by various other transliterations as Li Po, has been regarded as one of the greatest poets in China's Tang Dynasty, which is often called China's "golden age" of poetry. Thirty-four of his poems are included in the popular anthology *Three Hundred Tang Poems*. As regards to Chinese cultural influence, Li Bai's poetry has been much esteemed from his lifetime through the present day. Indeed, in China he has been known as the best of the Romantic Poets. In the West his influences include many translations, adaptations, and much inspiration.

And then three, i.e. the heaven, earth and man, is the first complete unit of the creation of the world. Therefore three is the foundation for the birth, growth and development of all things in the world.

Zuo's Spring Autumn Annals (*Zuo Zhuan* 左传, or *Zuo Shi Chun Qiu* 左氏春秋)[42] states that "Three is the number of the heaven, earth and man. 三者，天地人之数也." *Shuo Wen Jie Zi* or *The Origin of Chinese Characters* explains "three" as "the Dao (way) of Heaven, Earth and man 天地人之道也." *Shi Ji* or *The Historical Records* reads that "The numbers start at one, end with ten, and complete with three. 数始于一，终于十，成于三." *The Book of Changes* names the heaven, earth, and man as "Three *Cai*". The sinoram "才 Cai" is written as  in the oracle script, pictographic, in which the upper horizontal line stands for the soil, the part below it resembles the image of the tender shoot just sprouting from the seed but not coming up out of the ground, and so its original meaning is (of trees and grasses, or plant) newborn.

2.1.6.3 The Importance of "the Central and Harmonious *Qi*"

Let's now go back to *Lao Tzu. the 42nd Chapter.*

> "Dao begets the one,
> The one begets the two,
> The two begets the three,
> And the three gives birth to all things (in the world).
> All things in the world bear yin and embrace yang,
> where the central and harmonious *qi* makes them in harmony."
> 道生一，一生二，二生三，三生万物。万物负阴而抱阳，冲气以为和。

The relationship of "the central and harmonious *qi*" and "the Three Newborns" is just like that of "the soil" and "the five phases", where the soil is in the Center of the other four phases, i.e. Wood-East, Fire-South, Metal-West, and Water-North. If without the middle there would be neither Left Wing

---

42 It is the earliest Chinese work of narrative history and covers the period from 722 to 468 B.C. It is one of the most important sources for understanding the history of the Spring and Autumn Period. Together with the *Gong Yang Zhuan* 《公羊传》 and *Guliang Zhuan* 《谷梁传》, the work forms one of the surviving "Three Commentaries on the Spring and Autumn Annals".

nor Right Wing; if without the central and harmonious *qi* there would be neither Yin *qi* nor Yang *qi*.

Take the structure of an atom as an example. Its outer is the electrons (-), while its inner is composed of the protons (+) and neutrons. If without the neutrons, an atom could not be kept as a stable entity. It is clear that the central and harmonious *qi* bears the same importance as the neutrons. And Heaven – Earth – Man make up a holistic system, among which they are independent and closely related to each other and the man is the dominator.

2.2 *Tian Ren He Yi:* The World View of Chinese Culture

The idea of *Tian Ren He Yi* or the Unity of Heaven and Humankind first shows up in *Chuang Tzu*, which states that "The heaven and earth are father and mother of all things in the world. 天地者，万物之父母也。."

2.2.1 Dao 道: The Way of the Nature and Medicine

Actually there are two kinds of Daoism, i.e., *Dao Jia* or Daoist School 道家 and *Dao Jiao* or Daoist Religion 道教.

Daoist School 道家 is one of the major philosophical thoughts of school, stands for recluses' or hermits'[43] philosophy, and is named after its theoretical foundation and core concept – Dao 道, the source and rule of the nature. It has exerted deep influences on the development of Chinese philosophy as a whole, as well as almost every aspect of Chinese culture. It was initiated by Yang Zhu 杨朱 (?-?), founded by Lao Tzu 老子(580? – 500 B.C.?), further developed by Chuang Tzu 庄子(369? – 286? B.C.) and Lie Tzu 列子 (?-?). Its main works include *Lao Tzu* 老子, *Chuang Tzu* 庄子, *Lie Tzu* 列子, *Wen Tzu* 文子, *He Guan Tzu* 鹖冠子, *Huan Nan Tzu* 淮南子, and four chapters of *Guan Tzu* 管子 - *Xin Shu* 1 心术上, *Xin Shu* 2 心

43 Neither recluse nor hermit can convey the original connotations of the word in Chinese, i.e. "Yin Shi 隐士", which actually refers to talented people who are very capable in administering and running a country but not willing to do this. But persons who live a very simple life alone and like to avoid others are not always talented people.

术下, *Bai Xin* 白心, and *Nei Ye* 内业. Daoist school believes that Dao is the source and root of everything in the nature and that Dao creates everything in the nature in a complete natural way without any intervention, i.e. the nature of Dao is "Having Effortless Action", which is the fundamental rule of controlling everything in the nature. Daoist school observes the rule of the nature, and advocates a natural, simple, easy and free life. Some vital fundamental concepts such as *Dao* 道, *De* 德, *You* (有, Being), *Wu* (无, Non-Being), *Li* 理, *Qi* 气, *Tai Ji* 太极, and *Wu Ji* 无极 are all from Daoist school.

While Daoist Religion 道教 carried on the tradition of "Wu Dou Mi Dao 五斗米道", which was founded by Zhang Ling 张陵 (?-?). It was so named for whoever wanted to join the religion should donate five *dous* (*dou*, a measure for grain) of rice. The religion formed on the basis of ideas of Daoist school 道家 together with ways on how to become supernatural beings, popular worship of gods and ghosts, and witchcrafts. It regards Lao Tzu as the Guru, and has religious belief, worship of Gods, followers, organizations, as well as religious ceremonies and activities. It advocates being calm and "Having Effortless Action", pursuing immortality or eternal life, and finally achieving Dao and transforming into god. Zhang Lu 张鲁 (?-216), Zhang Ling's grandson, spread it through the country by the aid of his political influence.

Daoist school focuses on the study of "Dao", and *Lao Tzu* and *Chuang Tzu* are the most important classics of Daoist philosophy. "*Huang Di's Inner Classic* is the highest authority on philosophy of Chinese medicine, and also one of the most important classics on Daoism of Chinese philosophy."[44]

Dao 道 was originally written as «  «, following the part of "辵", which actually shows an image of a man walking on a way with his eyes big open, metaphorizing "the only way you must follow or take in order to go ahead" . Its original meaning is explained in *Shuo Wen Jie Zi* or *The Origin of Chinese Characters* as "the way to walk 所行道也", which indicates the direction for the walker, is the route to a certain destination, and then is metapharized to mean law, rule, or principle.

44 Ni, Maoshing. 1995: Back-Cover. Here Daoism refers to Daoist School not Daoist Religion.

Besides, Dao 道 in the ancient times had gained several other extended meanings: 1. "thinking system or theory" such as in *The Analects of Confucius · Living in brotherliness* that "My *thinking system* is run through by a central idea"; 2. "to govern or manage" explained in *Guang Ya · Shi Gu*《广雅 · 释诂》; 3. "way or method" such as in *Shang Jun Shu* or *The Book of Shang Yang's Ideas* that "There is not just one *way* to govern the society." Also, the sinogram 道 resembles the shape of 首 head, thereby bearing the meaning of start or beginning. You see that Dao 道 bears so many meanings, therefore, as a fundamental philosophical concept; its connotations are deep, subtle and complicated.

It is *Lao Tzu* that discusses Dao as an abstract concept and endows it with a philosophical meaning of "embracing all". *Lao Tzu· Chapter 25* states that "Therefore, Dao is great. Heaven is great. Earth is great. Man is great. In the country, there are four great things, and man is one of them. Man abides by the earth. Earth abides by the heaven. Heaven abides by Dao. Dao abides by the nature;" The Chapter 42 states that "Dao begets One (*Qi*). One begets Two (Yin-Yang). Two begets Three (the integration of Yin and Yang). Three begets all things. All things carry Yin and embrace Yang, where the central and harmonious *Qi* makes them in harmony.", which shows the generation of all things in the nature from Dao (*Wu* 无 or Non-Being) to all things (*You* 有 or Being). That is to say, Dao is the origin of all things in the nature and the Way which must be observed by all.

In Chinese medicine, *Huang Di's Inner Classic* states that "Yin and yang are Dao or the Way of the heaven and earth, the fundamental principles of the myriad things, the father and mother of all changes and transformations, the root and beginning of generating and killing, the palace of man's spirit" in *Basic Questions. Comprehensive Discourse on Images Corresponding to Yin-Yang.*[45] It also states that "Of all things in between the heaven and earth, nothing is more precious than man. Man lives on the *Qi* in between the heaven and earth, and grows in accordance with the laws of the seasons."

---

45 Note: The translations of the quotations from *Huang Di Nei Jing Su Wen* all accord with Guo Aichun's interpretation in his book "*Huang Di Nei Jing Su Wen* with Textual Criticisms, Annotations and Modern Language Interpretation 《黄帝内经素问校注语译》(2nd Ed.)", published by Tianjin Science and Technology Press (Tianjin, China) in 1999.

in *Basic Questions · Discourse on Protecting Life and Preserving Physical Appearance*. *The Origin of Chinese Characters · Man Part* also states that "Man is the most valuable being in between the heaven and earth."

Thereby, it can be seen from the above quotations that "Heaven", "Earth", and "Man" are independent from and closely related to each other, and they compose a whole system, in which man plays the leading role; and that the thinking way of the "heaven-earth-man" in *Lao Tzu* embodies the thinking way of the nature, which is specified in the *Inner Classic* as the thinking way of the Chinese medicine, which shows that the great progress of natural philosophy in the aspect of the nature replacing the God. In *Lao Tzu*, Dao abides by the nature; In the *Inner Classic*, medicine abides by the Dao; In essence, medicine abides by the nature. Holistic approach and individualized treatment based on pattern identification with the aim for the central and harmonious state in health care and disease treatment are all embodied in *Lao Tzu* and the *Inner Classic*.

Chuang Tzu carries on *Lao Tzu*'s Dao of the nature, and advocates that man was born in between the heaven and earth, and so should follow the way of the nature, i.e. the way of Yin-Yang and the seasons, in health care. It also states the way of cultivating the spirit - "to do nothing that is left undone" and "to be indifferent to any fame or gain." These ideas are all embodied in the *Inner Classic*.[46] Therefore, Dao abides by the nature, and medicine abides by Dao, and so medicine abides by the nature, which is the Dao of Chinese medicine.

2.2.2 *The Book of Changes: Tian Ren He Yi* as Philosophical Foundation of Dao of All Kinds in Chinese Culture

2.2.2.1 Viewpoint of Unity with Three Dimensions

> "In ancient times the holy sages made *The Book of Changes* to follow the order of their nature and fate. Therefore they determined the Dao of the heaven and named it yin and yang, determined the Dao of the earth and named it hardness and softness, and determined the Dao of man and

---

46 See the chapters of *Tian Shi* 天适 and *Ke Yi* 刻意 of *Chuang Tzu* 《庄子》, and the chapter *Discourse on the Prenatal True Qi of the Remote Antiquity* of *Basic Questions* 《素问 · 上古天真论》 for more details.

named it benevolence and upright. They combined these three fundamental powers and doubled them; hence in *The Book of Changes* a sign (*Gua* 卦 or Hexagram) is always formed by six lines."

昔者圣人之作易也，将以顺性命之理。是以立天之道，曰阴与阳；立地之道，曰柔与刚；立人之道，曰仁与义。兼三才而两之，故易六画而成卦。

- Shuo Gua, 说卦

The above quotation shows the viewpoint of unity with three dimensions in *The Book of Changes:*

Dao of Heaven: yin and yang to make all things begin;

Dao of Earth: hardness and softness to give birth to all things;

Dao of Man: benevolence and upright to complete all things.

And "the Three *Cai* 三才" or "the Three Newborns" are actually the symbol for the idea of "the Unity of Heaven and Humankind".

Viewpoint of unity with three dimensions also exists in Greek mythology. For example, there were three Goddesses for fate: One responsible for spinning the life line for a newborn baby, one determining the length of the life line, and one cutting off the life line when one was dying; three Goddesses for Opportunities to be in charge of good fate and opportunity; three Goddesses for Revenge to be in charge of punishing those who bore false witness, murdered family members, and maltreated non-natives respectively; and three Goddesses for Beauty and Wisdom, i.e. Zeus's three daughters - Aglaia for brightness and handsome, Euphrosyne for happiness and cheerfulness, and Thalia for vigour and youth; etc.

Viewpoint of unity with three dimensions is also available in Christian Belief. Comparative mythologists believed that the relationship among the Father, the Holy Ghost (Spirit), and the Son of God reflects the triangle relationship among Heaven Father, Earth Mother, and Man's Son.

Difference between the viewpoint of unity with three dimensions of Christian belief and Chinese philosophy reflects one major cultural difference between the two cultures. Christian belief focuses on the value of the belief of "One God", and thus its culture is a kind of God-based culture. While Chinese philosophy stresses the invaluable position of man 人, written as ? in the oracle script, who stands upright with one's two legs in between the heaven and earth, thus forming a situation of tripartite confrontation, like the three legs of a tripod, and therefore Chinese culture is a kind of Man-based culture. This has been very popular in almost every aspect of

Chinese culture, including ancient bureaucratic establishment, and Chinese medicine.

2.2.2.2 *Tian Ren He Yi* as Philosophical Foundation of Dao of Chinese Medicine

The Book of Changes establishes *Tian Ren He Yi* 天人合一 or the Unity of Heaven and Humankind by making a farfetched comparison between them. It states that "In the remote antiquity when Fu Xi 伏羲 ruled the country, he raised his head to observe images on the heaven, bowed his head to observe phenomena on the earth, observed images of birds and beasts and those of the earth, took near images from man and far images of other things from the nature, on the basis of which he then started to make the Eight Trigrams to illustrate the phenomena.", which lays the philosophical foundation for Dao of all kinds in Chinese culture and medicine, which formed through metaphorizing.

Here the formation of the Dao of Chinese medicine is the case in point. So, how the Dao of Chinese medicine formed? Or what is the relationship between *The Book of Changes* and Chinese medicine – one deals with *Xiang Shu* (images and numbers, 象数) and their implicit meanings in the nature, while the other talks about health and illnesses of man? Actually they are talking about the same thing in essence by applying metaphors or metaphorizing: life – one on the life of the cosmos and the other on the life of man. Both are open systems, both are communicated with and related to each other, and both should be in a state of harmony in itself and with the other, otherwise problems or illnesses will ensue, which is radically different from the strict divisions between the life and the inanimate, the subject and the object, the man and the nature etc. in the Western culture. Maybe it is fantastic for the Westerners that *The Book of Changes* and Chinese medicine do not reduce life or being to something material like cells, proteins, genes, etc., instead they understand life or being by establishing and interpreting something symbolic like *gua* 卦 and *yao* 爻, *Qi*, yin and yang, the eight trigrams, the five phases, the images and numbers, the visceral manifestation, and so on.

It's worth to note that most of the thinking ways of Chinese medicine originate from *The Book of Changes* and are established through metaphorizing:

1. The Thinking Way of *Xiang Shu* (images and numbers, 象数): The *Zang Xiang* (Visceral Manifestation, 藏象) theory is established on the basis of elementary understanding of the organs to explain physiological functions of man through *Qu Xiang Bi Lei* (taking image and analogizing, 取象比类); and "pattern identification and treatment" is set up by summarizing and generalizing various symptoms and signs into a certain "pattern image" also through *Qu Xiang Bi Lei*.

2. The Thinking Way of *Bian Yi* (changing, 变易): Chinese medicine regards life, health and illnesses as constantly changing processes, and stresses not only the transmission and transformation of illnesses, but also institutes corresponding treatments to meet the changes.

3. The Thinking Way of Holistic Approach: *The Book of Changes* establishes *Tian Ren He Yi* 天人合一 or the Unity of Heaven and Humankind, on the basis of which the theoretical system of Chinese medicine has formed. Chinese medicine regards man as an organic whole, and also studies the physiology and pathology of man in the unity and mutual relations of man, nature and society, thereby administers corresponding healthcare methods.

To sum up, *Tian Ren He Yi* is the philosophical foundation for Dao of all kinds in Chinese culture and science.

2.2.3 Dong Zhongshu[47]: Man Mirroring Heaven

Dong Zhongshu's proposal of "Proscribing all non-Confucian schools of thought and espousing Confucianism as the orthodox state ideology 罢黜百家，独尊儒术" was adopted by Emperor Han Wu Di 汉武帝 (live in be-

---

47 Dong Zhongshu 董仲舒 (179-104 B.C.) was a Han Dynasty scholar who was traditionally associated with the promotion of Confucianism as the official ideology of the Chinese imperial state. His thought integrated Yin Yang cosmology into a Confucian ethical framework. He is also considered the originator of the doctrine of Heaven and Man Being Mutually Responsive 天人感应. There are two works that are attributed to Dong Zhongshu: one is the *Countermeasures for Recommending Able and Virtuous Men* (*Ju Xian Liang Dui Ce*, 《举贤良对策》) in three chapters, preserved under "*The History of the Former Han Dynasty*" (*Han Shu*, 《汉书》); and the other that has survived to the present is the *Luxuriant Dew of the Spring and Autumn Annals* (*Chun Qiu Fan Lu*, 《春秋繁露》) in 82 chapters.

tween 156-87 B.C.; reign in between 141-87 B.C.). His thought integrated Yin Yang cosmology into a Confucian ethical framework.

He is also considered the originator of the doctrine of "Interactions between Heaven and Man", which mainly manifests in two parts: Chinese political philosophy and Chinese natural philosophy. From the standpoint of Chinese political philosophy, his proposal lays down rules for deciding the legitimacy of a monarch as well as providing a set of checks and balances for reining a monarch. Such a proposal legitimated the emperors' autocratic government for thousands of years since Emperor Han Wu Di in China.

While based on his natural philosophy, Chinese medicine, and Chinese astronomy, etc. came into being[48] and *Huang Di's Inner Classic* has still functioned as the highest authority on Chinese medicine since then. He said "To unite Heaven and Man into one by the way of analogizing.以类合一，天人一也。(From the chapter of *Yin Yang Yi* of *Chun Qiu Fan Lu*《春秋繁露·阴阳义》)."

Chun Qiu Fan Lu further states in the chapter of *Man Mirroring Heaven* (*Ren Fu Tian Shu*, 人副天数) that

> "The virtue of Heaven is to bestow, the virtue of Earth is to transform, and the virtue of Man is to be righteous. ... The essence of Heaven and Earth is to generate beings, among which Man is the most honored. ... In the nature only Man can be analogized to the Heaven and Earth. Man has 360 joints, analogizing the number of the Heaven; Man's body, bone and flesh analogize the thickness of the Earth. Ears and eyes on the head can listen and look, metaphorizing the sun and the moon; The orifices and vessels of the body are just like rivers and gorges; Happiness, anger, grief and joy of the heart (the gamut of human feeling) are similar to spirits (*SHEN Qi*). Man's body is so high, thus analogizes the Heaven. ... Therefore, Man's head is round, thus metaphorizing the appearance of the Heaven for the Heaven is also round; hair metaphorizes the stars; the ears and the eyes are bright, thus metaphorizing the sun and the moon; the exhalation and inhalation of the mouth and nose metaphorize the *qi* of the wind; the heart in the chest understands, thus metaphorizing the spirits and the gods; the emptiness or repletion of the organs in the abdomen symbolizes various things; various things is closest to the Earth, therefore the part below the lumbar is the Earth; the images of the Heaven and Earth are demarcated by the lumbar; the part above the neck is the place of the spirit and dignity,

48 Wei Zhengtong. 2003: 321-324.

thus showing the dignity of the Heaven; the part below the neck, some rich and thick, some poor and thin, analogizes the soil; the feet are square-shaped, analogizing the shape of the Earth. ... The symbols of the Heaven and Yin-Yang are complete in the body; the body is just like the Heaven, so its numbers accord with the numbers of the heaven; therefore the will of the Heaven (or God's will) makes them interrelate and interact with each other. The Heaven takes its numbers of a year to make a man; therefore, man has 366 small joints to accord with the days of a year, 12 big vessels to accord with the months of a year, 5 *zang* organs to accord with the five phases, and 4 limbs to accord with the four seasons; opening eyes and closing eyes accord with the days and the nights; hardness and softness accord with the winter and summer; grief and joy accord with yin and yang; the heart calculates to accord with moral standard or law; the behaviors observe moral principles to accord with the relationship between the Heaven and Earth. A man was born with all of the above mentioned, among which those countable take numbers of the Heaven and Earth and those uncountable analogize and metaphorize the Heaven and Earth. Anyway, man mirrors the Heaven."
天德施，地德化，人德义。…… 天地之精所以生物者，莫贵於人。…… 唯人独能偶天地。人有三百六十节，偶天之数也；形体骨肉，偶地之厚也。上有耳目聪明，日月之象也；体有空穹进脉，川谷之象也；心有哀乐喜怒，神气之类也。观人之礼一，何高物之甚，而类於天也。…… 是故人之身，首而员，象天容也；发，象星辰也；耳目戾戾，象日月也；鼻口呼吸，象风气也；胸中达知，象神明也，腹胞实虚，象百物也。百物者最近地，故要以下，地也。天地之象，以要为带。颈以上者，精神尊严，明天类之状也；颈而下者，丰厚卑辱，土壤之比也。足布而方，地形之象也。…… 天地之符，阴阳之副，常设於身，身犹天也，数与之相参，故命与之相连也。天以终岁之数，成人之身，故小节三百六十六，副日数也；大节十二分，副月数也；内有五藏，副五行数也；外有四肢，副四时数也；乍视乍瞑，副书夜也；乍刚乍柔，副冬夏也；乍哀乍乐，副阴阳也；心有计虑，副度数也；行有伦理，副天地也。此皆暗肤著身，与人俱生，比而偶之合。於其可数也，副数；不可数者，副类。皆当同而副天，一也。

Dong Zhongshu's thoughts on "Interactions between Heaven and Man"and "Man Mirroring Heaven" have been very influential to Chinese medicine. You may refer to the chapters of *Yin Yang Xi Ri Yue* 阴阳系日月 or *Yin-Yang Relating to the Sun & the Moon* and *Xie Ke* 邪客 or *Pathogens* of *Ling Shu* 《灵枢》 or *Miraculous Pivot* and *Qi Xue* 气穴 or *Acupoints* of *Su Wen* 《素问》 or *Basic Questions* of *Huang Di's Inner Classic*. By the way, *Huang Di's Inner Classic* can also be regarded as a philosophical classic, esp. in the fields of interpreting the nature, beings and life with *qi*, yin-yang and five phases, it is second to none although it is a well known classic on Chinese medicine.[49]

There are also some critical viewpoints on Dong Zhongshu's Interactions between Heaven and Man. Li Yangbo 李阳波 (1947-1991) commented that it is very difficult for the human society to mirror the nature, but the components of the nature such as plants, animals and human beings themselves as well as their growth, maturity, aging and death, can not escape from the rules dominated by the Heaven. Therefore, he advocated that the social part of Dong Zhongshu's "Interactions between Heaven and Man" should be discarded and the biological part should be preserved in Chinese medicine for man and the nature did not unit and resemble each other in the social structure, but only in physiological states, and believed that Chinese medicine is a system of transforming the relationships of *Shu Shu* 术数 among the heaven, earth and man, so he preferred the formulation: Perspective of "Nature and Living Beings" or Perspective of "Heaven and Man" instead of *Tian Ren He Yi*.[50]

As regards to how man mirrors the social structure, a chapter entitled *Ling Lan Mi Dian Lun* 灵兰秘典论 or *Discourse on Hidden Canons in the Numinous Orchid Chambers*[51] from *Huang Di's Inner Classic Basic Questions* analogizes *Zang Fu* with the ancient bureaucratic establishment, which reads that

> "The Heart is the official functioning as ruler. ...
> The Lungs are the official functioning as chancellor. ...
> The Liver is the official functioning as general. ...
> The Gallbladder is the official functioning as rectifier. ...
> The *Dan Zhong* or Thoracic Center is the official functioning as envoy. ...
> The Spleen and the Stomach are the officials responsible for grain storage. ...
> The Large Intestine is the official functioning as transmitter. ...
> The Small Intestine is the official functioning as recipient. ...
> The Kidneys are the official functioning as operator with force. ...

49 Ma Boying. 1994: 247.

50 Narrated by Li Yangbo, Systematized by Liu Lihong, et al. *Opening the Door of Chinese Medicine: Introduction to Doctrine of Periods and Qi*《开启中医之门：运气学导论》. Beijing: China Press of TCM, 2004.

51 The numinous orchid chambers are said to be Huang Di's library.

> The Triple *Jiao* is the official responsible for sluices. ...
> The Bladder is the official responsible for reservoirs. ...
> Hence, if the ruler functions efficiently, his subjects are in peace...
> If the ruler functions abnormally, then the twelve officials are in danger. ..."

You can see that this chapter discusses the importance of harmony of the internal environment of the human being from social and psychological aspects by metaphorizing the rules of administering a country, which is guided by "Man Mirroring Heaven" - it reflects some social problems by discussing physiological functions of organs on one hand, and improves understanding of the biological being by metaphorizing the rules of administering a country, social and psychological phenomena on the other. Thus it actually implies the biological-psychological-social medical mode.

Medical mode has evolved in the course of development of medical practice, which mainly reflects basic thinking and main methods when observing and dealing with medical problems. Medical modes have always existed and varied constantly with changes in thoughts of philosophy of medicine of different times. It's generally believed that the development of medical modes has gone through the following stages from god, natural philosophy, mechanism, biological to physiological – psychological – social medical mode. With the considerable progress in social medicine and medical psychology, the academic circle has come to know that the practice of traditional biological medical mode is just one-sided pursuit of well-being of human beings. The significant variations in disease spectrum also objectively require the transition of the medical mode to a comprehensive one, i.e. physiological – psychological – social medical mode, which regards the occurrence and development of diseases as the outcome of changes not only in biological and psychological states but also in social adaptability.[52]

A good social, political environment, the nature in an ecological balance, and a man who knows the importance of living harmony with the nature, are of vital significance not only in cultivating man's health in both mental and physical aspects but also in establishing a better world for all the living beings.

52 Sun Baozhi. 2003: 26, 29.

2.2.4 Connotations of *Tian Ren He Yi*

Tian Ren He Yi bears the following connotations: Man Mirroring Heaven, i.e. regarding the heaven as man, and man as the heaven; Harmony of Man and Heaven, i.e. Man and Heaven following the laws of the nature. *The Classic of Rites · The Doctrine of Mean* 《礼记·中庸》 states that "Sincerity is the way of the heaven; Sincerity is the way of man. 诚者，天之道也；诚之者，人之道也." That is to say, sincerity makes Man and Heaven unite. My understanding of "sincerity" is to be true to its original, to follow the way of the nature.

Lao Tzu. The 69th Chapter reads that

"Dao is great,
Heaven is great,
Earth is great,
Man is also great.
There are four great things in the country,
Man is one of them.
Man abides by the earth,
Earth abides by the heaven,
Heaven abides by Dao,
Dao abides by the nature."

2.3 *Tian Ren He Yi:* The Ontological Presupposition of Chinese Medicine

Tian Ren He Yi actually indicates that the heaven, earth, and man constitute in the same way, i.e. being composed of the same ingredient – *Qi*, in the same order. That is to say, the heaven is a bigger man, while the man is a smaller heaven; or the heaven is a macrocosm, while man is a microcosm.

Chinese medicine believes that all things in the world are related to each other, that the world is composed of the same constituent – *Qi*, and that the immense variety of things and phenomena in the world share some similar characteristics at different levels, different categories, and different aspects, and moreover, there exist many necessary relationships among them.

The theoretical system of Chinese medicine has formed on the idea of *Tian Ren He Yi* or the Unity of Heaven and Humankind. *Huang Di's Inner Classic ·Basic Questions· Discourse on Protecting Life and Preserving Physical Appearance* states that "Man is born on the earth, hanging his life to the heaven. The union of *qi* of the heaven and earth gives birth to man. Man can adapt himself to the seasons for the heaven and earth are his father and mother."

Tian Ren He Yi 天人合一 is the ontological presupposition of Chinese medicine. The classical Chinese "Dao-Qi" monism 道——气一元论 closes the incompatibilities between the nature and society, the heaven and man. That is the root reason why *Huang Di's Inner Classic · Basic Questions* emphasizes repeatedly the vital importance of "To know the line patterns in heaven above, to know the structures of the earth below, and to know the human affairs in the center 上知天文，下知地理，中知人事" in knowing medicine.[53]

Presupposed that the world is composed of the same constituent - *Qi*, analogies in Chinese medicine involve every aspect of human life – life in the nature, politics, society, astronomy, geography, military affairs, etc. Then what is *Qi*?

Chinese philosophy applies the concept of *Qi* to explain the nature of existence. *The Origin of Chinese Characters · Qi Part* states that "*Qi* refers to thin, floating clouds. The sinogram 气 [54] is a pictograph. 雲气也。象形。" The sinogram 气 in the oracle inscription of the Shang Dynasty (ca. 16th–11th century B.C.), was written as "  ", which resembles air current, evaporating and rising, whose image is just like cloud, will disappear very soon and become invisible. Therefore, *Qi* is invisible and formless, exists everywhere, can be gathered into a form, for instance, *Qi* can be condensed into water.

Soon afterwards, the *Qi* which surrounds and congests the man's space was abstracted into the *Qi* which bears a philosophical sense. Philosophers of the Spring Autumn and Warring States Periods (770-221 B.C.) believed that *Qi* is the basic ingredient constituting the world, and also the basic ingredient constituting the Man and that everything in the world comes into being by the movement and mutation of *Qi*, as stated in *The Book of*

---

53 See the chapter 69 "Comprehensive Discourse on Changes [resulting from] Qi Interaction" and chapter 75 "Discourse on Making Known the Perfect Teachings" for details.

54 The sinogram 氣 is not the original form of 气 but a mistake during the evolution of Chinese characters, which means "feed and grain for the guests" according to *Shuo Wen Jie Zi* or *The Origin of Chinese Characters · Rice Part.*

Changes that "Everything is transformed and generated by the enshrouding [*Qi*] of the heaven and earth. 天地氤氲，万物化生." As *Chuang Tzu* 莊子 comments that *The Book of Changes* talks about yin *qi* and yang *qi* from the beginning to the end.

Tian Ren He Yi actually indicates that the heaven, earth, and man constitute with the same ingredient – *Qi* in the same way. Therefore, *Qi* becomes the foundation of *Tian Ren He Yi*.

Later on, ancient Chinese medical experts introduced "*Qi*" into the medical field at the right moment. In the time of *Huang Di's Inner Classic*, "*Qi*" is regarded not only as the basic ingredient constituting the world, but also as the basic ingredient constituting the Man which can be transformed into blood, essence, and body fluid, etc., and the normal functional activities of the life which is governed by "*Qi*" is known as *Shen* 神 or spirit.

According to *A Concise Dictionary of Chinese Medicine*, *Qi* in Chinese medicine bears the following meanings: 1. nutritious, essential substance flowing inside the body, such as food *qi*, breathed air; 2. functional activities of the *zang fu* organs in a general sense, such as visceral *Qi*, i.e, the functional activities of the *zang fu* organs; *Qi* can also be classified into original *Qi*, nutritive *Qi*, defensive *Qi*, pectoral *Qi*, etc. according to its source, distribution, and function; 3. the location or stage of pattern identification of warm diseases.[55]

That is to say, *Qi* in philosophy of Chinese medicine is to make man become man, and the logic function implied in the *Wei* (Guard) – *Qi* – *Ying* (Camp) – Blood Pattern Identification for treatment of warm diseases is the condition of processes and activities of life, i.e. *Qi* is the condition for what it is conditioned, which is similar to Plato's ideas. Plato's ideas are the conditions of the understanding of things and of the beings of the things. Some conceptual aspects of *Qi* have the same argumentative function as Plato's theory of ideas.

Be aware, ancient Chinese philosophy regards *Qi* as the ontology of the nature, and stresses *Qi*'s material characteristics – the basic ingredient constituting the nature; while in philosophy of Chinese medicine, *Qi* is the unification of material aspect and functional activities – *Qi* is not only the basic

55 Li Jingwei, Ou Yongxin, Yu Ying'ao, et al. 2001: 173.

ingredient constituting the Man, but is also used to expound the dynamic processes and functional activities of the life.

Here is worth to note that the concept of *Qi* in Chinese culture is radically different from the concept of material in Western culture, a Chinese misinterpretation. *Guan Tzu* states that "*Qi* can be limitedlessly small and limitedlessly big." Therefore, *Qi*, the origin of the nature and life, is formless without any boundaries or any separation of two opposites (dichotomy). So man can feel *Qi* for man is a being of the integration of the body and mind, of the subject and object, of the material and function. The concept of material in the Western culture must be something with a form even with the rapid development of understanding the structure of materials. Materialism is a philosophical foundation of Western natural science, which stresses the separation and opposition of the body and mind, of the subject and object, and greatly promotes the development of modern Western science.

To sum up, the formless *Qi* explains the ontology of philosophy of Chinese medicine, i.e., in the structure of Chinese philosophy, *Qi* has the corresponding place of the Western ontology, and is also the foundation of the model of *Qi*, Yin-Yang, and Five Phases; *Tian Ren He Yi* 天人合一 is the ontological presupposition of Chinese medicine.

Language is metaphoric in its essence and nature. ...

- Ernst Cassirer[56]

Qu Xiang Bi Lei 取象比类 or Taking Image and Analogizing is the core methodology of Chinese medicine, and embodies the three key processes/elements of classical Chinese metaphor studies: "*Xiang* 象 or Imaging/Image – *Bi* 比 or Analogizing/Analogy – *Yu* 喻 or Metaphorizing/Metaphor" , finally forming metaphors in Chinese medicine, and guiding clinical practice, and developing Chinese medicine in both theoretical and clinical aspects.

- The Author

3 *Qu Xiang Bi Lei:* The Metaphorizing Process and the Way of Forming Metaphors in Chinese Medicine

Chinese medicine has been developed in the framework which the "Four Great Medical Classics" established around 2,000 years ago. Historical texts of Chinese medicine are full of metaphors: from terms to sentences, to paragraphs, to texts, and even to the whole system, which reflect the imaging thinking in Chinese medicine.

Metaphor is an important field of study shared in rhetoric, linguistics and philosophy. The nature of metaphor is to understand, analyze, perceive, and describe one category of things through another. *Qu Xiang Bi Lei* 取象比类 or Taking Image and Analogizing, the core, specific and major methodology of Chinese medicine, results in the formation of metaphors, and thus is the metaphorizing process and the way of forming metaphors in Chinese medicine. In order words, metaphorizing is the major way to form the ontological concepts, the fundamental theories, and to develop clinical explorations of Chinese medicine as well. And only by understanding the metaphors in Chinese medicine, we know that Chinese medicine is a different medical system incompatible with Western medicine, which weaves natural and social phenomena together with the basic correct understanding of the human being as an integrity, thus revealing its methodology "*Qu Xiang Bi Lei* or Taking Image and analogizing" under the guidance of "*Tian*

56 Translated into English from Chinese. Gan Yang, Translator; Ernst Cassirer, Author. 2004: 152.

Ren He Yi 天人合一 or and the Unity of Heaven and Humankind", the core idea of classical Chinese philosophy. By this way it becomes clear that Chinese medicine must not be taken as a natural science in the Western sense, but it goes closer to humanities (geisteswissenschaften).

Here it is worth to note that *Qu Xiang Bi Lei* is the core, specific and major methodology of classical Chinese science, and metaphorizations are the centre and of the most significance in Chinese scientific discourses, while induction and deduction are the core and major methodologies of modern Western science, and metaphorizations in Western scientific discourses are far away from being acknowledged compared to the so-called objective descriptive language.

The Chapter 25 of *Lao Tzu* states:

> "Therefore, Dao is great.
> Heaven is great.
> Earth is great.
> Man is great.
> In the world, there are four great things, and man is one of them.
> Man abides by the earth.
> Earth abides by the heaven.
> Heaven abides by Dao.
> Dao abides by the nature".

It is thus clear that metaphorizing is also the bridge in between the Dao (The Way) of the Nature and Medicine. "Heaven", "Earth", and "Man" compose a whole system; In *Lao Tzu*, Dao abides by the nature; In *Huang Di's Inner Classic*, medicine abides by the Dao; In essence, medicine abides by the nature.[57]

Qu Xiang Bi Lei is the core methodology of philosophy of Chinese medicine to know the cosmos and man, to construct and develop the theoretical system and clinical explorations of Chinese medicine. We can say that Chinese culture is *Xiang* culture, and Chinese science is *Xiang* Science, and Chinese medicine is a *Xiang* medicine, which stresses relationships among beings in the world.

---

57 Lan Fengli. Metaphorizing: The Way to Bridge *The Book of Changes* and Chinese Medicine. In Wallner F.G., Schmisberger F., Wimmer F.M. (eds). 2010: 177-192.

3.1 Metaphor West and East: Similarities and Differences

3.1.1 Metaphor West and East: Origins

The English word "metaphor" originates from the Greek word "metaphora", which means "carrying across", i.e. "from one to the other". Metaphor studies in the West can be traced back to Aristotle's works such as *Poetics* and *Rhetoric* (Aristotle, 384-322 B.C.) of the ancient Greek times. Later on, many philosophers, linguists and scholars of other disciplines have developed many different theories on metaphor in different times in the West.

Metaphor studies in China have a unique and original style, including important concepts such as "word-image-idea (*yan-xiang-yi*, 言—象—意)" in the field of philosophy, "*fu-bi-xing* (賦—比—興)[2]" in the field of poetics, "analogy-metaphor (*pi-yu*, 譬—喻)" in the field of rhetoric, "implication (yin xiu, 隱秀)" and "artistic conception [*qing jing*, 情景 (境)]" in the field of aesthetics, etc., thus running through classical Chinese philosophy, poetics, rhetoric, and aesthetics. Compared to metaphor studies in the West, they are not inferior at all no matter in the scope or the depth. Besides, they interpret "metaphor" from another specific angle of view, embodying the distinctive cultural and national features of China.

As early as in the Pre-Qin days (before 221 B.C.)[3], the ancient Chinese people did a deep-going research on "metaphor". Actually, *The Book of Changes*, which is composed of symbols (divinatory trigram image, *gua xiang*, 卦象) and interpreting words (*gua ci*, 卦辞 and *yao ci*, 爻辞), is a remarkable piece of writing on metaphor, and occupies an immeasurable place in the metaphor studies of China.

3.1.2 Metaphor West and East: Similarities

As we know, no matter in the West or in China, metaphor is an important field of study shared in rhetoric, poetry, linguistics and philosophy. As a rhetorical skill, metaphor is given a much more extensive meaning by logic pragmatics, referring to phenomena of meaning transfer of language in the course of expression and exchange; As a basic cognitive activity, metaphor is the medium as well as the result of man's metaphoric cognitive activities, and an indispensable means by which man cognizes the world; And besides, metaphor is an indispensable feature of poetry.

Language by itself contains a system of metaphor. This system is closely connected with man's thinking system. Language and symbol have formed a complete model that a nation cognizes and understands the world. Human beings have made themselves a whole. While metaphor is used, it brings back to life the image of human beings in the nature and the image of the nature of human beings as well.

3.1.3 Metaphors in Discourses of Western Science and Chinese Science: Similarities and Differences

Metaphors can be seen almost everywhere in seemingly objective scientific discourses[58] for metaphors play an absolutely necessary role in scientific exploration and dissemination of scientific thoughts.[59] In the recent years, studies on the essence, characteristics, methods, and principles of metaphors in Western scientific discourses have achieved important progress and gratifying outcome[60], but studies on metaphors in discourses of classical Chinese philosophy and science, which originated from *The Book of Changes*, are rarely seen. Among all the subjects of classical Chinese science, Chinese medicine remains to be the only one to survive up till today when facing the challenge from Western medicine; all the others like mathematics, astronomy, and engineering exist mainly in the field of study of history of science although they had gained splendid achievements before since corresponding Western sciences have been successfully transmitted to and disseminated in China.

Actually, agriculture, astronomy, geography, mathematics, and medicine of the ancient China were very advanced, and even more advanced than that of the West esp. before the 15th century. That is to say, Chinese philosophy of the nature and life in probing into the relationship between the Nature and Man produced all of the Chinese traditional natural sciences, which worked very well before or even have worked quite well until today.

For example, Du Jiang Yan 都江堰, a famous water control and irrigation dam, which has been listed in the World Inheritance Name List and was

58 "Scientific discourses" here refer to "discourses of Western science".

59 Dong Hongle. 2005: Synopsis.

60 Guo Guichun. Metaphor, Rhetoric, and Scientific Interpretation [M]. Beijing: Science Press, 2007.

designed and built in accordance with the classical scientific ideas, has been working so well in preventing serious flooding for over 2,000 years, and has even survived the Sichuan Earthquake in 2008; While cracks appeared in a modern big dam made of concrete mixer just after the earthquake in 2008, which was designed and built nowadays according to the modern science. So, it's clear that Classical Chinese sciences have their own unique values.

But why does only Chinese medicine survive up till today? My answer is that the philosophy of Chinese science fits much better to the dynamic living system than to the other systems, and the living system is the only one which is always in a state of constant changing and transforming.

What on earth is Chinese medicine? Is it just an indigenous folk art of healing, which has superficial understanding of human body and diseases and can be judged by Western scientific criteria? Or is it an independent, systematic, and complete medical system? My answer is: Chinese medicine originated from China, its concepts, theories and clinical explorations have been deeply rooted in and have been in perfect harmony with Chinese culture after going through thousands of years of development.

Western medicine is an applied science based on the achievements of modern Western science and technology. Metaphors exist almost everywhere in discourses of Western science and Chinese medicine, and the essence, characteristics, methods, and principles of which are exactly no different from each other.

The significant difference lies in that: What Western scientific discourse has been always seeking is objective description, Western science takes deduction and induction as its core methodologies, and the functions of metaphors in scientific cognition and exploration has always been in a marginal position in Western science; while Chinese medicine takes *Qu Xiang Bi Lei* or Taking Image and Analogizing as its core methodology, and is metaphorical from the formation of its concepts, construction of its theoretical framework, to the development of its clinical explorations, and even to the whole system. In other words, the functions of metaphors in scientific cognition and exploration have always been in the core position in Chinese medicine. I think that is the fundamental difference in between Western science and Chinese medicine, and that studies on metaphors in Chinese medicine can reveal true values of classical Chinese science.

The Table 1 shows that Chinese medicine is another complete medical knowledge system incompatible with Western medicine in ontology, methodology, way of thinking, theoretical structure, and practical experiences.

	Chinese Thinking	Western Thinking
Ontology	Phenomena: unstable, emerging, and disappearing	Unchangeable, universal basis of changing things (Plato: Being)
Methodology	*Qu Xiang Bi Lei* or Taking Image and Analogizing to govern changes: *Xiang* or Image & Phenomena as Reality → Metaphors	Deduction and Induction: Reality Beyong Phenomena → Universal rules
Way of Thinking	Circular reasoning: one point is explained by all the others (relationship)	Linear reasoning: reason and cause (causality)
Theoretical Structure	Unity and joint development of theory and practice	Separation of theory and practice; theory guiding practice
Practical Experiences	Result of interaction and unification between subject and object	A passive information reception; stressing objectivity, trying to reduce subjectivity to zero
Knowledge System	Forming a direct line of succession	Continuously renewing itself with new research findings along with achievements in modern science and technology

Table 1. The Incompatible Thinking of Chinese Medicine With Western Medicine[61,62]

61 Wallner, F.G.. 2009: 12.
62 Lan Fengli. 2010, 31 (7): 72-73.

3.1.4 Dao-Qi Monism: The Philosophical Foundation of *Tian Ren He Yi* and *Qu Xiang Bi Lei*

The theme of Chinese philosophy is to probe into the relationship between the "heaven (nature) and man", and classical Chinese philosophy believes that "The heaven (nature) and man unit each other, and resemble (mirror) each other". The *Tian Ren He Yi* or "the Unity of Heaven and Humankind" makes up the ontological presupposition of Chinese medicine.

Huang Di's Inner Classic states that "Man is born on the earth, hanging his life to the heaven. The union of *qi* of Heaven and Earth gives birth to Man. Man can adapt himself to the seasons for Heaven and Earth are his parents." It can be seen that Heaven, Earth and Man constitute with the same ingredient - *Qi* in the same way, thus Uniting and Resembling Each Other, which is abbreviated as "the Unity of Heaven (Nature) and Man".

The same constituent - *Qi* is the very basis of *Tian Ren He Yi* or "the Unity of Heaven and Humankind". The worldview determines the methodology. Chinese medicine believes that everything in the world is universally related to each other, that the world is composed of the same constituent, that the immense variety of things and phenomena in the world share some similar characteristics at different levels, different categories, and different aspects, and moreover, there exist many necessary relationships among them.

"Languages are metaphoric in its essence and nature...." "We should not content ourselves to the present state of language. We have to trace back to the origins of words if we want to discover the ties which link the words and their references." (Ernst Cassirer)

Chinese characters or sinograms are a kind of logographic writing based on pictographs, and *Qu Xiang Bi Lei* is the core methodology of Chinese medicine. Metaphor is universal in Chinese medical language from words, phrases to sentences, reflecting how basic Chinese medical concepts and theories were formed, stated, and constructed, and how Chinese medicine has been developed, determining that Chinese medicine is a metaphor system in its underlying structure. Therefore, the metaphor system formed by the way of *Qu Xiang Bi Lei* is the deep structure of Chinese medicine.

Based on *Tian Ren He Yi* or "the Unity of Heaven and Humankind", the ontological Chinese medical concepts and theories were formed, stated and constructed, and Chinese medicine has been developed by the way of Metaphorizing, or *Qu Xiang Bi Lei* or Taking Image and Analogizing:

Introducing and constructing the theories of essential *qi*, yin-yang, and five phases to explain physiological functions and pathological changes of human being, and to guide diagnosis and treatment of diseases in the clinical practice;

Constructing the Visceral Manifestation system to interpret functions of *zang fu* organs;

Inferring the flow of *qi* and blood to expound physiology of yang *qi*;

Constructing the *Jing-Luo* or Vessel theory to elaborate the amount of yin, yang, *qi* and blood in different meridian-vessels;

Constructing the theories of etiology and pathogenesis to interpret the onset and development of diseases;

Constructing the therapeutic system to interpret actions of acupoints and medicinals, and thus determining principles and methods of treatment.

3.2 Three Key Processes of *Qu Xiang Bi Lei*: Imaging – Analogizing – Metaphorizing[63]

Metaphors in Chinese medicine bear specific features of classical Chinese culture and science. Chen Kui 陈骙 (1128-1203) pointed out in his *Wen Ze* 《文则》 or *Writing Principles* that

> "*The Book of Changes* has *Xiang* or Image to fully express its ideas; *The Classic of Poetry* has *Bi* or Analogy to convey its feelings; and so how could the composition writing go if without *Yu* or Metaphor?"
> "《易》之有象，以尽其意；《诗》之有比，以达其情；文之作也，可无喻乎？"

Chen Kui showed clearly the three key elements of metaphor studies of Chinese tradition: "Image, Analogy, Metaphor", or rather, "Imaging, Analogizing, Metaphorizing". Thus metaphor is not only a kind of formless thinking process, but also a visible language form.

Qu Xiang Bi Lei or Taking Image and Analogizing is the core methodology of Chinese medicine. Its procedure "Observing Objects - Taking Image - Analogizing - Understanding Dao" runs through almost all the aspects of Chinese medicine from forming its fundamental concepts, elaborating its theories, to developing its clinical explorations, embodying the thinking

63 Lan Fengli. 2014, 36(2): 87-93.

process of "Imaging – Analogizing – Metaphorizing", finally forming metaphors in Chinese medicine, guiding clinical practice, and developing Chinese medicine as well. Based on the three key processes/elements i.e. "Imaging – Analogizing – Metaphorizing" in classical Chinese metaphor studies, I advance and demonstrate that *Qu Xiang Bi Lei* or Taking Image and Analogizing is the metaphorizing process and the way of forming metaphors in Chinese medicine.

3.2.1 "*Xiang* 象": From Elephant to Imaging

Xiang is an important concept of classical Chinese culture and philosophy. Compared to Western culture and philosophy, Chinese culture and philosophy stresses *Xiang*, relationships, and functions rather than causality (whys) and morphological structures, underlines circular reasoning instead of linear reasoning, focuses on understanding an entity from a holistic point of view (holism, integration, unity) rather than understanding it by breaking it down into its constituent parts (reductionism, separation, part), values changing process rather than the unchanged features, and emphasizes perceptual understanding rather than quantified measurement. All in all, *Xiang* is the key to understand Chinese culture and philosophy. Taking image and analogizing is a vital methodology of classical Chinese philosophy and of classical Chinese medicine as well.

Wang Fuzhi 王夫之 (1619-1692) said in his *Zhou Yi Wai Zhuan* 《周易外传》 or *Outer Interpretation of The Book of Changes* that

> "What fills the whole land under the heaven[64] is all *Xiang*. The rhetoric *Bi Xing* or Analogizing and Metaphorizing in *The Classic of Poetry*, political affairs in *The Book of Documents*, a person's fame, position, and status in *The Spring and Autumn Annals*, ceremonial rites in *The Book of Rites*, and melodies and rhymes in *The Classic of Music* are nothing but *Xiang*, while *The Book of Changes* gets all the principles together."
> "盈天下而皆象矣。《诗》之比兴，《书》之政事，《春秋》之名分，《礼》之仪，《乐》之律、莫非象也，而《易》统汇其理。"
> Then, what is "*Xiang*"?

64 The whole land under the heaven refers to the world.

3.2.1.1 The Original Meaning of "*Xiang* 象": Elephant

The original meaning of "*xiang* 象" is Elephant, as *Shuo Wen Jie Zi* or *The Origin of Chinese Characters* states that "*Xiang* 象, with long nose and teeth, a big mammal in the Southern Yue area, will be pregnant every three years. 象，长鼻牙，南越大兽，三年一乳。." See the Illus. 5, which shows how the sinogram "象" was conceived in the way of resembling the real image of an elephant, and the Illus. 6, which shows the evolution process of the sinogram "象 *Xiang*".

In the meanwhile, we can see that "*xiang*" originally evolved from "seeking similarities" between things from the angle of genetics, as stated in *The Book of Changes* "*Xiang* refers to something being like or resembling this thing." It is well known that Chinese characters are a kind of *Xiang Xing* 象形 writing, literally "resembling shape", or pictographic, ideographic, logographic writing in English. That is to say, sinograms are pictures, images, and surely suggest the imaging thinking of Chinese culture.

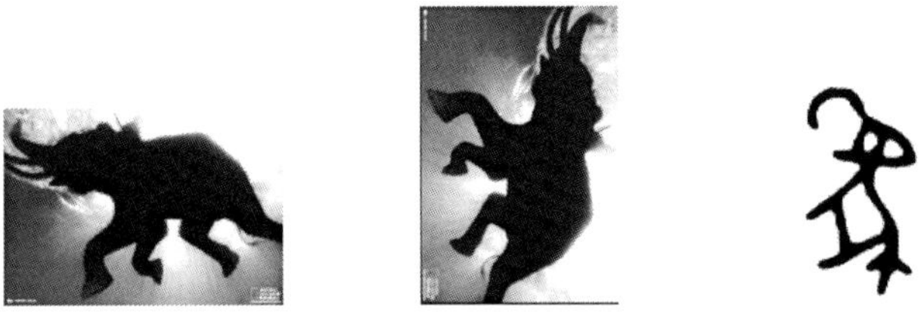

Illus. 5. A Swimming Elephant (Horizontal & Vertical) and "象" in Oracle Script[65]

Illus. 6. "Xiang 象" from Oracle, Bronze, Lesser-Seal to Regular Script

65 Here is worth to note that I cannot find a skeleton of a dead elephant in a lying position. The former two photos in the Illus. 5 are just used to illustrate the conceiving process of this character 象.

In the remote antiquity, the elephant had lived in the Central Plains of China. Later on, the elephant had to migrate south because of the changes in the weather, so the people in the Central Plains had few opportunities to see live elephants again. Han Fei 韩非 (280?-233 B.C.), a famous philosopher and the representative of the Legalists of the late Warring States Period (475-221 B.C.), said in the chapter of *Jie Lao Pian* of *Han Fei Tzu* 《韩非子·解老篇》 that

> "People seldom see a live elephant, but have gained the skeleton of a dead one, so they can imagine what it is like after investigating the picture or image of its skeleton. Therefore, all in people's imagination is known as '*xiang*'."
> "人稀见生象也，而得死象之骨，案其图以想其生也，故诸人之所以意想者，皆谓之象也。"

This quotation also reveals the mystery of the origin of the Chinese compound "*xiang xiang*" (想象，literally "thinking or imagining elephant", means "imaging or imagination"), setting off "*xiang* 象"'s "imagining" cultural connotations.

We can see that "*xiang*" originally evolved from "seeking similarities" between things from the angle of genetics, as stated in *The Book of Changes* "*Xiang* refers to something being like or resembling this thing". In the chapter of *the Fifteenth Year of Xi Gong's Reign* of *Zuo's Spring and Autumn Annals* it states that "Tortoise is *X*iang"; *The Book of Changes* states that "Change is *X*iang."

It is well known that Chinese characters are a kind of "*Xiang Xing* 象形" writing, which literally means "resembling shape", or pictographic, logographic, or ideographic writing in English. That is to say, the sinograms are based on pictures, images, and surely suggest the imaging thinking of Chinese culture.

It is thus clear that in classical Chinese thinking, "*Xiang* or Image" and the process of "*Xiang Xiang* or Imaging" are integrated as one. While in the background of Western thinking – Dichotomy, the Westerner makes a clear-cut division between the visible "*Xiang* or Image" and man's thinking process "*Xiang Xiang* or Imaging" because the subject is completely separated from the nature.

Ontologically, Western philosophy observes one in the two aspects or in the way of dichotomy, i.e. phenomenon and essence; while classical Chinese philosophy observes one in the three aspects, i.e. Dao or Way 道, *Xiang* or

Image 象, and *Qi* or Concrete Objects with Shape 器. *The Book of Changes* states that "The visible is *Xiang* 象, and the shapeable is *Qi* 器. 见乃谓之象，形乃谓之器"; And that "That which lies beyond shapes and features is Dao, and all things that lie within shapes and features are *Qi* 器. 是故形而上者谓之道，形而下者谓之器。". Pang Pu 庞朴 (1928–) made a penetrating analysis about this:

> "Dao, *Xiang*, and *Qi* 器 relate to each other step by step: Dao, without Image or Shape, but can govern *Xiang* or Image; *Xiang*, with Image but no Shape, but can signify Shape; *Qi* 器, with no Image but shape, but in the shape *Xiang* and *Dao* reside."; "Therefore, we can say that in between or the middle of 'That which lies beyond shapes and features is Dao, and all things that lie within shapes and features are *Qi* 器' is 'That which lies in the middle of Dao and *Qi* 器' should be named as '*Xiang*'!"[66]
> "道、象、器三者间，呈现为这样的梯形关系：道无象无形，但可以悬象或垂象；象有象无形，但可以示形；器无象有形，但形中寓象寓道。" "因此可以这样说， 在'形而上者谓之道，形而下者谓之器'之外或之间，更有一个'形而中'者，它谓之象!"

The division between phenomenon and essence, representation and reality is the outcome of artificial division between the subject and object in the Western thinking; while such a division does not exist in classical Chinese thinking. Actually, "*Xiang*" implies all the possibilities of reality, which explains why metaphors are so important for Chinese medicine; While Language can only provide one or two possibilities, so metaphors are much richer than language. In this sense, "metaphors" are "*Xiang*" in language.[67]

3.2.1.2 *Xiang* as Reality

First, let us distinguish three types of reality or three essential and fundamental dimensions of scientific work: "Wirklichkeit", "Life World", and "Realität". "Realität" and "Wirklichkeit" both mean "Reality" in English. Actually, they are very different from each other: "Wirklichkeit" refers to the

---

66 Pang Pu. 1995: 231.

67 Wallner F.G., Lan Fengli. Ontological Ambiguity and Methodological Circularity: *Qu-Xiang Bi-Lei*. In Wallner F.G., Schmisberger F., Wimmer F.M. (eds). 2010: 163-176.

being or the existence of the world, or "Reality as Environment and Condition for Living"; "Realität" refers to "Constructed Reality" or "Microworld"; in between is the "Life World", the world we live in.

Actually what the notions "Wirklichkeit", "Life World", and "Realität" name are three different dimensions in science and life. "Realität" describes the scientific microworld, the world that is constructed by selecting, excluding and reducing qualities of the object, a process that is guided by theory; "Wirklichkeit" describes the genuine world, the world that depicts the fundament for "Realität" and the basis for the selection, exclusion, and reduction; the "life world" describes the world the people live in, and people from different cultures have different life worlds. Both "Realität" and "Life World" take "Wirklichkeit" as the basis for their selection and reduction. The relationships among the three are different in different cultures.

For example, Western medicine is formed by a process of selecting, excluding, and reducing qualities of the object guided by Western thinking, the same as the way Western science is formed by; and both seek universality and objectivity. Western medicine can be considered as an artificial and constructed microworld that is based on selecting, excluding and reducing a world we name "Wirklichkeit". It is quite far away from the life world of the Western people. While Chinese medicine is formed by a process of selecting, excluding, and reducing qualities of the object guided by classical Chinese thinking, which focuses on constantly changing, flowing, emerging and disappearing phenomena or image. It can be considered as another artificial and constructed microworld that is based on selecting, excluding and reducing a world we name "Wirklichkeit". But Chinese medicine goes much closer to the "life world" of the Chinese people than Western medicine goes to the "life world" of the Western people. And all artificial and constructed microworlds make up the "Realität", the part all the human beings know by different approaches, the part which is still far smaller than the "Wirklichkeit".

Then it is not difficult to understand – there is manifoldness of perceiving the world, not just one way and not just one solution. There are several and different possibilities of referring to the world, different ways of selecting, excluding, and reducing the "Wirklichkeit" and/or the "life worlds". Based on this reductive reference and the legitimate manifoldness of different references we can propose that Chinese medicine can also be considered as a scientific system that has its own and alternative reference to the world and its own approach to its object. Thus it also has a legitimate claim for truth without getting into contradiction with other different systems like Western medicine. It can also be incompatible with Western medicine for both have different ways of constructing their microworlds.[68]

Actually it is very difficult to make a strict distinction between visible phenomena and man's imagination. And therefore it is very important to understand the differences between phenomena and noumena. Western science has always pursuing objectivity, and believes that what is left after removing all the subjectivities is the real. In the Western thinking, pictures and phenomena are all illusions, and cannot replace the thing. Friedrich Schiller (1759-1805), a great poet and philosopher of Germany, reflected this Western thinking on picture in his famous poem – "*The Veiled Statue at Sais*" – Uncover the veil (phenomena) and go beyond it to the essence.

We can see from the concept of *Xiang* that *Xiang* is not representation of reality, but an offer of reality itself. *Xiang* is another "Realität" based on the same "Wirklichkeit", but goes closer to the "life world" of the Chinese people, and thus is another reality. In one word, *Xiang* is the reality in classical Chinese culture and science.

3.2.1.3 The *Xiang* Taken: Image

The key of *Qu Xiang* or "Taking *Xiang*" is "*Xiang*", which exists in the following two forms:

One is the phenomena or image the object manifests itself outwardly, which can be perceived and caught by sense organs, as Wang Bing 王冰 (710-804) said that "*Xiang* is what manifests outwardly and can be seen. 象，谓所见于外可阅者也。."

The other is moving *Xiang*, a kind of dynamic functional pattern in the world, which is constantly emerging, disappearing, and changing; it lays particular emphasis on function but not shape or material, as *The Book of Changes* states that "The changes and transformations of the heaven and earth is what the sages follow 天地变化，圣人效之;" "*Yao*, the line in the Eight Diagrams, follows moving images of the land under the heaven (i.e. the world). 爻也者，效天下之动者也."

68 Wallner, Friedrich. How to Research TCM. In Wallner F.G., Kubiena G., Jandl M.J (eds). 2009: 22-45.

The whole process of *Qu Xiang* lies in observing *Xiang* and taking *Xiang*. The following four concepts indicate the progressive process of *Qu Xiang* or Taking image, i.e. the imaging process.

- *Wu Xiang* 物象, refers to the appearance, phenomena, manifestations the object manifests itself outwardly, and is the existing or being form of the object itself, only after it is internalized as human conceptual image can it enter the thinking process.

- *Zhi Jue Xing Xiang* 知覺形象, literally means "perceptual image", comes directly from *Wu Xiang*, referring to the intuition image the subject produces when the *Wu Xiang* acts on human sense organs, which can not go into the thinking process for it cannot depart from the direct action of the *Wu Xiang* on the sense organs. But it is a necessary step in the process of internalization of the *Wu Xiang*. After the perception caused by the *Wu Xiang* disappears, there remains more or less trace of the perceptual image or *Zhi Jue Xing Xiang* in human brain, such trace left in human memory is known as *Biao Xiang* or external image.

- *Biao Xiang* 表象, literally means "external image", is the internalized *Wu Xiang*, and refers to the image of the object taken, stored and reflected by human brain after repeatedly feeling, perceiving the *Wu Xiang* many times.

- *Yi Xiang* 意象, literally means "imagery image" or "image in imagination", is usually translated into "image" and is defined differently by different scholars of the same or different disciplines. It is generally believed that *Yi Xiang* refers to the result of generalizing and abstracting the image information of the common characters of the objects of the same category, and is the rational image generalized from *Biao Xiang* or the external image, is the unity of the external image of the object and the subject's deep understanding of it. *Yi Xiang* is the cell of the imaging thinking, running through the imaging thinking process from the beginning to the end.[69]

In fact, what is finally taken is *Yi xiang* 意象 or image. Wang Yuxiong 汪裕雄 (1937–) pointed out that

> "Image has been held in high esteem in Chinese culture, which is the so-called 'esteeming image'. This is a fact that every person gradually influenced by this culture will agree with. *The Book of Changes* applies the

69 Xing Yurui. 2004: 196-198.

> method of observing phenomena & image (*guan xiang*, 观象) and making instruments (*zhi qi*, 制器) to explain the origin of Chinese culture; Sinograms take 'resembling image or pictographic' as the foundation of their etymologies; Chinese medicine advances Visceral Manifestation Theory; classical Chinese astronomy and calendar system stresses observing phenomena & image (*guan xiang*, 观象) and issuing an official calendar (*shou shi*, 授时); Chinese aesthetic tradition takes image as its central domain, and regards full, rich image as its general appreciation of the beauty … Image, just like a huge net, encompasses all the fields of Chinese culture."[70]
> "中国文化推重意象，即所谓'尚象'，这是每个接受过这一文化熏染的人都不难赞同的事实。《周易》以'观象制器'的命题来解说中国文化的起源；中国文字以'象形'为基础推演出自己的构字法；中医倡言'藏象'之学，天文历法讲'观象授时'；中国美学以意象为中心范畴，将'意象具足'作为普遍的审美追求 … 意象，犹如一张巨网，笼括着中国文化的全副领域。"

In one word, *Xiang* is an all-embracing symbol in Chinese culture and philosophy. In Chinese traditional culture, all of the sceneries, the stars, even man's pulses, tongues and viscera are termed together with *xiang* like "jing (scenery) xiang 景象", "xing (star) xiang 星象", "mai (pulse) xiang 脉象", "she (tongue) xiang 舌象" and "zang (visceral) xiang 藏象"; Dao or Dao 道, the primitive motive force of the origin of everything in the universe, is also known as *xiang*, the big *xiang*. *Xiang* has a very strong adhesive power, and is a vital part of a series of compounds, including everything from the concrete *xiang* of objects which can be felt and the metaphysical subtle *xiang* which is difficult to grasp, thus possessing both perceptual and rational ingredients, and also indicating relationships.

In fact Chinese medicine is the product of the integration of Chinese understanding of the human being and classical Chinese philosophy, and is an image medicine, which accords with the Dao of Chinese Natural Philosophy. For example, its fundamental theories such as *Qi*, Yin-Yang, Five Phases, Visceral Manifestation Theory, Vessel Theory, and Herbal Theory are all formed by mirroring similarities between the Nature and Man; In its clinical practice, diagnosis is made according to patient's outward manifestations, including tongue Image, pulse image, and so on, and finally is given as

70 Wang Yuxiong. 1996:4.

a certain "Pattern Image"; its development is based on image or phenomena observation, and the ability of relating the image in the nature to man.

To sum up, *Xiang*, an all-embracing Chinese cultural and philosophical symbol, runs through almost every aspect of Chinese culture, such as its origin – Observing Phenomena and Making Instruments, its logographic writing – with pictographs as its foundation, literature – being composed of Word, Image and Idea, arts of painting – stressing the beauty of image rather than the reality, Calendar – Observing Phenomena and Issuing an Official Calendar, medicine – based on understanding of the dynamic living being instead of the dead body, and also implies a vital methodology of classical Chinese sciences – *Qu Xiang Bi Lei* or Taking Image and Analogizing. Therefore, we can say that classical Chinese culture is a kind of *Xiang* culture, classical Chinese science a kind of *Xiang* science, and classical Chinese medicine a kind of *Xiang* medicine.

3.2.2 "*Bi* 比": From "Shoulder to Shoulder" to Analogizing

The sinogram "比 *Bi*", an associative compound, follows 二 and 匕, and the 匕 also indicates pronunciation. It is written as  in the oracle script, which resembles the image of two persons keeping in step with each other and walking shoulder to shoulder or side by side. The shape is just like another sinogram "从 *Cong* or to follow" written as  in *Shuo Wen Jie Zi* or *The Origin of Chinese Characters* but just in the opposite direction. *Shuo Wen Jie Zi* or *The Origin of Chinese Characters* reads that "Two persons make up '*Cong* 从'; Reversing '*Cong* 从' is '*Bi* 比'二人为从，反从为比." The original meaning of "*Bi* 比" is "shoulder to shoulder"; "side by side."

3.2.2.1 *Bi Lei*: Analogizing

Zhu Xi 朱熹 (1130-1200) explained "*Bi* 比", one of the three formulas for the creation of *Shi Jing* or *The Classic of Poetry*, as "to compare that thing with this thing 比者，以彼物比此物也", which basically accords with what Huang Che 黄彻 (1093-1168) said that "*Bi* is to quote one thing with reference to other things of the same category. 比者，引物连类。."

Bi Lei 比类 in the context of *Qu Xiang Bi Lei* refers to *Bi Xiang* 比象, i.e. to analogize with the taken image, and thus can be translated into "Analogizing". *Bi Xiang* actually refers to a method of comparing the thing which needs to be known with the image which has already taken to catch and find similarities between them, and then migrating, transferring, and inferring the knowledge from the already known image to the thing which needs to be known, and so to understand its qualities or functions.

There are some common features in between *Bi Lei* or Analogizing in Chinese culture and Analogy in Western culture although both bear specific features of their own. As regards to analogy in Western culture, Johannes Kepler (1571-1630), a famous astronomer of Germany, pointed out that "What I respect most – Analogy, the teacher to be trusted, knows all the mysteries of the nature ..."[71]

In the chapter 76 "*Shi Cong Rong Lun* 示从容论 or *Discourse on Demonstrating a Natural Approach*" of *Huang Di's Inner Classic ·Basic Questions*, *Bi Lei* or Analogizing in Chinese culture is regarded as the most brilliant way of knowing (明引比类、从容，是以名曰诊经，是谓至道也), and the ability of *Bi Lei* or Analogizing can enable a physician to achieve mastery of all the medical principles (及于比类，通合道理) and to adjust himself to the changing circumstances (援物比类，化之冥冥)."

Qu Xiang Bi Lei, the core methodology of Chinese medicine, is summarized into the following four steps according to *The Book of Changes:* (1) Observing the object 观物: directly observing the object or phenomenon; (2) Taking image 取象: summarizing and refining the image of the object after repeatedly observing and feeling it; (3) Comparing and Analogizing 比类: comparing the things which need to understand or know with the "image (*xiang*, 象)" just taken; (4) Understanding Dao or the Way, the Rule 体道: finding the rules through the above comparing and analogizing activities.

The prominent characteristics of this methodology are as follows: (1) "*Xiang*" or Imaging/Image is its foundation with observing *xiang* and taking *xiang* as key steps; (2) The thinking manifests as transformation and flow of "*xiang*" as well as the contradictory movement between "*xiang*" and intuition; (3) *Bi Lei* or Analogizing is to compare, find, and catch the simi-

71 Here is quoted from a secondary source: Chinese translation of Методологический анализ процесса открытияи иэобретения: [苏联] P·3·吉江 著；徐明泽, 魏相 译．发现与发明过程方法学分析[M]．广州：广东人民出版社，1988: 99.

larities between the two different kinds of things, then migrate and infer the knowledge of one thing to the other.

Qu Xiang Bi Lei is an immanent methodology which is given by the activity. It holds that things present themselves with phenomena or images, and abstractions and concepts which are not illustrative do not exist in classical Chinese thinking. This is similar to the core idea of phenomenology: to go back to the things as they are.

3.2.2.2 The Ontological Presupposition of *Bi Lei* or Analogizing: *Tian Ren He Yi*

The theme of Chinese philosophy is to probe into the relationship between "Heaven and man", or the relationship between "the Way of Heaven and the Way of man", regarding the Heaven as man's Heaven and the man as Heaven's man.

The Book of Changes establishes *Tian Ren He Yi* 天人合一 or Unity of the Heaven and Humankind by metaphorizing, where Heaven and humankind are mutually responsive 天人相应. Actually, *The Book of Changes*, which is composed of symbols (divinatory trigram image, *gua xiang*, 卦象) and interpreting words (*gua ci*, 卦辞; *yao ci*, 爻辞), is a remarkable masterpiece on metaphor. Then what is the relationship between *The Book of Changes* and Chinese medicine – one deals with *Xiang Shu* (images and numbers, 象数) and their implicit meanings, while the other talks about health and illnesses? Actually they are talking about the same thing in essence by metaphorizing: life – one on the life of the Heaven and the other on the life of man.

Tian Ren He Yi 天人合一 is the cultural presupposition of analogizing. *Huang Di's Inner Classic · Basic Questions· Discourse on Treasuring Life and Preserving Physical Appearance* states that "Man is born on the earth, hanging his life to the heaven. The union of the heaven *qi* and earth *qi* gives birth to man. Man can adapt himself to the seasons for Heaven and Earth are his parents."

Tian Ren He Yi actually indicates that Heaven and Humankind are composed of the same ingredient – *Qi*. That is to say, the Heaven is a bigger man – the macrocosm, while the man is a smaller Heaven – a microcosm.

The classical Chinese "Dao-Qi" monism closes the incompatibilities between the nature and society, the Heaven and man. That is the root reason why *Huang Di's Inner Classic · Basic Questions* emphasizes repeatedly the vital importance of "To know the line patterns in heaven above, to know the structures of the earth below, and to know the human affairs in the center" in knowing medicine.[72]

Presupposed that the world is composed of the same constituent - *Qi*, analogies in Chinese medicine involve every aspect of human life – life in the nature, politics, society, astronomy, geography, military affairs, etc. Then how to analogize?

3.2.2.3 Chief Procedure of *Bi Lei* or Analogizing: Joint Application with Other Method(s)

There are two possibilities to apply *Bi Lei* or Analogizing: independent and joint applications with other method(s). *Bi Lei* or Analogizing in Chinese medicine, in most cases, is jointly applied with other method(s), and thus improving and ensuring the rationality and reliability of the outcome of analogizing. Due to the limited space, here we take just one example – the construction of the *Zang Xiang* or Visceral Manifestation Theory to illustrate this point.

The *Zang Xiang* or Visceral Manifestation Theory is a *Zang Fu*-centered basic theory with vital significance in Chinese medicine. *Zang Fu* 脏腑 was originally written as 藏府 in Chinese.

The sinogram "脏 *Zang*" underwent such an evolution process "臧—藏—臟—脏". "Zang 藏" originally refers to "a place to store precious things or treasure house". *Shuo Wen Jie Zi* or *The Origin of Chinese Characters* reads that "藏 zang4 is used to store (藏 cang2)", which was annotated by Duan Yucai 段玉裁 (1735-1815) that "*Zang* 藏" is the place to store valuable and precious things 凡物善者，必隐于内也, i.e. "storehouse". In the remote antiquity, *Zang* 藏 was a specialized establishment for storing imperial mandates, files, gold, jades and other precious things, and all the things inside the storehouse "*Zang* 藏" were extremely precious or invaluable, which were generally stored inside and not allowed to be taken out.

72 See the chapter 69 "Comprehensive Discourse on Changes [resulting from] Qi Interaction" and chapter 75 "Discourse on Making Known the Perfect Teachings" for details.

Fu 腑 was originally written as "府". One of the earliest meanings of "*fu* 府" refers to a storing system established by kings of the remote antiquity to govern six kinds of money and goods, known as "Six Materials", i.e. water, fire, metal, soil, wood, and grain. What were stored in the "*Fu*" were daily consumed and of course needed corresponding fresh supplies on daily bases and indispensable to ancients' life.

The formation of the concept of *Zang Fu* 藏府 in Chinese medicine was first based on a roughly correct anatomical knowledge of the human body. *Ling Shu · Jing Shui* or *Miraculous Pivot · Rivers and Meridians* describes the procedure of dissecting a dead body, which reads that

> "Regard the body of an eight *chi* (feet) man, when alive, take his measurement, feel his pulses; when dead, dissect his body and regard the strength of his *zang* organs, the size of his *fu* organs, the volume of the trunk cavity and the organs within it, then the length of the vessels, the clarity of the blood and the state of the *qi* ... All are shown to conform to a standard."
> "（若夫）八尺之士，皮肉在此，外可度量切循而得之，其死可（解剖）而视之。其藏之坚脆，府之大小，谷之多少，脉之长短，... 皆有大数。"

Anatomical knowledge is the foundation to construct the Visceral Manifestation Theory of Chinese medicine. Actually there are some more accurate anatomical records in the *Huang Di's Inner Classic.* For example, the ratio of the esophagus and the intestinal canal of human beings was 1.6 *chi* : 55.8 *chi*, i.e. 1: 34.87, which is very close to 1:34 in the modern anatomy.[73] The procedure of dissecting the dead body is just like to open a mysterious precious deposit, from which the concepts of exterior-interior and *Zang Fu* were formed, and the physical structure level – skin, vessel, flesh, sinew, and bone was understood. Then the further anatomical practice showed shapes or structures of internal organs, helped build the concepts of concrete organs, including Triple *Jiao* and its relative theory, learned relationship among internal organs, and discovered basic physiological functions of internal organs.

73 Wang Hongtu. 2004: 245.

Take the nomenclature of concrete organs for example. The sinogram for *heart* evolved from a direct vision of the organ, which underwent from  in the oracle script through 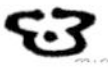 in the bronze script and  in the lesser seal script to 心 in the regular script; others like the sinogram  in the lesser seal script and 肺 in the regular script for the *lungs*, and the sinogram  in the bronze script,  in the lesser seal script, and 胃 in the regular script for the *stomach*, etc. all embody the *Xiang* or Images of corresponding substantial internal organs.

Basic physiological functions of some concrete organs were also cognized and discovered by dissecting dead bodies. For example:

1. The heart governs blood and vessels, and the vessels are the residence of the blood;
2. The lungs govern *qi*, perform respiration, open at the nose, relate to all the vessels, and help the heart to move the blood;
3. The kidneys govern water metabolism;
4. The major physiological functions of the stomach, the small intestine, and the large intestine: The stomach governs food intake and decomposition, then sends the decomposed food down to the small intestine, where it is separated into the clear and the turbid; Then the clear is absorbed and distributed throughout the body, while the turbid is further passed down to the large intestine, through which it becomes the waste and is discharged from the body through the anus.

Then, based on accumulation of anatomical knowledge and long-term observation of physiological and pathological phenomena, ancient Chinese analogized the organs stored deeply inside the body as the storing systems established by kings of the remote antiquity. Thereby, the unique concept of *Zang Fu* and cognition of their functions came into being in Chinese medicine: Five "*Zang* 藏" were taken and analogized to the five organs in the body which are said to store the essential *qi* but not discharge it – Heart, Liver, Spleen, Lungs, and Kidneys; Six *Fu* were taken and analogized to the organs in the body which are said to receive, transform, move water and grain and discharge the waste out of the body but not to store – Gallbladder, Stomach, Large Intestine, Small Intestine, Bladder, and Triple *Jiao*.

The entire above mentioned take the anatomical knowledge as their background and foundation. Because of the limited anatomical knowledge, *Huang Di's Inner Classic* interprets the life phenomena and constructs its own system by integrating the philosophical theories of the essential *qi*, yin-yang, and five phases with the accumulation of practical knowledge together with the limited anatomical knowledge also by metaphorizing.[74]

Besides, with the cognition of the functions of *Zang Fu*, *Huang Di's Inner Classic · Basic Questions · Discourse on the Hidden Canons in the Numinous Orchid [Chambers]* analogizes *Zang Fu* with the ancient bureaucratic establishment, which reads that

> "The Heart is the official functioning as ruler. …
> The Lungs are the official functioning as chancellor. …
> The Liver is the official functioning as general. …
> The Gallbladder is the official functioning as rectifier. …
> The *Dan Zhong* or Thoracic Center is the official functioning as envoy. …
> The Spleen and the Stomach are the officials responsible for grain storage. …
> The Large Intestine is the official functioning as transmitter. …
> The Small Intestine is the official functioning as recipient. …
> The Kidneys are the official functioning as operator with force. …
> The Triple *Jiao* is the official responsible for sluices. …
> The Bladder is the official responsible for reservoirs. …
> Hence, if the ruler functions efficiently, his subjects are in peace…
> If the ruler functions abnormally, then the twelve officials are in danger. …"

The Visceral Manifestation Theory takes *Zang Fu* as its core. Presupposed that "The interior must manifest itself outwardly 有诸内，必形诸外" and based on the method that "Inspecting the exterior to predict the interior 司外揣内", the cognition of *Zang Fu* was formed first on the basis of ancient anatomical knowledge, then through long-term observation of human physiological and pathological phenomena as well as repeated medical practice, by analogizing the storing system and bureaucratic establishment of the remote antiquity. The *Zang Xiang* or Visceral Manifestation is actually the unity of the external image with the subject's deep understanding of *Zang Fu*.

To sum up, the Visceral Manifestation Theory experiences evolution from substantial organs to functional entities and then to the final establishment of its theoretical system, during which analogizing plays a vital role.

74 Lan Fengli. 2012: 321-327.

In this case, analogizing is jointly applied with ancient dissection practice, observation of life phenomena and repeated medical practice, as well as classical philosophical thoughts such as the theories of the essential *qi*, yin-yang, and five phases, and thus greatly improving and ensuring the rationality and reliability of the Visceral Manifestation Theory with notable features of Chinese culture.

3.2.3 "*Yu* 喻": Metaphor and Metaphorizing

"*Yu* 喻" is a signific-phonetic sinogram and originally means "to inform" as explained in *Guang Ya*[75]. The last step of *Qu Xiang Bi Lei* is "Understanding Dao". Briefly speaking, this Dao is "*Yu* 喻", which is both a gerund – metaphorizing, a formless thinking process, and a noun – metaphor, a concrete language form. Therefore, I advance that *Qu Xiang Bi Lei* is the metaphorizing process and the way to form metaphors in Chinese medicine. Specifically speaking, it manifests in the following three aspects in Chinese medicine:

1. Constructing Theoretical System (Theory): Forming systematic metaphors - image-taking based nomenclature to name basic concepts, stating and constructing the theoretical system of Chinese medicine;
2. Guiding Clinical Practice (Practice): Grasping the hidden essence or telling the interior through observing the external image or manifestations such as in the processes of making diagnosis and identifying pattern in the practice, which is also a metaphorizing process;
3. Gaining New Knowledge through Metaphorizing (Development): Inferring the unknown through the known image, such as developing new theories and therapeutic methods.

3.2.3.1 Constructing Theoretical System

The theoretical system is constructed by forming systematic metaphors, i.e. image-taking based nomenclature. *Qu Xiang Bi Lei* extensively embodies in

75 *Guang Ya* 《广雅》, the earliest encyclopaedia dictionary in China with the aim to explain sinograms in ancient books, was compiled by Zhang Yi 张揖 (?-?) of the Three Kingdoms Period (220-265).

the nomenclature of core concepts of Chinese medicine, which I name it as "Image-Taking Based Nomenclature to Form Systematic Metaphors" – and thus constructing the theoretical system in Chinese medicine from understanding of the human being, the onset and development of a disease, making diagnosis, to instituting corresponding treatment based on pattern identification.

For example, "*Qi* 气", originally means "cloud, a pictographic sinogram", an image taken from the nature, and is used to name "the essential nutrient substance flowing in the body"; "*Zang Fu* 藏府", originally means "depots and palaces", a pair of images taken from life and official system, and is used to name the organs of the human body; the meridians of the human being are named by metaphorizing the rivers of the earth, an image taken from the nature; the weight and graduated arm of a steelyard as well as a pair of compasses and carpenter's square are used to describe the pulse images of the four seasons, which are images taken from everyday life; "closing door to keep the invader" – e.g. administering tonics for a patient with externally contracted febrile disease will keep external pernicious influences inside the body, and"struggle between the Upright and the Evil" – i.e. the fight between the healthy *qi* and pathogenic agents, which will determine whether a person will catch a disease or not, are named by metaphorizing events of military affairs; "Monarch, Minister, Assistant, and Envoy", images taken from political affairs, are used to name the principles and strategies of composing a prescription; and so and so forth. Here I just give you one detailed example, *Jing Luo* 经络.

Several translations are available for "經絡系統": "Meridian System" is the standard translation approved by WHO, but the word "Meridian" only indicates a two-dimensional grid while *Jing Luo* system is supposed to carry *qi* and blood, and thus must be a three-dimensional system; "Channel System" is the most popular translation in the English literature on Chinese medicine, but the word "Channel" is polysemous; "Vessel System", a translation in *Huang Di Nei Jing Su Wen* by Paul U. Unschuld in 2003 is the best translation if we take into account the origin and development of the concepts of *Mai* (脈, vessel) and *Jing-Luo* (經絡).

Based on some anatomical knowledge on *Mai* (脈, vessel) and medical practice esp. the application of acupuncture, moxibustion, *tuina* or Chinese massage, and *qigong* or breathing exercise, the concepts of *Jing-Luo* (經絡) are actually metaphors formed in the way of observing, taking images of and analogizing the water flow in the rivers under the earth and the longitudinal lines of the textiles, which are embodied in their writing forms. The chapter *Water & Earth* of *Guan Tzu* states that "Water is the *qi* and blood of the earth, running on (under) the earth just like *qi* and blood flowing in the vessels."

The simplified form of "*mai* 脉" has 4 variant original complex forms.[76]

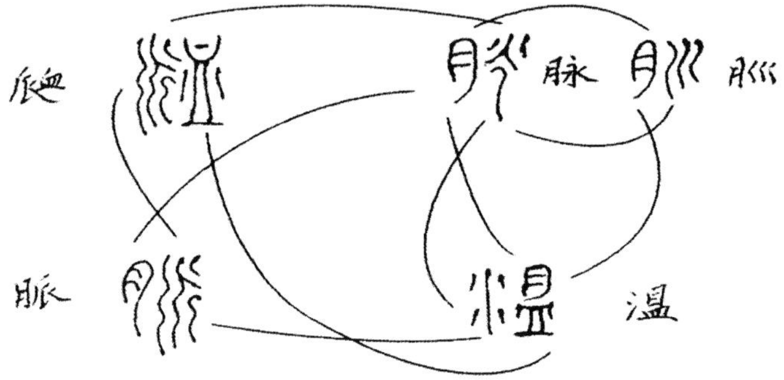

Illus. 7. Variant Original Complex Forms of "*Mai* 脉"

脈 and 衇 are its common original complex forms. Its lesser seal script is  . This sinogram is a signifc-phonetic compound: the left part is its signific component 月 (flesh moon) or 血 (blood), indicating that *mai* (脈) functions to carry and move blood and is a part of the human body; And the right part is its phonetic, indicating both pronunciation and meaning at the same time. In medical books unearthed from Mawangdui Han Tomb, most writing forms of "*mai* 脈" were written as "温". "水" is the variant form of " 氵 ", "目" the variant form of "月 (flesh moon)", "皿" the variant form of "blood 血". The structure of the sinogram has clearly illustrated that ancient Chinese analogized or metaphorized water flow with blood flow.[77] It is thus clear that "*mai*" of the early days referred to blood vessel, so "*mai* 脉" is also known as "blood vessel 血脈", as stated in *Huang Di Nei Jing Su Wen · Mai*

76 Li Ding. Rationality of Acupuncture: The Origin and Development of Theories of Vessels and Acupoints. In Lan FL, Wallner F. G., Wobovnik C. (eds). 2011: 191.
77 Li Ding. 1998: 2-3.

Yao Jing Wei Lun 脉要精微论 or *Huang Di's Inner Classic · Basic Questions · Discourse on Subtleties and Essentials of Vessels* "The vessels 脈 are the residence of the blood. 脉者，血之府也." Be aware, *Qi* does not show up in this quotation.

The concepts "*jing*" and "*luo*" appeared later than "*mai* or vessel". *Jing* and *luo* are further divisions of "*mai* or vessel", i.e. "*jing*" vessel and "*luo*" vessel, which was first recorded in the *Huang Di Nei Jing Ling Shu. Mai Du* 脉度 or *Huang Di's Inner Classic · Miraculous Pivot · On Vessels* "*Jing* vessels reside in the interior; their branches running transversely are known as *luo* vessels; the branches of *luo* vessels are known as grandchild vessels. 经脉为里，支而横者为络，络之别者为孙."

The sinograms "經 *jing*" and "絡 *luo*" share the same radical – the silk part "糸", which is originally used in the textiles.

The concept "*jingmai* 經脈" is a metaphor formed in the way of *Qu Xiang Bi Lei* or taking images and analogizing. The right part of "經" is "巠", indicating both pronunciation and meaning, which is interpreted in *Shuo Wen Jie Zi* or *The Origin of Chinese Characters* as "water vessels, following (川, pictographic, indicating rivers), under the 一; 一, refers to the earth 水脉也，从巛（川）在一下；一，地也", that is to say, "巠" refers to the water vessels running under the earth. *Jing* 經 is explained in *Shuo Wen Jie Zi* or *The Origin of Chinese Characters* as "the longitudinal lines of the textiles or the warps 织纵丝也." The reason that "*Jing* 經" is used to name the main stems of the vessels is closely related to the origin of the sinogram "*jing* 經", which contains two images and reflects the similarities between the longitudinal lines of the textiles, the rivers running under the earth and the running routes of the main stems of the vessels.

Another part of "luo 絡" is "各", indicating both pronunciation and meaning, which is interpreted in *Shuo Wen Jie Zi* or *The Origin of Chinese Characters* as "divergent views being different 异辞也." Another interpretation of *Luo* 絡 is that "It originally meant unreeled silk, hemp, or cotton fiber, and from its association with stringy fibers came to be used in Chinese medicine as a noun that means network and as a verb that means to net."[78] Anyway, 絡 is used to name divergent branches of the vessels.

78 Wiseman Nigel, Zhang Yuhuan. 2003: 174.

Huang Di Nei Jing Ling Shu. Ben Zang 本藏 or *Huang Di's Inner Classic · Miraculous Pivot · On Viscera* states that "*Jing* vessels 經脈 function to move *qi* and blood, nourish yin and yang, moisten tendons and bones, and lubricate joints. 经脉者，所以行血气而营阴阳，濡筋骨，利关节者也." Compared to the statement that "The vessels 脈 are the residence of the blood.", quite a lot new contents were supplemented to *jing* vessels, among which the most remarkable point is that the function of moving *blood* was extended to moving *qi and blood*.

"*Xue mai* 血脈", "*jing* 經" and "*luo* 絡" appeared together in the *Han Shu·Yi Wen Zhi* or *Treatise on Literature* of *The History of The Former Han Dynasty* 《汉书·艺文志》,"Medical classics explore the origins of *blood vessels* 血脈, *jing-luo* 經絡, bone marrow, yin-yang, exterior and interior in order to treat various diseases from the root.", where blood vessels seemed to be differentiated from *jing-luo*.

Jing-luo 經絡 functions to carry and move *qi* and blood in the body. *Guan Tzu · Water & Earth* states that "Water is the *qi* and blood of the earth, running on the earth which is just like *qi* and blood flowing in the vessels." Judged from the cognizing order, the flow of *qi* and blood in man is analogized and inferred from the natural phenomenon of water flow in the rivers under the earth. The extensions from "vessel 脈" to "*jing-luo* 經絡" and from "blood" to "*qi* and blood" are also closely related to the application of acupuncture, moxibustion, *tuina*, *qigong*, etc., which explore the phenomenon of *qi* and blood flowing in the body, thus enriching the understanding on the "vessels".

Seeing that "*jing* 經" and "*luo* 絡" are subdivisions of "*Mai* 脉" or Vessel, i.e. *Jing* Vessel and *Luo* Vessel, *Jing-Luo* system is surely the "Vessel system" – being mainly composed of *Jing* Vessels and *Luo* Vessels.

To sum up, the concepts and theory of *jing-luo* were formed first on the basis of some anatomical knowledge on "vessel 脈"; then by the way of *Qu Xiang Bi Lei*, i.e. observing and taking images of the water flow in the rivers on/under the earth and the longitudinal lines of textiles, then analogizing, enlightened by the idea of *Tian Ren He Yi*; and then have been proved and modified in the medical practice esp. the application of acupuncture, moxibustion, *tuina*, and *qigong*. That is to say, *jing-luo* or the vessels are metaphors, referring to the circular round pathways of the living system.

Therefore, I believe that it will take forever to find any three-dimensional structure of *jing-luo* 經絡 through dissecting dead human bodies.

Jing-luo 經絡 system or the vessel system is more like a functional concept reflecting a certain image, which is embodied in their writing forms. As stated in the *Huang Di's Inner Classic · Basic Questions · Discourse on Leaving and Uniting of True Qi and Evil Qi* (*Huang Di Nei Jing Su Wen·Li He Zhen Xie Lun*) that "The sages formulated principles, which must conform to the heaven and earth. Therefore, the heaven has 365 degrees and 28 constellations, the earth has 12 *jing* rivers, and man has 12 *jing* vessels. 夫圣人之起度数，必应于天地，故天有宿度，地有经水，人有经脉."

3.2.3.2 Guiding Clinical Practice

Lakoff and Johnson clearly pointed out in their monograph *Metaphors We Live By*[79] that metaphor is not only a rhetoric figure of speech, but rather a way of cognition or even a way of behavior deeply rooted in the thinking. They defined metaphor as using one thing to understand another, and applied existence of concept metaphors to prove this point. Man's conceptual system controls man's thinking and behaviour. So if concepts are metaphorical then thinking and action will be surely metaphorical.

The diagnosing and treating procedure, in brief, is to synthesize the information and data from the four examinations – inspection, listening and smelling, inquiry, and palpation, then to diagnose which disease the patient suffers and which pattern the patient is identified, and then to institute treatment. Metaphor thinking or metaphorizing, intentionally or subconsciously, guides the whole process of "diagnosing disease, identifying pattern and instituting treatment".

For example, "Insomnia. Pattern of Liver Stagnation Transforming into Fire" presents with the following symptoms as described in the 5th edition textbook of *Chinese Internal medicine*[80]: Insomnia, irritability, bad temper, no desire for food, thirsty with desire for drink, reddish eyes, bitter mouth, dark yellow urine, constipation, red tongue with yellowish coating, wiry and rapid pulse, among which the "fire" symptoms are very prominent – bitter

79 Lakoff, George & Johnson, Mark. Metaphors We Live By [M]. Chicago: The University of Chicago Press, 1980.
80 The description of this disease pattern is taken from the textbook of the fifth edition *Chinese Internal Medicine*. See Zhang Boyu. 1989: 113-116. But the interpretation afterwards is from the author.

mouth, thirsty with desire for drink, red tongue with yellowish coating, and reddish eyes are caused by "fire flaming upwards" to the mouth, the tongue, and the eyes; dark yellow urine and constipation result from "fire disturbing downward"; irritability, bad temper, wiry and rapid pulse arise for this fire is not other kinds of fire but "liver fire". Therefore, in the clinical practice, a practitioner of Chinese medicine will naturally relate the above mentioned symptoms to the fire and liver fire in particular, and thus diagnose a patient with these symptoms as "Insomnia. Pattern of Liver Stagnation Transforming into Fire" after long-term learning, studying, and practicing Chinese medicine, and then institute corresponding treatment of herbal medication or acupuncture or other kinds of treatment. In the whole process the practitioner naturally or subconsciously applies the metaphorizing thinking, and here "fire" is the key metaphor to reveal the intrinsic relationships among all the pathological phenomena simultaneously happening to the patient. That is to say, metaphor reveals relationships between the phenomena - clinical manifestations and the object - patient, and makes the practitioner diagnose and treat the disease properly, and thus guiding the clinical practice.

3.2.3.3 Making New Explorations

"In the beginning, metaphors in scientific discourse may be not a kind of standardized scientific language, but can produce important scientific findings or even lead to the occurrence of scientific revolutions. Metaphorization stands for an approach which frees from the shackles of a kind of literal meaning, and being divergent and being creative constitute its intrinsic essence. In the scientific activities, scientists use metaphors mainly for the purpose of theoretical innovation not out of their interest of appreciation of the beauty."[81]

In Chinese medicine, *Qu Xiang Bi Lei* or Taking Image and Analogizing, the metaphorizing process, not only states, constructs its theoretical system, guides its clinical practice, but is also a very important way to develop the system. Chinese medical experts are good at taking image and analogizing, and applying metaphorizing to make new explorations so as to develop Chinese medicine. Here I give you three examples:

81 Guo Guichun. 2007: 36.

A *Ti Hu Jie Ga* or
Carrying a Kettle and Uncovering Its Lid to Treat Dysuria

Zhu Danxi 朱丹溪 (1281-1358), a famous physician and the founder of Yin-Nourishing School of the Jin-Yuan Dynasties (1115-1368), gained inspiration from a phenomenon in daily life that uncovering the upper lid of a kettle filled with boiling water can make the water be poured out, and then inferred a treating method named after this phenomenon "*Ti Hu Jie Gai* 提壶揭盖", which literally means "carrying a kettle and uncovering its lid (in order to pour out water)". What does this mean? The story reads that:

One day, a male patient with dysuria visited Zhu Danxi, who was formerly treated by other physicians with diuretics of Chinese medicine, which did not relieve but aggravated his condition instead. Zhu Danxi felt that his right *cun* pulse (indicating the condition of the lungs) was quite wiry and slippery, and then treated the patient with the method of dispersing the lung *qi*, then diuresis was successfully induced, and finally the patient was cured of the disease.

Zhu Danxi pointed out that the disease is caused by accumulation of phlegm in the lungs, and that the lungs are located in the upper *jiao* and the urinary bladder is located in the lower *jiao*, and that when the upper *jiao* is blocked the lower *jiao* will surely be obstructed, just like a kettle, only after the lid is uncovered, can water be poured out. This therapeutic method is known as *Ti Hu Jie Gai*, which literally means "carrying a kettle and uncovering its lid (in order to pour out water)", and actually refers to the method of dispersing the lung *qi* to induce diuresis, which is usually used to treat edema, dysuria, or anuria when the patient does not respond to the routine therapeutic methods.

B *Ni Liu Wan Zhou* or
Saving the Boat in an Adverse Current to Treat Dysentery

Yu Jiayan 喻嘉言 (1585-1664), a famous physician in the early Qing Dynasty (1644-1911), created a therapeutic method termed as *Ni Liu Wan Zhou* 逆流挽舟 or saving the boat in an adverse, swift current to treat enduring dysentery. He believed that the dysentery caused by an external pathogen sinking into the interior should be treated by lifting the external pathogen out of the exterior from the interior, just like saving a boat in an adverse and swift current to make the boat move upward. Accordingly, he formulated a formula named "Ginseng Toxin-Vanquishing Powder 人参败毒散" to treat the disease. Afterwards, physicians of Chinese medicine usually apply this method and the formula to treat the dysentery with external pattern complicated with dampness.

C *Zeng Shui Xing Zhou* or
Increasing Water to Move the Boat to Treat Constipation

The phrase *Zeng Shui Xing Zhou* 增水行舟 or Increasing Water to Move the Boat implies that: When the river flow cuts off for the lack of water, then boat will surely run aground; When the water is supplied and rises, then the boat will move in it easily.

Wu Jutong 吴鞠通 (1758-1836), a distinguished expert in warm diseases of the Qing Dynasty (1644-1911), created a treating method termed as *Zeng Shui Xing Zhou* or Increasing Water to Move the Boat to treat constipation caused by humor insufficiency or heat drying the humor, which is just like the boat running aground for the lack of water. Accordingly, he also formulated a formula named "Humor-Increasing Decoction 增液汤" to treat this condition, which has become a famous and effective formula to treat constipation of this kind.

Besides, many other effective treating methods created by the way of *Qu Xiang Bi Lei* or Taking Image and Analogizing or metaphorizing, have been still in use in the clinical practice, such as:

Yin Huo Gui Yuan 引火归源 or Conducting Fire Back to Its Origin: a therapeutic method of leading the rising fire to the kidney, used in the treatment of declining fire of the life gate with floating of deficient yang;

Fu Di Chou Xin 釜底抽薪 or Taking Away firewood from under the Cauldron: a therapeutic method of clearing heat or fire by purgation;

Zi Shui Han Mu 滋水涵木 or Enriching Water to Moisten Wood: a therapeutic method of nourishing kidney yin to subdue liver yang for hyperactivity of liver yang due to liver kidney yin deficiency, which presents with such symptoms as dizziness, red complexion due to rising fire, and hypertension in some cases.

There are still many other methods or theories in Chinese medicine created by the way of *Qu Xiang Bi Lei*. We can see that the process of constructing and understanding metaphors is a typical example for creativity. The creative nature of metaphor is to find new relationships in two or more existing concepts or phenomena so as to explore new mental spaces and advance new theories, thus developing Chinese medicine in both theoretical and clinical explorations.

Qu Xiang Bi Lei or Taking Image and Analogizing is the core methodology of Chinese medicine. Its procedure "Observing Objects - Taking Image - Analogizing - Understanding Dao" runs through almost all the aspects of Chinese medicine from forming its fundamental concepts, elaborating its theories, to developing its clinical explorations, embodying the thinking process of "Imaging - Analogizing - Metaphorizing", finally forming metaphors in Chinese medicine, guiding clinical practice, and developing Chinese medicine as well. *Qu Xiang Bi Lei* is the metaphorizing process and the way of forming metaphors in Chinese medicine, and metaphor is its deep structure. In real fact, Chinese medicine is a Linguistic medical system for it forms in the way of linguistication and metaphorization. Interpreting metaphors in Chinese medicine is a key to understand, reconstruct, inherit and develop Chinese medicine.

Chinese medicine is formed in the way of linguistication and metaphorization for it is recorded in self-interpreting sinograms and full of metaphors: from terms to sentences, to paragraphs, to texts, and even to the whole system. Chinese medicine is just like a text full of metaphors. The text offers so much on knowledge, on information, on relationships among its constituent parts by metaphorizing, much more than the stabilized objects of the Western medicine. That is the source of the exactness of Chinese medicine.

- The Author

4 Metaphors in Chinese Medicine: Revealing Relationships and an Exact Thinking

Compared to Western medicine, an applied science based on achievements of Western science and technology, Chinese medicine is a typical linguistic metaphorical medical knowledge system in essence for it is formed in the way of linguistication and metaphorization, and is recorded in self-interpreting sinograms. Therefore Chinese medicine can be regarded as a linguistic metaphorical medical system being composed of its logographic language writing forms, systematic metaphors (concepts & terminology), formulations, sentences, and their logic relationships.

Metaphors in Chinese medicine reveal relationships, and metaphor thinking is an exact thinking.

4.1 Metaphors in Chinese Medicine: Revealing Relationships

As we have discussed before, metaphor is far more than a rhetoric figure of speech. Metaphor is not a description by a vivid picture but an exact description to show relations. The relations are described by the metaphor. So, metaphor does not describe objects. Metaphor reveals relations, relations done by actions. Therefore metaphor has the function of relating different phenomena. Here I give you three examples to illustrate this point of view: Fire, Tongue Diagnosis and Heart Fire Blazing.

4.1.1 Example 1: Understanding Fire in Chinese Medicine

The core knowledge of Chinese medicine is from classical Chinese medical texts, which are written in self-interpreting characters, or more exact, sinograms. Compared to phonetic writing forms, Chinese language (logographic writing) is more stable and accumulative. In Chinese language, giving the original sinogram new meanings by the way of metaphorizing instead of creating new sinograms is the major way to reflect the changes and developments of the world and the means and process of Chinese people cognizing, understanding and stating the world. After tracing back to the original meanings of sinograms, concepts and statements are not difficult to understand in their contexts in a broad sense, which also provide us extensive but close links among different disciplines of Chinese science and culture. Therefore, etymology investigation is of vital significance for etymology of a sinogram can unify all the migrating meanings of concepts based on the one sinogram with the same etymology. The theoretical system of Chinese medicine is stated and expressed in a natural language with the two major characteristics: being polysemous and ambiguous, which can also be clarified and unified by etymology investigation and metaphor understanding.

Fire in Chinese medicine comes from the fire in the common sense or from the fire in everyday life.

1. Etymology – Fire in Everyday Life: "Huo 火" or Fire, as stated in *Shuo Wen Jie Zi* or *The Origin of Chinese Characters* that "火 *Huo*, the phase of the South, flaming upward, is a pictograph." The ancient Chinese people observed that fire is warm, hot, red, burning, and flaming, bearing the characteristics of being bright, rising and upbearing.

2. Fire in the Five Phases: In the five phases, fire represents not only the real fire, but also the substances and qualities bearing characteristics of fire – "Fire is the flaming upward." And then the south, summer, summer-heat, red, bitter in the nature, and the heart, small intestine, vessel, tongue, sweat, joy, laugh of the human beings are all attributed to fire in the five phases.

3. Fire as One of the Six *Qi* or Six Climatic Factors: In the philosophical context that *qi* is the basic substance or the source constituting everything in the world, the fire is also a kind of "*qi*", a form of object in a specific state, also known as "fire *qi*". Six *Qi* is the summarization of six kinds of weather in three categories in the nature: the flow of air - wind, or wind *qi*; changes in temperature (*qi wen* 气温) – cold or cold *qi*, heat or heat *qi*, summer-heat or summer-heat *qi*; and moisture - dampness or damp *qi*, dryness or dry *qi*. The heat *qi* and summer-heat *qi* pertain to fire in the five phases for they all indicate being high in temperature. The *Huang Di's Inner Classic* names the "heat *qi*" "the monarch fire", "summer-heat *qi*" "the primer fire".

4. Fire as One of the Six Excesses or Six Climatic Pathogenic Factors: Pathogenic fire pertains to yang, flaming upward, rising, dispersing, burning, having heat manifestations, consuming liquid, damaging *qi*, harming the upper part of the human beings, tending to produce wind, stir blood, disturb the heart spirit, etch flesh, form pus, cause sores, which should be treated by reducing fire, clearing heat and resolving toxin with medicinals of bitter and cold in property.

5. Fire in the Four Properties of Medicinals: Every medicinal is said to be cold, cool, hot, or warm (the four properties) in property. Hot and warm pertain to fire. Warm medicinals are regarded as "lesser fire", being bland in taste, can engender *qi*; hot medicinals are regarded as "vigorous fire", being rich or thick in taste, can consume *qi*.

6. Fire in the Yin-Yang Theory: In the philosophical context of *qi* and yin-yang theory, it is believed that water and fire can fully embody the most essential characteristics of yin and yang, as stated in *Huang Di's Inner Classic* that "Water is yin, fire is yang;" "Water and fire are the symbols of yin and yang."

7. Fire Functions as the Physiological State of Yang *Qi*: For fire being warm, giving heat to people (the original recognition of fire and direct experience of fire), *qi* being classified into yin and yang and the abstraction of the things with yang characteristics and functions, as well as analogizing the normal state of yang *qi* with the function and characteristics of fire, Chinese medicine calls the physiological state of yang *qi* of the human being "fire" or "lesser fire". Wang Bing's 王冰 (710-804) annotations of *Su Wen* or *Basic Questions* reads that "to supplement the source of fire to eliminate the yin shading 益火之源以消阴翳." Zhang Jiebin 张介宾 (1563-1640) regarded the heart yang as the monarch fire, the kidney yang as primer fire, which together fulfill the function of warming, activating all the organs of the human being, maintaining the flow and distribution of the essence, blood, and body fluid for all liquid substances prefer warm and dislike cold, and warm activates them to flow, while cold causes them to stagnate.

8. Fire as a Pathological State when Yang *Qi* Functions Abnormally: *Huang Di's Inner Classic* states that "All fever with impaired consciousness and convulsion is ascribed to fire," "All trismus with shivering chills and delirium is ascribed to fire," "All disorders with upward perversion are ascribed to fire," "All states of agitation and mania are ascribed to fire," "All illnesses with swelling and aching of the instep and mental strain are ascribed to fire." Later on, Liu Wansu 刘完素 (?1110-1200) developed and enriched the

pathological connotations of fire, advanced that "The six *qi* can all transform into fire," "*Qi* in its surplus will become fire."

Finally, the pathological fire bears 3 connotations:

The first is "vigorous fire", referring to excessive pathological conditions of exuberance of yang *qi*, also known as "excessive fire, excessive heat", which should be treated by medicinals of cold and bitter in property to clear heat and reduce fire, including such conditions as flaming upward of heart fire, flaming upward of liver fire, exuberance of stomach fire, and fire toxin of sores and carbuncles, etc;

The second is the "ministerial fire", resulting from the deficient pathological condition of relative exuberance yang *qi* due to yin deficiency failing to control yang *qi*, also known as "deficient fire, deficient heat", which should be treated with enriching yin and reducing fire, mainly including "frenetic stirring of ministerial fire", manifesting in dizziness, headache, tinnitus, irritability if the liver is chiefly involved, and feverish feeling in the chest, palms of the hands, and soles of the feet, aching in the loins, and hyperaphrodisia if the kidney is chiefly involved;

The third is the "yin fire", referring to the spleen heat caused by irregularities in diets and physical overstrain as well as the heart fire caused by excessive joy, anger, or anxiety.

It is thus clear that etymology investigation of "Huo 火" or Fire is of vital significance for it can unify all the migrating meanings of the related concepts based on the same sinogram.

4.1.2 Example 2: Tongue Diagnosis: A Metaphorizing Process

Tongue reading and pulse taking are two essential steps to diagnose a disease and identify a pattern in Chinese medicine. The tongue coating in Chinese medicine is formed by the way metaphorizing, and tongue reading is also a metaphorizing process.

As regards to the formation of the tongue coating, Zhou Xuehai 周学海 (1856-1906) said that "The coating is the result of the fuming or steaming of the stomach *qi*. All of the five *zang* organs rely on nutrients from the stomach, hence the tongue coating can be used to diagnose the conditions of the five *zang* organs, such as heat or cold, deficiency or excess."

Wu Kun'an 吴坤安 of the Qing Dynasty (1644-1911) explained that "The coating of the tongue is just like the moss of the earth. The moss of the earth results from the upgoing of the dampness, while the coating of the tongue results from the upgoing of the spleen dampness steamed by the stomach. That is why it is named as *Tai* or Moss."

It is thus clear that the *Tai* 苔 or Moss or Coating of the tongue is formed by metaphorizing the moss of the earth, which is clearly embodied in the sinogram "*Tai* 苔". The sinogram "*Tai* 苔", a signific-phonetic, following 艸 (grass) and pronounced as "*Tai* 台", originally means moss, a very small green plant which grows on damp soil, or on wood or stone. Many moss plants usually grow close together in a clump.

Tongue reading is also a metaphorizing process.

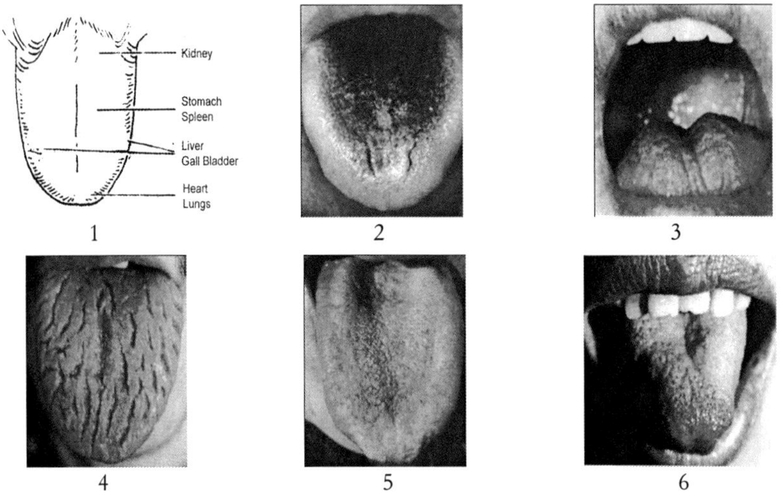

Illus. 8. Tonge Reading

Illus. 8-1 shows that the tip of the tongue reflects conditions of the heart and lungs, the middle reflects conditions of the spleen and stomach, the root reflects conditions of the kidneys, and the two sides reflect conditions of the liver and gallbladder, which results from metaphorizing the locations of the organs in the body in Chinese medicine.[82] In Chinese medicine, the result of

---

82 Chinese medicine views every single separate part as a part with the information of all the parts of the body. Some are significant in diagnosing and treating certain diseases while some others are not. The typical example is the ear acupuncture ther-

tongue inspection is usually described from the following three aspects: the body, coating, and shape of the tongue, which are collectively known as the "tongue image". The normal tongue image is usually described as "red tongue with thin whitish coating". Now let us read some tongues and practice metaphorizing thinking in this process.

The tongue image of the Illus. 8-2 can be generally described as "a pale tongue with burnt-black coating". In details, the color of the tongue proper is pale, indicating blood deficiency; the shape is corpulent or swollen with tooth-prints, indicating *qi* deficiency; and the coating is burnt-black, indicating extreme fire flaming upward. So, in Chinese medicine, this tongue image usually indicates extreme fire flaming upward and deficiency of *qi* and blood.[83]

The tongue image of the Illus. 8-3 can be generally described as "red atrophy tongue with yellowish greasy coating". In details, the color of the tongue proper is red, quite normal; the shape is atrophy, indicating that phlegm-heat stagnates in the network vessels; and the coating is yellowish greasy, indicating accumulation of damp-heat in the body.[84]

The tongue image of the Illus. 8-4 can be generally described as "light-red tongue with fissures and little coating". In details, the color of the tongue proper is light-red, indicating deficiency of blood; the shape: there are many longitudinal fissures distributed on the tongue, indicating deficiency fire flaming upward; the coating is very little, indicating extreme deficiency of yin. So, in Chinese medicine, this tongue image usually indicates deficiency of yin and blood and deficient fire flaming upward.[85]

---

apy, which is used to treat diseases of various parts of the body for the ear resembles an inverted fetus and thus has points corresponding to most important parts of the body.

83 The tongue with burnt-black coating is known as black hairy tongue in Western medicine, which is most often seen in acute pyogenic infections such as pyemia, gangrenous appendicitis, peritonitis, and cholecystitis, and may also occur in diseases such as chronic bronchitis and uremia. Western medicine explains that it may result from growth of bacteria after long administration of antibiotics, high fever, dehydration, absorption by the tongue coating of iron present in blood from minor bleeding in the oral cavity, etc.

84 The atrophy or shrinkage of the tongue in Western medicine can be seen in patients with pulmonary tuberculosis or advanced carcinoma.

85 Fissures in Western medicine are chiefly associated with chronic glossitis, and 0.5% of the cases with fissures on the tongue are wholly unrelated to disease.

The tongue image of the Illus. 8-5 can be generally described as "light-red tongue with white greasy coating on the edge and greenish coating in the middle". In details, the color of the tongue proper is light-red, indicating deficiency of blood; the Shape is corpulent or swollen, indicating *qi* deficiency; the coating is white, greasy, but yellow-green in the middle, indicating fire-transmission from long-term cold-damp due to yang deficiency, and damp-heat retention and evaporation.[86]

The tongue image of the Illus. 8-6 can be generally described as "light-red tongue with red spots and white, light yellow, greasy coating". As you know, the color of the tongue proper is light-red, red on the tip, indicating deficiency of blood and heat in the heart; the shape: there are many red-spots at the tip and the right side of the tongue, indicating heat-fire in the heart, lungs and stomach; the coating is full of white, light yellow, greasy coating, indicating the heat in the Ying-Camp phase in externally contracted febrile diseases.[87]

You see that the tongue reading process is in essence a metaphorizing process.

Here the subjects of the five photos of the tongues are Chinese patients. It is worth to note that the result and clinical significance of tongue reading are not influenced by differences in races. If you are interested in this topic, you can read further a monograph by Giovanni Maciocia "*Tongue Diagnosis in Chinese Medicine*", in which 59 colored plates and accompanying case histories are from the author's own practice.

Tongue examination provides some of the most important data for disease diagnosis and pattern identification esp. of externally contracted febrile diseases, so the "Tongue Inspection and Pattern Identification Songs" by Wu Kun'an 吴坤安 reads that

Exterior white, interior yellow,
Decide sweating or purgation.
Camp crimson, Guard white,

86 The corpulent or swollen tongue, also known as tongue enlargement, in Western Medicine, may be seen in myxedema, chronic nephritis, and chronic gastritis, and is attributed to hyperplasis of the connective tissue, tissue edema, or blood and lymphatic drainage disturbances.

87 The red spots in Western medicine result from an increase in the size or number of fungiform papillae.

Refine therapeutic differentiations.
Then check fluids for further information.
Moist, no damage; dry, depletion.

"Exterior white, interior yellow" refers to the color of the tongue coating: if the coating is white, this disease will be identified as exterior pattern, and thus should be treated by sweating; if the coating is yellow, this disease will be identified as interior pattern, and thus should be treated by purgation. A crimson tongue indicates that pathogenic heat penetrates to the Camp phase. External pathogens at the Guard phase still indicate the disease can be identified as exterior pattern. The moistness of the tongue indicates the state of the fluids.

4.1.3 Example 3: Heart Fire Blazing

When you see the formulation "Heart Fire Blazing", you may think it is ridiculous, and ask "How do we know there is fire in the heart?", "Is the temperature in the heart higher than that in other organs?", "How can we measure it?", etc. Actually, fire in Chinese medicine is a metaphor, and metaphorizing is the key to understand it.

Fire is the extreme state of heat. The external pathogenic wind, cold, summer-heat, dampness, and dryness can all transform into fire when they penetrate through to the interior of the body; disorders of functions of *zang fu* organs, and internal depression of the seven affects, i.e. joy, anger, melancholy, anxiety, sorrow, fear and fright, can also transform into fire.

Fire, a yang pathogen in nature, is characterized by "flaming upward". In the case of heart fire blazing, if fire flames upward, symptoms of red complexion, thirsty, sores on the tongue or in the mouth, red tongue[88] will show up; if fire disturbs the spirit, symptoms like vexation, insomnia, manic episodes, delirious speech, and unconsciousness will show up; fire consumes fluids, symptoms like thirsty with desire for drink, dry tongue and mouth, constipation, scanty dark yellow urine will show up; the pulse is usually rapid. Accordingly, the therapeutic principle should be "clearing the heart fire"; and then corresponding treatment of medication and/or acupuncture can be prescribed.

88 "Tongue is the signal orifice of the heart."

It is thus clear that "Heart Fire Blazing" says nothing about the temperature in the heart, but connects the concept of the heart identified in Chinese medicine with a series of phenomena of fire, such as thirsty with desire for drink, insomnia, vexation, constipation, scanty dark yellow urine, red tongue, rapid pulse, and so on. Therefore "Heart Fire Blazing" is identified by all of these phenomena which relate to each other by metaphorizing the fire and the heart.

In Western medicine, the heart is identified by its location, functions, and some possible related diseases of the organ heart which are clearly defined, and all the other aspects or body happenings are not interesting. While in Chinese medicine, oral ulceration and frequent, difficult and painful urination with passage of dark yellow urine (which can be seen in acute urinary tract infection in Western medicine) can be both cured by clearing the heart fire with the corresponding formula *Dao Chi San* 导赤散 or Redness-Removing Powder.

It is thus clear that metaphors in Chinese medicine reveal relationships.

4.2 Metaphorizing in Chinese Medicine: An Exact Thinking

It is worth to note that, when talking about differences between Chinese medicine and Western medicine, people generally believe that Western medicine is exact, while Chinese medicine is vague. Based on the common sense and general knowledge, it is obvious that data from lab is indeed much more precise than a pattern of disharmony. But the answer is not so simple if we see this question from the perspective of metaphor cognition. We have already known that the metaphor system of Chinese medicine is the deep structure of Chinese medicine, and the key to understand Chinese medicine. In fact, metaphors in Chinese medicine not only reveal relationships, but are also a kind of exact thinking - metaphorizing. Here I give you three examples to illustrate this point of view.

4.2.1 Example 1: Stomach pain in 6 people

Clinical studies Kaptchuk applied to illustrate difference between Western and Eastern perceptions of medicine can also demonstrate that metaphorizing in Chinese medicine is an exact thinking.

Six patients with stomach pain were all diagnosed as having peptic ulcer disease by using upper-gastrointestinal X-ray or endoscopy by means of a fiberscope. But these six patients diagnosed as having the same disease in Western medicine were identified as having six different patterns of disharmony: "Damp Heat Affecting the Spleen", "Deficient Yin Affecting the Stomach", "Exhausted Fire of the Middle Burner", "Excess Cold Dampness Affecting the Spleen and Stomach", "Disharmony of the Liver Invading the Spleen", and "Disharmony of Congealed Blood in the Stomach" by a practitioner of Chinese medicine.

From the perspective of Western medicine, the six patients suffered from the same disease, and so if they were treated by this doctor they would have accepted more or less the same treatment. While if they were treated by a practitioner of Chinese medicine they would have accepted different individualized treatments based on their specific patterns. Obviously, six individualized treatments provided by Chinese medicine are more exact than one treatment provided by Western medicine, which is based on the same diagnosis in Western medicine - the six different patients suffer from the peptic ulcer disease.

4.2.2 Example 2: High Blood Pressure

"Persistently high systemic arterial blood pressure. Based on multiple readings (blood pressure determination), hypertension is currently defined as when systolic pressure is consistently greater than 140 mm Hg or when diastolic pressure is consistently 90 mm Hg or more."

Hypertension, also known as high blood pressure, will be treated by antihypertensive pills of different kinds such as diuretics, beta blocker, ACE inhibitor, angiotensin receptor blocker, etc. in Western medicine. The effect can be checked by a sphygmomanometer. If the blood pressure is lowered down and kept at the normal level, the treatment will be evaluated as effective. Generally speaking, doctors do not care so much the other aspects of patients, or backgrounds of different patients with high blood pressure.

While practitioners of Chinese medicine identify patients with hypertension as having different patterns such as "hyperactivity of liver fire", "yin deficiency and yang hyperactivity", "pattern of phlegm turbidity", "pattern of phlegm and blood stasis", etc., and then give them individualized treatments based on different specific patterns. Chinese medical treatments may not directly lower the blood pressure, but can be used as auxiliary treatments for relieving common symptoms of hypertension patients such as headache, vertigo, insomnia, tinnitus, and so on, in stabilizing the blood pressure, softening the blood vessels, and preventing the situation from deteriorating.

4.2.3 Example 3: Inflammation and Fire

Another common example is the inflammation in Western medicine and fire in Chinese medicine. Inflammation is a pathological condition in Western medicine, manifesting in local redness, swelling, pain, ulcer and dysfunction as well as fever of different degrees, leukocytosis, fatigue, poor appetite, and so on, which is usually treated by antibiotics. This pathological condition is generally known as "fire" in Chinese medicine. But you may ask what is the difference between Chinese understanding and Western understanding of the same or similar pathological condition for inflammation with the "flame" as its root is also a kind of fire.

The concept of fire in Chinese medicine comes from *Huo* 火 or Fire, as stated in *Shuo Wen Jie Zi* or *The Origin of Chinese Characters* that "火 *Huo*, the phase of the South, flaming upward, is a pictographic character." The ancient Chinese people observed that fire is warm, hot, red, burning, and flaming, bearing the characteristics of being bright, rising and upbearing.

Fire as a pathological condition in Chinese medicine can be caused by eight kinds of pathological agents – warm heat, damp heat, fire toxin, yin deficiency (deficient fire caused by yin deficiency), wind cold or cold dampness, phlegm fluid (with edema), deficient cold (cold is caused by yang deficiency), stagnation of *qi* and blood (with pain). These agents are not fixed, may vary according to the progression or retrogression of the disease. But anyway, practitioners of Chinese medicine prescribe different formulas to fit different patterns, i.e. identifying patterns and applying proper treatments. It is really amazing for Chinese medicine does not yield drug resistance like antibiotics do, and it works even when the agent(s) of a disease cannot be identified.

The above examples show that Chinese medicine is even more exact than Western medicine in the clinical practice. Besides, Dichotomy is like "1", while *Tiao Ji Tu* 太极图 or Yin-Yang Diagram is like "S" (See Illus. 12 Yin-Yang Diagram and Dichotomy), much more complicated than dichotomy, therefore more exact and fitting to the dynamic living system. *Tiao Ji Tu* 太极图 or Yin-Yang Diagram, one of the vital philosophical foundations of Chinese medicine, is also more exact than one of the vital philosophical foundations of Western science – Dichotomy. You know Chinese medicine is constructed under the guideline of *Tian Ren He Yi*, and the object of Chinese medicine is the live dynamic human being, composed of the body, mind and other aspects, which can explain why Chinese medicine can usually achieve desired therapeutic effects in treating psychosomatic diseases. While Western medicine is an applied science based on achievements of Western science and technology, and is practiced mainly based on understanding of the dead bodies – a very detailed and precise understanding of the physical structure of the body, and thus has achieved amazing revolutionary developments in surgery, and even organ transplantation.

Metaphor thinking is an exact thinking. Chinese medicine is formed in the way of linguistication and metaphorization for it is recorded in self-interpreting sinograms and full of metaphors: from terms to sentences, to paragraphs, to texts, and even to the whole system. Chinese medicine is just like a text full of metaphors. The text offers so much on knowledge, on information, on relationships among its constituent parts by metaphorizing, much more than the stabilized objects of the Western medicine. That is the source of the exactness of Chinese medicine.

The Book of Changes deals with *Xiang Shu* (images and numbers, 象數) and their implicit meanings, while Chinese medicine talks about health and illnesses. But metaphorizing bridges them for they both actually talk about the same issue in essence – life: one on the life of cosmos and the other on the life of man.

- The Author

5 Metaphorizing: The Way to Bridge *The Book of Changes* and Chinese Medicine

Qu Xiang Bi Lei 取象比类 or Taking Image and Analogizing is the metaphorizing process and the way to form metaphors in Chinese medicine, i.e., bireifly speaking, *Qu Xiang Bi Lei* actually means metaphorizing. Metaphorizing is also the way to bridge *The Book of Changes* and Chinese medicine.

5.1 *The Book of Changes* and Chinese Medicine Being of the Same Origin: Shamans' Practice

5.1.1 The Origin of "*The Book of Changes*"

In the remote antiquity of China, shamans applied special instruments like the stone, tree, tortoise or other animals to communicate with the heaven and earth. Among so many ways to communicate with the heaven and earth *bu* 卜 and *shi* 筮 were two popular ones. *Bu* 卜 with the tortoise shell and *shi* 筮 with the stalk of *shi* 蓍 grass, were mainly supposed to foretell good or ill luck, good fortune or misfortune in the future for the tortoise (shell) and *shi* grass not only have long lives but also bear strange shapes or patterns and thus were considered as god-created beings. The images of *gua* 卦 and *yao* 爻 were created at the inspiration of cracks on tortoise shells, while the numbers of *gua* 卦 and *yao* 爻 (nine and six) were attached to them at the inspiration of numbers of stalks of *shi* grass in divining activities. That is to say, *Xiang Shu* (images and numbers, 象數) originated from *bu* 卜 with the tortoise shell and *shi* 筮 with the stalk of *shi* grass respectively. Therefore, it is clear that *The Book of Changes* originates from shamans' divining activities: *bu* 卜 and *shi* 筮.

5.1.2 The Origin of Chinese Medicine

What is the origin of Chinese medicine? The circle of medical history of contempory China generally holds that Chinese medicine originated from the summarization of ancient people's living, producing and laboring experiences for such a viewpoint is believed to accord with the historical standpoint of Marxism and scientific materialism. But first of all, let's go back to the original forms of the sinogram 医 (medicine or medical practitioner): 毉 and 醫.

The sinogram 毉, appearing in *Guan Tzu* 管子 and *Guang Ya* 廣雅, is composed of 医 *(yi*, medicine or medical practitioner) and 巫 (*wu*, shaman or shamans' practice), thus showing the close relationship between them. *Shuo Wen Jie Zi* or *The Origin of Chinese Characters* explains 醫 as "the practitioners who specialize in treating illnesses. The upper part 殹 means bad postures. Their treating behaviors were driven by wine (酉→酒), therefore following the wine part 酉. ... Wine was applied to treat illnesses. According to the records of *Zhou Li* or *The Rites of Zhou [Dynasty]* there existed medicinal wine in the Zhou Dynasty (ca.11th century-256 B.C.), and the Shaman Peng 巫彭 was one of the first medical practitioners of the remote antiquity. 治病工也。殹，惡姿也；醫之性然。得酒而使，从酉。... 酒所以治病也。《周禮》有醫酒。古者巫彭初作醫."

Illnesses are man's diseased states, as explained in *Shuo Wen Jie Zi* or *The Origin of Chinese Characters. Disease Part* 《说文解字. 疒部》 that "疒, leaning on or against something. Whenever man has illnesses, his posture is like leaning on something. All disease-related sinograms follow 疒. 倚也。人有疾病，象倚箸之形。凡疒之屬皆从疒."

It's interesting that shamans' extraordinary behaviors' driven by the wine could treat man's extraordinary states: illnesses, which can also be regarded as a kind of metaphorizating. Wine may influence man's consciousness, which can be regarded as the bridge between psychotherapy and Chinese medicine. Here is an explanation of the parts to make up 毉 and 醫:

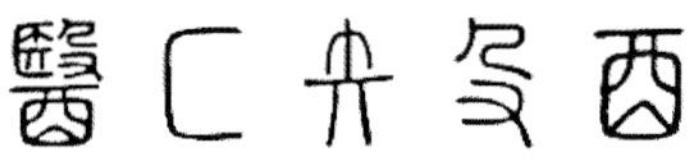

- 匚：Principles of medicine should be upright and foursquare;
- 矢：arrow; acupuncture;
- 殳：hand feeling in the water of a pond; massage;[89]
- 酉：wine;
- 巫：shaman; shaman's practice.

Besides, there are many records on witchdoctors or shamans of the remote antiquity such as in *The Classic of Mountains and Seas* (shan hai jing, 山海經)[90] and *The Historical Records* (shi ji, 史記)[91].

Actually, the formulation that "Medicine originates from shamans' practice" was put forward long ago in China. With the rising of anthropology in the 19th century, many scholars at abroad also insist on this point of view. This formulation includes the following three aspects:

Medicine grew out of shamans' practice;

The earliest medical practitioners were shamans; and

Shamans' practice was the earliest method to treat illnesses.

This is indeed the case as regards to the origin of Chinese medicine.

5.1.3 *The Book of Changes* and Chinese Medicine Being of the Same Origin: Shamans' Practice

Then what is the relationship between *The Book of Changes* and Chinese medicine – one deals with *Xiang Shu* (images and numbers, 象數) and their implicit meanings, while the other talks about health and illnesses? Actually they are talking about the same issue in essence by metaphorizing: life – one on the life of the cosmos and the other on the life of man. Both are open

89 A Chinese idiom 手到病除 relates to this sinogram, which means "Illness departs at a touch of the hand."

90 *Shan Hai Jing* or *The Classic of Mountains and Seas*, is a classical Chinese text of at least 2,000 years old. It is largely a fabled geographical and cultural account of Pre-Qin China as well as a collection of mythology.

91 *Shi Ji* or *The Records of History*, written by Sima Qian 司馬遷 (145 or 135? – ca. 86 B.C.) of the Western Han Dynasty, recounts over 3,000 years of Chinese history from Huang Di's era to his own time. As the first systematic Chinese historical text, the records profoundly influenced Chinese historiography and prose. In its effect, the work is comparable to Herodotus and his Histories.

systems, both are communicated with and related to each other, and both should be in a state of harmony in itself and with the other, otherwise problems or illnesses will ensue, which is radically different from the strict divisions between the life and the inanimate, the subject and the object, the man and the nature etc. in the Western culture. Maybe it is fantastic for the Westerners that *The Book of Changes* and Chinese medicine do not reduce life or being to something material like cells, proteins, genes, etc., instead they reduce life or being to something symbolic like the *gua* 卦 and *yao* 爻, yin and yang, eight trigrams, five phases, images and numbers, visceral manifestation, and so on.

5.2 *Qi* and *Xiang*: Fundamental Metaphors to Bridge *The Book of Changes* and Chinese Medicine

Ernst Cassirer defined man as a symbolic animal (or animal symbolicum) instead of a rational animal. He said: "Only by such a definition can we point out the specific features of man and can we understand the new way open to the man – that is the way into the culture."[92]

Chinese people created specific cultural symbols like *qi* 气 and *xiang* 象, which are the fundamental metaphors of Chinese culture and medicine.

5.2.1 *Qi*: A Metaphor as Foundation of *Tian Ren He Yi*

Chuang Tzu 莊子 comments that *The Book of Changes* talks about yin *qi* and yang *qi* from the beginning to the end. Actually, "*Qi*" is a metaphor, and its formation is a process of metaphorization.

Shuo Wen Jie Zi or *The Origin of Chinese Characters · Qi Part* 《说文解字. 气部》 states that "*Qi* refers to thin, floating clouds. The sinogram 气 is a pictograph." The sinogram 气 was written as "  " in the oracle script, which resembles air current, evaporating and rising, whose image is just like cloud, will disappear very soon and become invisible. Therefore, *qi* is invisible and formless, exists everywhere, can be gathered into a form, for instance, *qi* can be condensed into water. *Qi* at this moment actually referred to air or vapor.

92 Author: Cassirer Ernst. Translator: Gan Yang. 2004: 37.

Soon afterwards, the *qi* which surrounds and congests the space of the man was abstracted into the *qi* which bears a philosophical sense. Philosophers of the Spring Autumn and Warring States Periods (770-221 B.C.) believed that *qi* is the basic ingredient constituting the world, and that everything in the world comes into being by the movement and mutation of *qi*. For example, *The Book of Changes* states that "Everything is transformed and generated by the enshrouding [*qi*] of the heaven and the earth."

Later on, ancient Chinese medical experts introduced "*qi*" into the medical field at the right moment. And then, "*qi*" became a medium to bridge the natural philosophy of the Pre-Qin Days (before 221 B.C.) and Chinese medicine. The concept and theory of "*qi*" gradually formed in Chinese medicine.

In the time of *Huang Di's Inner Classic*, "*qi*" is regarded not only as the basic ingredient constituting the world, but also as the basic ingredient constituting the man which can be transformed into blood, essence, and body fluid, etc., and the normal functional activities of the life which is governed by "*qi*" is known as *Shen* 神 or spirit. *Huang Di's Inner Classic · Basic Questions · Discourse on Protecting Life and Preserving Physical Appearance* states that "Man is generated by *qi* of the heaven and earth, and is completed by the law of the four seasons;" and that "The union of *qi* of the heaven and earth gives birth to man."

That is to say, Heaven, Earth, and Man constitute with the same ingredient in the same way – *Qi*. That is to say, the heaven is a bigger man, while the man is a smaller heaven; or the heaven is a macrocosm, while man is a microcosm. And therefore, *Qi* is a metaphor functioning as the ontological foundation of *Tian Ren He Yi* or the Unity of Heaven and Humankind in Chinese culture and medicine.

5.2.2 *Xiang*: A Metaphor as Foundation of *Qu Xiang Bi Lei*

Xiang 象, another very important metaphor of Chinese culture and medicine, implies the core methodology of Chinese medicine – *Qu Xiang Bi Lei* or Taking Image and Analogizing, the metaphorizing process and the way of forming metaphors. See *3.2.1 "Xiang 象": From Elephant to Imaging* for details.

Qu Xiang Bi Lei or Taking Image and Analogizing, the core methodology of Chinese medicine, plays a vital role in constructing and developing the theoretical system and clinical explorations of Chinese medicine.

5.3 Metaphorizing: The Way to Bridge Specific Symbols of *The Book of Changes* and Metaphors of Chinese Medicine

Metaphorizing is the way to bridge specific symbols of *The Book of Changes* and metaphors of Chinese Medicine. Let's take "—" and "- -" and yin-yang, the eight trigrams and the five phases, the five phases and the visceral manifestation theory as examples to illustrate this point of view.

5.3.1 "—" and "- -" and Yin-Yang

The two symbols "—" and "- -" are the basic lines to compose the eight trigrams and the sixty-four hexagrams. The Fu Xi's Eight Trigrams stand for the eight basic phenomena in the nature (See Illus. 9), which are grouped into four pairs of opposites - *Qian* 乾 and *Kun* 坤, *Kan* 坎 and *Li* 离, *Gen* 艮 and *Xun* 巽, *Zhen* 震 and *Dui* 兑. Double the Eight Trigrams to get the Sixty-Four Hexagrams, which are used to symbolize various phenomena in the nature and the society.

- *Qian* 乾 for Heaven
- *Dui* 兑 for Lake or Marsh
- *Li* 离 for Fire
- *Zhen* 震 for Thunder
- *Xun* 巽 for Wind
- *Kan* 坎 for Water
- *Gen* 艮 for Mountain
- *Kun* 坤 for Earth

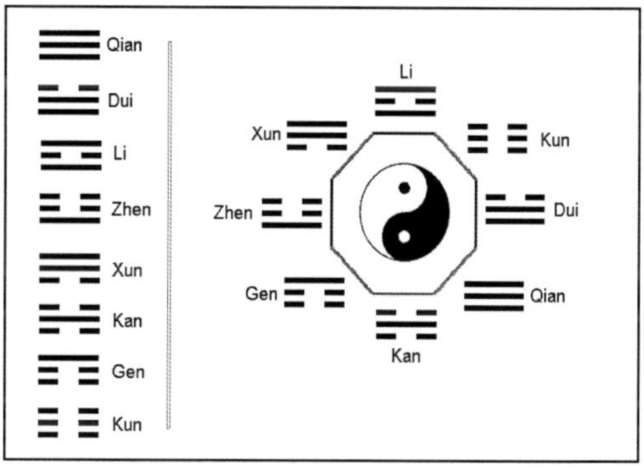

Illus. 9. Fu Xi's Eight Trigrams

There preserves a precious original manuscript in the *Schlossbibliothek zu Gotha* of Freistaat Thüringen in Germany, which is entitled "1 and 0, the magical origin of all the numbers, and mystical and wonderful paragons of the Nature for all comes from nowhere but the God." [93] This is Gottfried Wilhelm Leibniz's (1646-1716) original handwriting. But have you ever known this? His great discovery of binary system was enlightened by two illustrations of the Sixty-Four Hexagrams. The two symbols "—" and "- -" stand for "1" and "0" respectively. But then how did they evolve from?

The Book of Changes sums up the origin or ontology of man and everything in the world as the outcome of the interaction between the heaven and earth, yin and yang, which all apply the two symbols "—" and "- -" to stand for and interpret. The Eight Trigrams are also composed of the two symbols. Where are they from or what do they mean? Guo Moruo 郭沫若 (1892-1978) believed that they are the outcome of worshipping the male's and female's genitals. According to his understanding, the following quotation from *The Book of Changes* can be interpreted in this way: *Qian* 乾, "—", the heaven or yang, symbolizes the male's penis, which can curl up or be erectile; *Kun* 坤, "- -", the earth or yin, symbolizes the female's perineum, which can open or close. The interaction of them can produce everything in the world.

The concepts of yin and yang are metaphors formed in the way of observing and taking the image of directions of a mountain or a river in the nature and then analogizing – yin refers to the northern side of a mountain or the southern side of a river, and yang the southern side of a mountain or the northern side of a river. Later on, the meanings of yin-yang are summarized as "the side facing the sun being yang and the reverse side being yin." Then, things that are mobile, external, upward, ascending, warm, hot, bright, hyperactive, or pertaining to functional activities are classified as *Yang*; those that are unmoving, internal, downward, descending, cold, dull, hypoactive, or pertaining to materials (or structures) are classified as *Yin*. Thus, yin and yang has become a pair of philosophical concepts to summarize the dynamic images of things or phenomena in the world.

The Book of Changes advances that "One yin and one yang makes Dao," which abstracts yin-yang to the extensive universality and regards yin-yang as the fundamental rule of the world for the first time.

The *Chun Qiu Fan Lu* or *The Luxuriant Dew of the Spring and Autumn Annals* by Dong Zhongshu states that "The heaven has yin-yang, the man

93 Translated from Chinese translation into English.

also has yin-yang. Yin *qi* of the heaven rises and yin *qi* of the man will respond it to rise, while yin *qi* of the man rises and yin *qi* of the heaven will respond it to rise too. The principles or ways are the same."

On one hand, Chinese medicine discards the symbols (*gua xiang*, 卦象) and interpreting words (*gua ci*, 卦辭; *yao ci*, 爻辭) of *The Book of Changes*; on the other hand, absorbs the ideas on "—" and "- -" and yin-yang in it, and makes a systematic and definite expression on the ideas of interdependence, waning-waxing, transformation, counterbalance of yin-yang implied in it, then developing these ideas in combination with medical practice, and thus making yin-yang theory become a guiding theory of Chinese medicine.

To sum up, "—" and "- -" came from the image of the male's and female's external genitals, and *The Book of Changes* is a book on the philosophy of life or being. Then, "—" and "- -" evolved (or integrated with yin-yang) into the yin-yang theory, thus becoming a vital part of philosophy of Chinese medicine on the man.

5.3.2 Eight Trigrams and Five Phases

The five phases do not show up in the general version of *The Book of Changes*, but they do appear in its silk version which was unearthed in 1973 from Mawangdui Han tomb. It's generally believed that the five phases were the worldview of the people of the Yin Dynasty (ca. 16th – 11th century B.C.) and the eight trigrams were the worldview of the people of the Zhou Dynasty (ca. 11th century – 256 B.C.). But they both were well-developed in about the same era, sharing the common and typical features and viewpoints of inland culture, expressing by means of taking image and metaphorizing, thus laying the foundation for their integration.

The Book of Changes states that, of the eight trigrams, "*Qian* 乾 is metal, *kun* 坤 is earth (soil), *zhuan* 巽 is wood, *li* 離 is fire, *kan* 坎 is water, *gen* 艮 is mountain (soil), *zhen* 震 is east (wood), *dui* 兌 is west (metal) ;" and that "The heaven has 5 numbers, the earth has 5 numbers, then they integrate into five pairs," which was explained by Zheng Xuan 鄭玄 (127-200) as "matching the numbers of the heaven and earth 1, 2, 3, 4, 5 with water and north, fire and south, wood and east, metal and west, soil and middle respectively. The numbers of 1, 2, 3, 4, and 5 are regarded as solitary yin or yang, do not change, and therefore are known as generating numbers (*sheng shu*, 生數); They can generate only together with the soil, that is to say, only after they plus 5 (the number of soil), can they start to generate and transform, thus becoming round numbers (*cheng shu*, 成數). Obviously, the numbers of 8, 7, 9, and 6 are the round numbers of the wood, fire, metal and water respectively, while the soil only takes the generating number 5 not the round number 10, which is the general viewpoint of the *Xiang Shu* (images and numbers, 象數) theory. Thus, the *He Tu* 河圖 could be evolved when matching the generating numbers and round numbers with the five phases, five directions, five seasons, and so on. That is to say, the *He Tu* is the outcome of the integration of the five phases and the numbers in *The Book of Changes*.

Yin-yang, five phases, and eight trigrams are all subdivisions of *Qi* of different levels from the viewpoint of *Qi*, which indicates a gradual generating and dividing process from *Qi* to Yin-Yang then to the Five Phases then to the Eight Trigrams.

The Book of Changes states that "The changes have *Tai Ji* or the Supreme Ultimate (the Absolute in ancient Chinese cosmology, presented as the primary source of all created things, i.e. *qi*), *Tai Ji* generates yin and yang, yin and yang generate the four images, i.e. the greater yang, the greater yin, the lesser yang, and the lesser yin, and the four images generate the eight trigrams." That is to say, *qi* can generate and transform into yin and yang, yin and yang can generate and transform into the five phases which are composed of two pairs of yin and yang (water and fire, wood and metal) plus one middle soil. Actually, the four images and the eight trigrams indicate the five phases although the term "five phases" does not appear in this quotation: The four images can be regarded as four phases, i.e. water, fire, wood, and metal; the eight trigrams can be regarded as water, fire, wood (yin wood and yang wood), metal (yin metal and yang metal), and soil (yin soil and yang soil).

The theory of five phases influences almost every aspect of classical Chinese social and natural sciences, esp. Chinese medicine. *Huang Di's Inner Classic* establishes the theory of *Zang Xiang* or Visceral Manifestation on the basis of the five-phase theory, which is mainly used to explain the physiological functions, pathological changes of the internal organs and their relationships, formulating therapeutic principles according to the engendering and restraining relationships among them, thus constructing a dynamic model of the holistic human being, and thus bearing practical significance in clinical sense as well.

5.3.3 Five Phases and Visceral Manifestation (*Zang Xiang*)

All of the knowledge related to *zang fu* organs in Chinese medicine were summarized and systematized as the theory of *Zang Xiang* or "Visceral Manifestation". "*Zang Xiang* 藏象" reflects the integration of the *zang-fu*'s external images and the subject's deep understanding of them, which were gained by means of metaphorizing on the basis of the idea of *Tian Ren He Yi*.

The formation of the theory of *Zang Xiang* was a process of integrating knowledge on the man and Classical Chinese philosophy: first anatomical knowledge, then the attributes of the organs to the yin-yang and five phases in the way of *Qu Xiang Bi Lei* or metaphorizing guided by the idea of *Tian Ren He Yi*, then the theory being proved and modified in the clinical practice.

Huang Di's Inner Classic. Miraculous Pivot. Rivers and Vessels states that "Regard the body of an eight *chi* (feet) man; when alive, take his measurement, feel his pulses; when dead, dissect his body and regard the strength of his *zang* organs, the size of his *fu* organs, the volume of the trunk cavity and the organs within it, then the length of the vessels, the clarity of the blood and the state of the *qi* ... All are shown to conform to a standard." This quotation shows that the ancient Chinese people had got a rough idea on the positions of the organs of the body. For example, the lungs were analogized as the "canopy" for their uppermost position in *Huang Di's Inner Classic*. The ancient drawings on the organs also show the almost correct positions of the organs in the body such as the liver at the right side and the spleen at the left side.

Huang Di's Inner Classic. Basic Questions. On Contraindications in Acupuncture started with Huang Di's question "Can you tell me the areas that are contraindicated in acupuncture? 願聞禁數。" Qi Bo answered that "The five *zang* organs are the vital parts of the body, so you should be very careful in acupuncture treatment as so to avoid damaging them. The liver grows at the left, while the lungs store at the right. 藏有要害，不可不察。肝生於左，肺藏於右..." It is clear that what they were discussing is the areas contraindicated in acupuncture, so the positions of the organs should be their real locations in the body. But why here is quoted as the liver at the left and the lungs at the right?

There were two versions as regards to the attributes of the five *zang* organs to the five phases in the ancient times. One is recorded in *Lü Shi Chun*

Qiu or *Lyu's Spring Autumn Annals*[94], which attributes the spleen to wood (east, left), the lungs to fire (south, upper), the heart to soil (middle), the liver to metal (west, right), and the kidneys to water (north, lower). The other is the same as that stated in the *Huang Di's Inner Classic*, which attributes the spleen to soil (middle), the lungs to metal (west, right), the heart to fire (south, upper), the liver to wood (east, left), and the kidneys to water (north, lower). In the two versions, only the attributes of the kidneys to water are identical with each other. Then some scholars believe that the positions of the five *zang* organs in the *Huang Di's Inner Classic* do not refer to their real positions but imagery positions instead. But *Huang Di's Inner Classic · Basic Questions · Discourse on Contraindications in Acupuncture* talks about which areas should be avoided in acupuncture, so the positions of the five *zang* organs in it should refer to their actual positions in the body.

Li Ding 李鼎 holds that the former version accords with their actual positions of the back view which was arranged according to the order of animals' internal organs in the offer sacrifices to the gods or ancestors; While the latter accords with their actual positions of the front view for the doctor sits face to face to the patient when diagnosing and treating him. Therefore the left and the right in the formulation "The liver grows at the left, the lungs store at the right" do not conform to the patient's left and right hand respectively, but refer to the opposites. The *He Tu* 河圖 and *Luo Shu* 洛書, the two mysterious patterns of numbers of the Bearings of the Eight Trigrams (*Li* 離-South, *Kan* 坎-North, *Zhen* 震-East, *Dui* 兌-West) also takes the East as the left and the West as right.[95] I agree with this explanation.

That is to say, the theory of *Zang Xiang* established in the *Huang Di's Inner Classic* is first of all based on the ancient anatomical knowledge; then, on the attributes of the organs to the yin-yang and five phases in the way of *Qu Xiang Bi Lei* or metaphorizing guided by the idea of *Tian Ren He Yi*, and then has been proved and modified in the clinical practice.

---

94 *Lü Shi Chun Qiu* or *Lyu's Spring Autumn Annals*, is an encyclopedic Chinese classical text compiled around 239 B.C. under the patronage of the Qin Dynasty Chancellor Lü Buwei 呂不韋 (?-235 B.C.).

95 Li Ding. 1998: 99-191.

To sum up, *The Book of Changes* and Chinese medicine are of the same origin: shamans' practice; *Qi* and *Xiang* are the fundamental metaphors to bridge *The Book of Changes* and Chinese medicine; *Tian Ren He Yi* is the cultural presupposition for metaphorizings of Chinese medicine; *Qu Xiang Bi Lei* is the metaphorizing process and the methodology to form metaphors of Chinese medicine; and metaphorizing is the way to bridge *The Book of Changes* (the philosophy of Chinese medicine) and medicine. Therefore, the metaphors of Chinese medicine are systematic, carrying unique Chinese cultural and philosophical characteristics, and embodying the core methodology of Chinese medicine.

Yin and yang are
the Way of the Heaven and Earth,
the fundamental principles [governing] the myriad beings,
the father and mother of all changes and transformations,
the basis and beginning of generating and killing,
the palace of spirit brilliance.

- *Huang Di's Inner Classic Basic Questions · Comprehensive Discourse on Images Corresponding to Yin-Yang*

The five phases are the root and source of the Creator[96], the endowment and beginning of the human relations. Emergence, change, and extinction of all the qualities result from the inter-actions among them. ... Therefore, Heaven has the five phases to reveal *Xiang* or Images, Earth has the five materials available to use, and Man has the five constant virtues – benevolence, righteousness, propriety, knowledge (or wisdom), and sincerity (or faith) to show his moral integrity. The myriads of beings take five as the limit. Beyond five, the essence of the numbers changes.
五行者。盖造化之根源。人伦之资始。万品禀其变易。... 故天有五度以垂象。地有五材以资用。人有五常以表德。万有森罗。以五为度。过其五者。数则变焉。

- The Preface of *The Great Connotations of Five Phases*[97]

6 Metaphorizing: A Vital Approach to Understand Yin-Yang and Five Phases

6.1 The Yin-Yang Theory

There is no way available to investigate when the concepts of "yin and yang" were transmitted to the West. Let's take a look at how Ilza Veith translated "阴阳yin-yang" in *Huang Di' s Inner Classic* in the 1940s[98]:

96 Creator refers to the Nature.
97 *Wu Xing Da Yi* 《五行大义》 or *The Great Connotations of the Five Phase*, the most important work on five phases of the middle ancient times written by Xiao Ji 萧吉 in 594 for his emperor. A comment from Joseph Needham (1900-1995): It not only epitomizes the thoughts on five phases theory before its time, but is also a must for studying the entire developing course of the five phases theory in China.
98 Veith, Ilza. 1949; 1966, 1972: 97-253.

"Yin and Yang [the male and female elements in nature];
Yang, the element of light; Yin, the element of darkness;
Yin and Yang, the negative and positive principles in nature;
The element of light; the element of darkness;
Yang, the lucid element of life; Yin, the turbid element of darkness;
Yang, the male element; Yin, the female element;
Yin and Yang [the two elements in nature];
Yang, the lucid element; Yin, the turbid element;
Yin and Yang [the two opposing principles];
Yang (the male principle of light and life); Yin (the female principle of darkness and death);
..."

It is thus clear that the Westerner did not fully understand the meanings of "yin and yang" at Veith's time: "阴阳 Yin and Yang" were occasionally translated into the element of light and the element of darkness; in most cases, they were pinyin transliterated with a concrete explanation.

You see, long before, "yin" had been translated into the female or feminine, negative, inactive, dark, or turbid principle or element, and "yang" into the male or masculine, positive, active, bright, or lucid principle or element in the West. As time went by, people came to find out that no such a pair of opposites available can cover all the philosophical meanings implied in "yin-yang", finally accepted the two loan words: yin and yang. Actually, the words "yin and yang" have already been included as word entries into English dictionaries such as *Webster's*, *Longman* and *The Oxford Dictionaries*, etc. For example,

Longman Dictionary of Contemporary English: "yin, the female principle in Chinese PHILOSOPHY which is inactive, dark, negative, etc. and which combines with YANG (= the male principle) to form the whole world"; "yang, the male principle in Chinese PHILOSOPHY which is active, light, POSITIVE, etc. and which combines with YIN (= the female principle) to form the whole world."[99]

Webster's Encyclopedic Unabridged Dictionary of the English Language: "Yin and Yang (in Chinese philosophy and religion) two principles, one

99 *Longman Dictionary of Contemporary English* [Z]. 1998: 1789, 1787.

negative, dark and feminine (Yin), and one positive, bright, and masculine (Yang), whose interaction influences the destinies of creatures and things."[100]

Actually, yin and yang have already gone beyond concrete meanings and have become philosophical concepts with broad and abstract senses. Then what are the original meanings of yin and yang?

6.1.1 The Original Meanings of Yin and Yang

The sinogram "阴 Yin" was originally a pictophonetic. See Illus. 10 for the evolution of its writing forms.

The first one is the writing form in the oracle script with the upper as "今" for pronunciation and the lower as "隹（鸟） bird" for the shape, which means it is going to be cloudy and the bird is unceasingly crying;

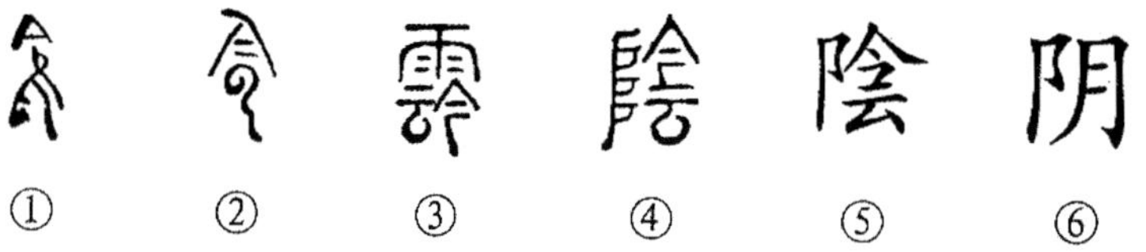

Illus. 10. The Sinogram "Yin 阴" from Oracle to Simplified Regular Script

The second is the ancient writing form in *Shuo Wen Jie Zi* or *The Origin of Chinese Characters* with the lower part changed into "云 cloud", which is still very reasonable for being cloudy indicates that there must be dense clouds;

The third, the lesser seal script, is composed of three parts "雨 rain", "今 Jin" – the phonetic part, and "云 cloud", which apparently shows the intimate relationship between "阴 Yin" and "雨 rain";

The fourth is a variant writing form of the lesser seal script;

The fifth is the original complex writing form in regular script;

And the sixth is the simplified writing form of the sinogram.

100 *Webster's Encyclopedic Unabridged Dictionary of the English Language* [Z]. 1994: 1656.

Shuo Wen Jie Zi or *The Origin of Chinese Characters* interprets "yin 陰" as "dark", "the northern side of a mountain or the southern side of a river"; interprets "yin 霒" as "clouds covering the sun". Now there is just one sinogram "阴" for both. The original meaning of "阴 Yin" is cloudy. "The northern side of a mountain" and "the southern side of a river" are termed yin for they shelter from the sun. *Han Fei Tzu · Shuo Lin Shang* states that "夏居山之*阴*", which means "In the summer [it is advisable to] live at *the northern side* of a mountain." *Lie Tzu · Tang Wen* states that "达于汉*阴*", which means "Arrive at *the southern side* of Han(shui) River."

The sinogram 阳 Yang was originally an associative compound and a pictographic character as well. See Illus. 11 for the evolution of its writing forms.

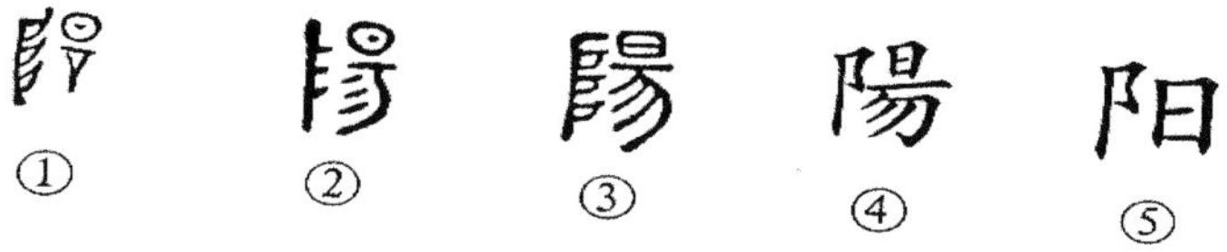

Illus. 11. The Sinogram "Yang 阳" from Oracle to Simplified Regular Script

The first one is the writing form in the oracle script with the left as "阜 fu", which means "going up"; with the right as a bright lamp, which means "extreme bright";

The second is the writing form in the bronze script, which is similar to that in the oracle script, supplemented with the three left falling strokes at the lower left part to indicate "the light glittering in all directions";

The third is the writing form in the lesser seal script, which is identical with that in the bronze script;

The fourth is the original complex writing form of Yang in regular script;

And the fifth is the simplified writing form of the sinogram yang in regular script.

Shuo Wen Jie Zi or *The Origin of Chinese Characters* interprets yang as "high bright". It is later extended to refer to "the sun", as stated in *The Classic of Poetry· Xiao Ya ·Zhang Lu* that "匪阳不晞," which means "If without the sun [it] would not have dried;" Then it is extended to mean "warm", as stated in *The Classic of Poetry· Bin's Tone ·July* that "春日载阳，有鸣仓庚，"

which means that "Spring days are warm, yellow warblers are singing." "The southern side of a mountain" and "the northern side of a river" are generally facing the sun and thus warm, so are termed as "Yang". *The Book of Documents · Yu Gong* states that "岷山之*阳*，至于衡山," which means "from the southern side of Minshan mountain to Hengshan Mountain." *The Classic of Poetry · Qin's Tone · Weiyang* states that "我送舅氏，日至渭*阳*," which means "I see my uncle, to the northern side of Wei(shui) River in the daytime."

Now the question is why the northern side of a mountain or the southern side of a river is Yin 闇 or dark, the southern side of a mountain or the northern side of a river is Yang 阳 or high bright? Actually this is decided by the geographical location of China.

China is located in the Northern Hemisphere. The core area of Chinese culture – Yellow River Valley is at the north of the Tropic of Cancer, where the sunshine is all from the south through the four seasons of a year. Hence the southern side of a mountain is "high bright" because of being exposed to the sunshine, while the northern side of the mountain is "dark" because of too less being exposed to the sunshine. Thereby the southern side of a mountain is yang while the northern side of the mountain is yin.

The Changjiang River (or the Yangtze River) and Yellow River, the two major rivers inside China, run generally from the west to the east. That is known as "a river of spring water rolling towards the east 一江春水向东流." And so the northern side of a river being exposed to the sunshine is therefore "high bright", while the opposite side being sheltered from a mountain ridge and thus being kept out of the sunshine is therefore "dark". That's why the northern side of a river is yang while the southern side of the river is yin.[101]

And then, the meanings of yin and yang are summarized as "the side facing the sun being yang and the reverse side being yin". Later on yin-yang are extended to mean the cold and warm of weather conditions, the upward and dawnward, the left and right, and inward and outward of the directions, etc. All in all, yin is the opposite of yang, and yin-yang has become a pair of basic concepts in classical Chinese philosophy. Ancient Chinese philosophers believed that everything in the world contains two facets, i.e. yin and

101 Zhu Anyi. 2005, 21（3）: 47-48.

yang, and that changes and transformations of yin and yang account for the onset and development of things.

6.1.2 Exploring the Origin of Yin-Yang in Chinese Medicine

It was "Bo Yang Fu 伯阳父" of the last years of Western Zhou Dynasty (ca. 1100-771 B.C.) that first used the words of yin and yang, gave them the abstract meaning of opposition, and used them to explain natural phenomena. He believed that "Yang hides [inside] and can not come out, yin is forced and can not ascend, and then earthquake ensues 阳伏而不能出，阴迫而不能蒸，于是有地震 (*Guo Yu · Zhou Yu*)."

Fan Li 范蠡 (536-448 B.C.) of the last years of Spring Autumn Period (770-476 B.C.) said that "Yang in its extreme becomes yin, and yin in its extreme becomes yang; the sun in the end rises again, and the moon in the full wanes. 阳至而阴，阴至而阳；日困而还，月盈而匡 (*Guo Yu · Yue Yu*)." This quotation was the first and earliest formulation of waxing-waning and transformation of yin and yang.

Lao Tzu · the 42nd Chapter states that "All things in the world bear yin and embrace yang, where the central and harmonious *qi* makes them in harmony. 万物负阴而抱阳，冲气以为和." This quotation affirms that the contradictory qualities of yin and yang are intrinsic attributes of everything.

The Book of Changes further advances that "One yin and one yang makes Dao 一阴一阳之谓道," which abstracts yin and yang to the extensive universality and regards yin and yang as the fundamental rule of the world for the first time. *The Book of Changes* also uses yin-yang to make a comparison with social phenomena, and yin-yang has by extension come to imply the relationship between the upward and downward, monarch and ministers, wife and husband, etc. Joseph Needham (1900-1995) held that yin and yang as definite philosophical terms appear in *The Book of Changes*. The *Chun Qiu Fan Lu* or *Luxuriant Dew of Spring-Autumn Annals* by Dong Zhongshu 董仲舒 (179-104 B.C.) states that "The heaven has yin and yang, the man also has yin and yang. Yin qi of the heaven rises and yin qi of the man will respond it to rise, while yin qi of the man rises and yin qi of the heaven will respond it to rise too. The principles or ways are the same. 天有阴阳，人亦有阴阳。天之阴气起，而人之阴气应之而起。人之阴气起，而天之阴气亦宜应之而起。其道一也."

Chinese medicine inherits and develops the ideas of yin-yang in *The Book of Changes*. Not all the yin-yang in ancient medical texts is abstract in the philosophical sense. For example, among the medical books unearthed from the Mawangdui Han Tomb[102], *Shi Wen* 《十问》 or *Ten Questions* discusses the way of meeting yin [the female's genitals]; *He Yin-Yang Fang* 《合阴阳方》 or *Methods of Integrating Yin and Yang* on the methods of copulation of the male and female; *Tian Xia Zhi Dao Tan* 《天下至道谈》 or *The Supreme Way of the Land under Heaven* on harms and benefits of sexual intercourse; *Yang Sheng Fang* 《养生方》 or *Ways of Cultivating Health* and *Za Liao Fang* 《杂疗方》 or *Miscellaneous Therapies* on functions of sexual intercourse and antenatal instructions.

The theory of yin-yang is easy to tally with the male and female in the sexual intercourse. So, it is very natural to use the principles of yin-yang to explain the sexual intercourse or even use yin-yang as a synonym or euphemism of the sexual intercourse in the above-mentioned works. These works on sexual intercourse press close to the philosophy of yin-yang on one end and to the medical life on the other, so yin-yang can be regarded as a bridge between philosophy and medicine. Thus, it is very common in ancient Chinese medical texts to adopt yin-yang to represent the male and female or sexual intercourse as stated in the Mawangdui medical books.

---

102 The medical manuscirpts unearthed from the Mawangdui Han Tomb in December 1973, Changsha, Hunan Province, include 11 silk manuscripts and 4 manuscripts written on bamboo slips. The time of the tomb is 168 B.C. The manuscripts were copied around 3 B.C., and were the oldest documents on Chinese medicine extant in China. Most of them are stray fragments of text without a title, and then they were entitled according to their contents by modern Chinese scholars: *Prescriptions for 52 Diseases*, *Classic of Moxibustion with 11 Vessels of Arms and Feet*, *Classic of Moxibustion with 11 Yin-Yang Vessels*, *Methods of Pulse-Taking*, *Manifestations of Yin-Yang Pulse Indicating Death* (with one volume of silk manuscript); *Que Gu Shi Qi* 却谷食气, *Classic of Moxibustion with 11 Yin-Yang Vessels* (B ed.), *Illustrations of Daoist Breathing Exercises* (with one volume of silk manuscript); *Methods for Cultivating Health*, *Miscellaneous Therapies, On Obstetrics* (with one volume of silk manuscript); *Ten Questions* (bamboo slips), *Methods of Integrating Yin and Yang* (bamboo slips), *Miscellaneous Contraindications* (wood slips), and *Supreme Way of the Land under Heaven* (bamboo slips). The first five manuscripts and related research outcome were published with the title *Prescriptions for 52 Diseases* by Cultural Relics Publishing House in 1972.

Moreover, ancient Chinese medical classics have applied yin-yang theory extensively into the medical field in accordance with *Qu Xing Bi Lei* or taking images and analogizing. For example, yin-yang in concrete medical texts may refer to some specific medical meanings, such as the male and female, sex or sexual activity, yin and yang meridians, yin and yang pathogens, yin and yang *qi*, *cun* and *chi* pulse, etc.

In *The Book of Changes*, yin-yang is mainly used in the field of natural philosophy; while in Chinese medicine, yin-yang is used not only in the philosophical field, but also in the medical field, and yin-yang is an ingenious unification of philosophical and medical senses. *Huang Di's inner Classic* makes a more systematic and definite expression on the ideas of interdependence, waning-waxing, transformation, counterbalance and harmony of yin-yang implied in *The Book of Changes*, develops these ideas by integrating them with the medical practice, and thus makes yin-yang theory become the guiding theory of Chinese medicine.

6.1.3 Understanding Yin-Yang in the Way of *Qu Xiang Bi Lei*

As a pair of philosophical concepts, yin-yang in essence is to summarize the dynamic images of things or phenomena. Generally speaking, things that are mobile, external, upward, ascending, warm, hot, bright, hyperactive, or pertaining to functional activities are classified as *Yang*; those that are unmoving, internal, downward, descending, cold, dull, hypoactive, or pertaining to materials (or structures) are classified as *Yin*. See Table 2.

	Yin	Yang
Examples From The Nature To The Man	the earth	the sky
	the moon	the sun
	Water	Fire
	Night	Day
	Cloudy	Clear
	dark (dull)	Bright
	cold (cool)	heat (warm)
	Heavy	Light
	Still	Move
	Internal	External
	Downward	Upward
	Hypoactive	Hyperactive
	structure (material)	Function
	Negative	Positive
	Descending	Ascending
	Female	Male
	Death	Life
	Abdomen	Back
	Blood	Qi
	Five *zang* organs	Six *fu* organs

Table 2. Examples of *Yin-Yang*

Based on different characteristics of images of *Yin* and *Yang*, all things in the world can be classified as one or the other in accordance with the way of *Qu Xiang Bi Lei*. The attribute of yin or yang has nothing to do with concrete materials or shapes, but is only determined by their dynamic functions, actions and relationships instead. For example, water pertains to yin for the image of water being cool, moistening and flowing downwards is of yin; fire to yang for the image of fire being warming and rising is of yang. Heaven pertains to yang for the image of the heaven *qi* being light, lucid, ascending and floating is of yang; earth to yin for the image of the earth *qi* being heavy, turbid, descending and sinking is of yin.

Similarly, Chinese medicine often regards *qi*, which has a propelling and warming function, as *Yang;* blood, which has a nourishing and moistening function, as *Yin*. The organic structure, the physiological functional activities of the body, as well as the signs and symptoms of pathological changes, can all be differentiated on the basis of the characteristics of the images of *Yin* and *Yang*. See Table 3.

Yang Pattern	*Yin* Pattern
1.Fever, perspiration, hyperfunction	Chills or aversion to cold, hypofunction
2. Raised basal metabolic rate	Reduced basal metabolic rate
3. High temperature	Low temperature
4. Profuse perspiration	Reduced perspiration
5. Raised systolic blood pressure	Low systolic blood pressure
6. Raised diastolic blood pressure	Low diastolic blood pressure
7. Increased gastric peristalsis	Reduced gastric peristalsis
8. Sympathetic hyperactivity	Parasympathetic hyperactivity
9. Intolerance of heat	Intolerance of cold
10.Red or rosy complexion	Pale complexion
11.Desire for cold drink and food	Desire for hot drink and food
12.Dry tongue , with thirst	Moistened tongue, without thirst
13.Yellow urine	Clear urine
14.Normal quantity of saliva, normal salivation	Much saliva, hyper-salivation
15.Constipation	Diarrhea

Table 3. Pattern Identification According to Yin and Yang[103]

Therefore, in short, the meanings of Yin and Yang are extremely simple, yet very profound. One can seemingly understand them on a rational level, and yet, continually find new connotations or expressions of them in the theoretical system and clinical practice of Chinese medicine, and, indeed, in life as well for the concepts and theory of yin-yang have formed and will continually gain their new connotations in accordance with the way of *Qu Xiang Bi Lei* or Taking Image and Analogizing, as stated in the *Huang Di's Inner Classic · Basic Questions · Comprehensive Discourse on Images Corresponding*

103 Quoted from a secondary source. See Li Lei. New Century TCM English Course. 2006: 18.

to Yin-Yang states that "*Yin and yang* are the Way of the Heaven and Earth, the fundamental principles [governing] the myriad beings, the father and mother of all changes and transformations, the basis and beginning of generating and killing, and the palace of spirit brilliance."

6.1.4 Translation of Yin-Yang in Classical Chinese Medical Texts

In classical Chinese medical texts, yin-yang bears rich and varied meanings. How to translate the two concepts in classical Chinese medical texts into other languages – to consistently use their pinyin transliterations or make their translation accord with their actual contextual meanings they have acquired? My opinion is that "yin-yang" can not all be pinyin transliterated, its translation should be determined by its concrete and specific meanings in the different contexts; when there are different interpretations of yin and yang, it is advisable to give the pinyin transliteration in the text and explanations in the related notes afterwards. Here I give you some examples:

6.1.4.1 Original Text: 丈夫八歲，腎氣實，髮長齒更；二八，腎氣盛，天癸至，精氣溢寫，*陰陽和，故能有子*。（《素问·上古天真论》）

Translation 1 (Lan Fengli, 2007) [104]: In the male, at the age of eight the boy's kidney *qi* is abundant, his hair grows and his baby teeth are replaced by permanent ones. At the age of 16 his *tian gui* or sex-stimulating essence matures, he begins to secrete semen; if at this point *the male and female unite in harmony*, a child may be conceived.

Note: My translation accords with Guo Aichun's interpretation of the text. Here, "yin-yang" refers to the female and male. "实" should be "盛". "肾气盛" is redundancy. "和" should be "和合", i.e. unite in harmony.

Translation 2 (Unschuld, 2011):

In a male,
at the age of eight,
the *qi* of the kidneys is replete;
his hair grows and

104 Lan Fengli. 2007, 28(4): 69-72.

the [initial] teeth are substituted.
With two times eight,
the *qi* of the kidneys abounds;[52]
the heaven *gui* arrives and
the essence *qi* flows away.
Yin and yang find harmony.[53]
Hence, he can have children.

Footnotes:

52 Gao Jiwu/236: "Guo Aichun-92 considers the three characters 腎氣盛 to be a later addition."

53 Most Chinese authors interprete 陰陽和 as a reference to the sexual union of man and woman. In contrast, the Japanese commentator 喜多村: "That is to say, in males, with two times eight [years], yin and yang, that is, *qi* and blood, are blended harmoniously." 925 agrees.[105]

Comments: As Prof. Unschuld said in his footnote 53, most Chinese authors interprete 陰陽和 as a reference to the sexual union of man and woman, and so do most translators. But such an interpretation writes off the other possibilities of understanding and interpreting 陰陽和, such as "*Qi* and blood are blended harmoniously." Thus, I think Prof. Unschuld's translation is more faithful to the original.

6.1.4.2 Original Text: 冲任之脉既起于胞内，*阴阳*过度，则伤胞络，故风邪乘虚而入于胞，损冲、任之经，伤太阳、少阴之血，致令胞络之间，秽液与血相兼，连带而下。(《诸病源候论·妇人杂病诸候·带下候》)

Translation (Lan Fengli, 2007) [106]: The controlling and thoroughfare vessels both originate from the uterus. Excessive *sexual activities* harm uterine network vessels, and then pathogenic wind invades the uterus, impairing the two vessels, damaging blood of Taiyang and Shaoyin, causing turbidity and blood in the uterine network vessels, together with vaginal discharge, flowing down out of the body.

Note: Here, no doubt, "yin-yang" refers to the sexual activity.

---

105 925 refers to the No. 925 reference after the text: Li Guoqing et al. 李国卿 等 1988. *Su wen* yi nan qian shi 《素问》疑难浅识. *Zhong yi yao xue bao* 中医药学报 3, 11-14.

106 Lan Fengli. 2007: 69-72.

6.1.4.3 Original Text: 百病之始生也，皆生于风雨寒暑、*阴阳*喜怒、饮食居处、大惊卒恐。(《灵枢·口问》)

Translation (Lan Fengli, 2007) [107]: Various diseases are caused by exposure to wind, rain, cold or summer-heat, or excess sex, or a lack of harmonious emotions, or improper diet, or a lack of regularity in lifestyle, or great fear or sudden fright.

Note: Here, no doubt, "yin-yang" refers to excessive sexual activities or excess sex.

6.1.4.4 Original Text: 粗工治之，亟刺*阴阳*，身体解散，四支转筋，死日有期。(《素问·疏五过论》)

Translation (Lan Fengli, 2007) [108]: A careless doctor treats it by pricking the *yin and yang meridian vessels* time and again, thus causing the patient getting emaciated, having crumps in the limbs and coming closer to the death day.

Notes: Here, "yin-yang" refers to yin *Jing* and yang *Jing*. The standardized translation for "经脉" approved by WHO（World Health Organisation) is meridian, which implies a two-dimensional grid. Seeing that "*Jing Mai* 经脉 " can carry and move *qi* and blood and so must be a three-dimensional tube, and that "Channel", a popular translation in the West indicating a three-dimensional tube, is a polysemant, whose meaning is not clear and definite, and that "*Jing Mai*" and "*Luo Mai*" are further divisions of "*Mai* or Vessel", "Vessel" can refer to a three-dimensional tube of the human being. And therefore, "meridian vessel", a strict and proper translation for *jing mai*, is worth to be popularized in the future.

6.1.4.5 Original Text: 夫*陰*與*陽*，皆有俞會，陽注於陰，陰滿之外，*陰陽*勻平，以充其形，九候若一，命曰平人。夫邪之生也，或生於*陰*，或生於*陽*。其生於陽者，得之風雨寒暑；其生於陰者，得之飲食居處、*陰陽*喜怒。(《素问·调经论》)

---

107 *Ibid.*
108 *Ibid.*

Translation (Lan Fengli, 2007) [109]: The *yin and yang meridian vessels* possess acupuncture points, where transportation and convergence of *qi* and blood occur. Blood and *qi* of the yang meridian vessels will transport to the yin meridian vessels. Blood and *qi* then fill the yin meridian vessels and flow to other parts of the body. Then *yin and yang* are balanced, the body becomes robust, the nine indicators of the body's pulses will also be concert. This occurs in a normal, healthy person. The pathogens may attack the body. There are *internal damages caused by yin pathogens* and *external contractions caused by yang pathogens*. The external contractions caused by yang pathogens may result from exposure to rain, wind, cold, or summer-heat; while the internal damages caused by yin pathogens may arise from improper diet, a lack of regularity in lifestyle, *excessive sexual activities*, or a lack of harmonious emotions.

Note: "Yin and yang" in "夫阴与阳" refers to the yin and yang meridian vessels; "yin-yang" in "阴阳匀平" refers to the abstract yin-yang in general sense, thus should be pinyin transliterated into "yin and yang"; as to "yin and yang" in "或生于阴，或生于阳", Zhang Qi 张琦 said that "there are internal damages caused by yin pathogens, and there are external contractions caused by yang pathogens"; "yin-yang" in "阴阳喜怒" refers to "the female and the male", or "the sexual activity", here refers to excessive sexual activities. Undoubtedly, such explanation is correct in view of medical principles.

6.1.4.6 Original Text: 蘖木， 味苦，寒。主治五脏、肠胃中结热；黄疸；肠痔；止泄痢；女子漏下赤白；*阴阳伤*；蚀疮。(《神农本草经卷三·中品》)

Translation (Lan Fengli, 2007) [110]: Phellodendri Cortex (Huang Bai), bitter in flavor and cold in property. Indications: accumulated heat in the five *zang* organs, the stomach and intestines; jaundice; perianal abscess; arresting diarrhea and dysentery; spotting with red or light-colored discharge in women; *hypersexuality*; sores resistant to healing.

Note: Here, "yin-yang" refers to female's and male's genitals. The sinogram "伤" is interchangeable with "壮". "Yin-Yang Shang 阴阳伤" refers

109 *Ibid.*
110 *Ibid.*

to “the sexual desire of female’s and male’s genitals being exuberant”, i.e. both the female and male having strong lust for sex, i.e. hypersexuality. In the quotation “望卿走，自投井死，昭信出之，椓杙其阴中” from *Han Shu* or the *History of the Former Han Dynasty* (《汉书·景十三王传·广川惠王刘越》), yin refers to the female’s genitals; in the quotation “囝生南方，闽吏得之乃绝其阳” from *Nan* or *Boys*, by Gu Kuang of the Tang Dynasty (唐·顾况《囝》), yang refers to the boy’s genitals. *Guang Ya* (《广雅·释诂四》) states that “ 壮 is 伤”. Yu Xinwu 于新吾 explains “伤 in the quotation “带甲婴马害歌於行伍，使人身伤” from *Xun Tzu* (《荀子·乐论》) as “壮”.

6.1.4.7 Original Text: 伤寒之脉，*阴阳*俱盛而紧涩；热病之脉，*阴阳*俱浮，浮之而滑，沉之散涩。(《难经·五十八难》)

Translation (Lan Fengli, 2007) [111]: The pulse of cold-induced diseases: both *the yin (chi) and yang (cun) [sections of the pulse]* are strong, tense, and choppy. The pulse of febrile disease: *both sections* are floating; the pulses are slippery when felt slightly, and scattered and choppy when felt heavily.

Note: Here, “yin-yang” refers to *chi* and *cun* section of the pulse respectively for *chi* pertains to yin and *cun* pertains to yang.

6.1.4.8 Original Text: *阴阳*相搏，名曰动。*阳*动则汗出，*阴*动则发热。(《伤寒论》)

Translation: When *yin [qi] and yang [qi]* wrestle with each other, the pulse is throbbing. When *the yang (cun) [section of the pulse]* is throbbing, sweating results; when *the yin (chi) [section of the pulse]* is throbbing, fever ensues.

Note: “Yin-yang” in “阴阳相搏” refers to “yin *qi* and yang *qi*”; “yang” in “阳动” refers to “the *cun* pulse”, and “yin” in “阴动” refers to “the *chi* pulse”.

Undoubtedly, ancient Chinese medical texts are of vital importance to study Chinese medicine. In the modern society, most of the readers of these ancient texts are practitioners of Chinese medicine who want to draw on Chinese medical knowledge from the texts and apply the knowledge to clinical practice. So I advocate that translators should choose and follow

111 *Ibid.*

what is good about the existing critical commentaries and various annotations made through the ages on the texts to make the translation reflect a generally recognized reasonable explanation; and that "yin-yang" can not all be pinyin transliterated, its translation should be determined by its concrete and specific meanings in the different contexts; when there are different interpretations of yin and yang, it is advisable to give the pinyin transliteration in the text and explanations in the related notes afterwards.

6.1.5 The Application of Yin-Yang Theory in Chinese Medicine

The Yin-Yang Theory runs through almost every aspect of Chinese medicine - it is applied to explain the organic structure, physiological activities, and pathological changes of the human body in the theoretical system, and to guide diagnosis and treatment of dieases in the clinical practice as well.

6.1.5.1 Yin-Yang Theory is used to analyze the organic structure

"The physical appearance of human life cannot go without yin and yang." (*Su Wen. Bao Ming Quan Xing Lun* or *Basic Questions. Discourse on Protecting Life and Preserving Physical Appearance*)

"Yin is in the inner body and protects yang; yang is in the outer body and moves yin." (*Su Wen. Yin Yang Ying Xiang Da Lun* or *Basic Questions. Comprehensive Discourse on Yin-Yang Corresponding to Images*)

Chinese medicine is a holistic medicine, which treats the whole person, not just the diseased part. In other words, Chinese medicine is based on holistic approach, or holism. Chinese medicine sees the human body as a whole, the component parts of which may all be analyzed in terms of yin and yang. As *Su Wen. Jin Gui Zhen Yan Lun* or *Basic Questions. Discourse on the True Words from the Golden Chamber* states that

"As to the yin and yang of the human body, the outer part is yang and the inner part is yin. As to the trunk, the back is yang and the abdomen is yin. As to the organs, the *zang* organs are yin whereas the *fu* organs are yang. The liver, heart, spleen, lungs, and kidneys are yin; while the gallbladder, stomach, large intestine, small intestine, bladder, and triple *Jiao* are yang."

6.1.5.2 Yin-Yang Theory is used to analyze physiological activities.

Yin and yang provide a general method of analyzing the functions and activities of the human being, which can be seen in terms of upbearing, downbearing, inward and outward movements. Upbearing and outward movement are yang, while downbearing and inward movement are yin. These movements serve to explain the interactions between blood and *qi*, and the organs and the meridian vessels. The normal life activities result from the counterbalance in between yin and yang. For example, functions pertain to yin, while materials pertain to yang. The life activities are based on materials. There would be no physiological functions if without materials. And physiological functions promote metabolism of materials as well. As *Su Wen. Sheng Qi Tong Tian Lun* or *Basic Questions. Discourse on How the Generative Qi Beats as One with Heaven* states that "If one keeps yin even and yang firm, one's spirit will be in order; If one's yin and yang fail to communicate, his essential *qi* will be exhausted."

6.1.5.3 Yin-Yang Theory is used to analyze pathological changes.

In Chinese medicine, morbidity (unhealthy states) is explained in terms of yin-yang imbalance, relative predominance or decline of yin or yang. The occurrence and development of illnesses relate to two aspects, i.e. healthy *qi* and pathogenic factors. Both healthy *qi* and pathogenic factors can be analyzed in terms of yin and yang - Healthy *qi*, the body's health-maintaining force, comprises two aspects, yang *qi* and yin humor; There are both yin and yang pathogenic factors, e.g. among the six external pernicious influences, pathogenic cold and damp being yin; while pathogenic wind, summer-heat, heat or fire, and dryness being yang. The process of illnesses is actually the process of the healthy *qi* fighting against pathogenic factors.

"When yin prevails there is cold, when yang prevails there is heat; when yang is deficient there is cold, when yin is deficient there is heat." These can be regarded as the general principle of pathogenesis of Chinese medicine.

6.1.5.4 Yin and Yang are the general principles of diagnosis.

Imbalance of yin and yang accounts for the emergence and development of diseases. The essential nature of any disease may be analyzed in terms of yin and yang, despite the infinite number of possible clinical manifestations, as

Su Wen. Yin Yang Ying Xiang Da Lun or *Basic Questions. Comprehensive Discourse on Yin-Yang Corresponding to Images* states that "Proper diagnosis involves inspecting the appearance and feeling the pulse, first differentiating yin and yang."

As regards to pattern identification, yin and yang form the basic principles of eight-principle pattern identification - exterior, heat and excess disorders being yang; while interior, cold, and deficiency disorders being yin.

As regards to the color and luster, being bright and lustrous is yang; while being dark and gloomy is yin.

As regards to breathing and speaking sounds, being loud, sonorous, talkative, and restless is yang; while being low, weak, and silent is yin.

As regards to pulse image, *cun* is yang, while *chi* is yin (location); being rapid is yang, while being slow is yin (the number of beats); being floating, surging, flooding, and slippery is yang, while being sunk, small, thin, and choppy is yin.

All in all, the four examinations should take differentiating yin and yang as the primary task.

6.1.5.5 Yin and Yang are the foundation of treatment and medication.

Because imbalance of yin and yang accounts for the emergence and development of diseases, treatments must involve restoring the balance between yin and yang. *Su Wen. Zhi Zhen Yao Da Lun* or *Basic Questions. Comprehensive Discourse on Essentials of Diseases and Therapies* states that "One must carefully observe the positions of yin and yang, and apply proper treatment until they are balanced."

The general treating principle is to reduce what is in excess and to supplement what is in deficiency. Besides, yin-yang is also used to generalize properties, flavors, and actions of Chinese medicinal agents.

As to the properties, cool and cold are yin, while warm and hot are yang; As to the flavours, sour, bitter and salty are yin, while acrid, sweet and bland are yang; As to the actions, astringing, descending and sinking actions are yin, while dispersing, ascending and floating actions are yang.

To sum up, for the purpose of treating an illness, the treating principle should be determined first, and then corresponding medicinal agents are chosen according to their properties, flavors, and actions to correct the imbalanced state of yin and yang, and finally cure the illness.

6.1.6 Yin-Yang Diagram and Dichotomy

How do you appraise the Yin-Yang theory? You must be very familiar with these two illustrations. One is *Tiao Ji Tu* 太极图 or Yin-Yang Diagram, one of the vital philosophical foundations of Chinese medicine, while the other is one of the vital philosophical foundations of Western science – Dichotomy.

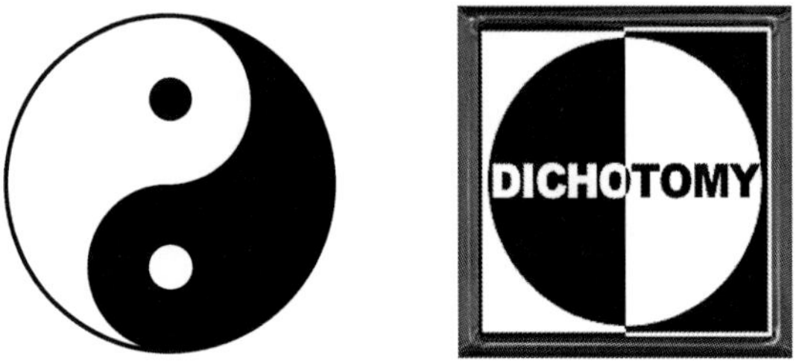

Illus. 12. Yin-Yang Diagram and Dichotomy

As you know, a dichotomy is any splitting of a whole into exactly two non-overlapping parts. In other words, it is a bipartition of elements which are mutually exclusive, nothing can belong simultaneously to both parts, and everything must belong to one part or the other. Dichotomy is directly applied in mathematics, philosophy or linguistics. For example, if there is a concept A, and it is split into parts B and not-B, then the parts form a dichotomy: they are mutually exclusive, since no part of B is contained in not-B and vice-versa, and they are jointly exhaustive, since they cover all of A, and together again give A.[112] In the anthropologic field of theology and in philosophy as well as in the Western medicine, dichotomy is the belief that human beings consist of a soul or mind and a body, which is a vital cultural presupposition of Western medicine. Western medicine focuses on studying the morphological structure of the human body from a system to separate organs, to cells, to genes, and so on, therefore is good at treating body diseases; it views the body like a machine, and so surgery, even organ

112 http://en.wikipedia.org/wiki/Dichotomy

transplantation, is so advanced; but as regards to psychosomatic diseases it cannot achieve satisfactory therapeutic effects.

Tiao Ji Tu or Yin-Yang Diagram shows that in Chinese thinking everything in the world has two facets: one yin aspect and one yang aspect; yin contains the seed of yang, and vice versa; yin and yang create, counterbalance (or wax and wane), transform into each other. The two parts in the illustration of dichotomy is like "1", while that of *Tiao Ji Tu* or Yin-Yang Diagram is like "S", much more complicated than dichotomy, therefore more exact and fitting to the complicated dynamic living system. You know Chinese medicine is constructed under the guideline of *Tian Ren He Yi*, and the object of Chinese medicine is human being, composed of the body, mind and other aspects. Chinese medicine can usually achieve desired therapeutic effects in treating psychosomatic diseases. You know now why Chinese medicine is more exact than Western medicine in this sense.

Here I could make this much clearer by another example. For Western medicine the body is a cooperation of genes, cells, organs, tissues, systems, and so on; For Chinese medicine the living system is just like a text full of metaphors, like a composition of words and every word can be understood by the other words. And you cannot fully understand one word if you don't know all the other words; You cannot understand the meaning of the text if you just check the letters and words. You must care the relations among them and interprete the metaphors for the purpose of understanding the text. Now you can see the source of the exactness of Chinese medicine. The text offers so much knowledge, information, much more than the stabilized objects of Western medicine.

In Western medicine – referring to the example – the lungs are an object which is clearly defined by its place and its functions, and there are some diseases possible which are clearly defined and all other things are uninteresting. For example, in Chinese medicine, constipation caused by the heat in the lungs can be effectively relieved by the therapeutic method of clearing the heat in the lungs; but in Western medicine, constipation is not associated with and treated through treating the lungs. This reduces so much the possible information that a living system can offer. In a difficult text in the field of Philosophy or Poetry you can understand a word only if you understand the full text. You must go always around. You cannot read the full text at the beginning, you must read word by word and then you must find out what is the meaning of the word of this text.

"We think this is fascinating. This is the motivation for us to study Chinese medicine because it is incredible fascinating – what can be done in interpreting a text".[113]

6.2 The Theory of Five Phases

In actual fact, the concept and theory of five phases were put forward earlier than that of *qi* and yin-yang as first stated in the *Shang Shu· Hong Fan* or *The Book of Documents · The Fundamental Principles*, which comes from observing and taking the images of the five materials: wood, fire, soil, metal and water in the nature, and analogizing.

6.2.1 The Origin and Background of *Wu Xing*

The concept of five phases in classical Chinese philosophy evolved from the ancient concepts: "five directions" and "five materials". Now let us take a look at the unique background of the five phases in China:

Firstly, the land of China has been vast with clear definition of the five directions. According to the records of oracle inscriptions of the Yin-Shang Dynasty 殷商 (ca. 16th-11th century B.C.) on the tortoise shells or animal bones, the people of Yin Dynasty 殷人 termed the Shang's territory "Center Shang", being juxtaposed to "East Land", "South Land", "West land", and "North Land". Thereby, the whole territory was divided into five parts, and then the concept of "five directions" formed.

Secondly, China is located in the North Temperate Zone with clear division of the four seasons - hot summers, freezing winters, and regular floods. If the location of China were in or around the Equator or the Polar Regions, terribly hot or freezing cold all year round, how could the ancient Chinese develop the system of the five phases – generating in spring, growing in summer, transforming in the late summer, reaping in autumn, and storing in winter?

Thirdly, in the remote antiquity, China had quite well developed agriculture and metallurgical engineering, which resulted in philosophical understanding of the five materials – wood, fire, soil, metal, and water. In the late period of Western Zhou Dynasty and Spring-Autumn Period

113 Wallner F.G., Lan Fengli. Researching Chinese Medicine: Methods and Problems. In Wallner F.G., Lan FL, Jandl M. J. (eds). 2011: 171-182.

(ca.1100-476 B.C.), theory of "the five directions" was followed by the theory of "the five materials". Shi Bo 史伯 of the late period of Western Zhou Dynasty said that "The metal, wood, water, fire and soil are mixed to generate one hundred items (*Guo Yu · Zhen Yu*)." Zi Han 子罕 of the Spring-Autumn period said that "The heaven gives birth to the five materials. People use them together. Either can not be disposed with (*Zuo Zhuan · The 27th Year of Xiang Gong's Reign*)."

Fourthly, China had been in relative isolation – bounded by Pacific, Himalayas, and deserts. Hence Chinese thinking is quite conservative, and the theory of five phases independently evolved from the concepts of "five directions" and "five materials", thus being radically different from the Greek system of the four elements from the very beginning. The Greek system of the four elements was abolished in Greek medicine as the Greek culture has been continuously exchanged with and influenced by other cultures.

Fifthly, as we know, Chinese characters or sinograms are logographic writing. The two sinograms 五行 embody cultural connotations of the five phases:

, the oracle script of *Wu* 五. *Shuo Wen Jie Zi* or *The Origin of Chinese Characters* interprets that "[It refers to] the *wu xing*. [It] follows 二, indicating that yin and yang interact in between the heaven and earth. All of the fives follow it." "二" is interpreted by Xu Xuan 徐铉 (916-991) as "the heaven and earth".

, the oracle script of *Xing* 行; , the Lesser Seal Script of *Xing* 行. It is a pictographic sinogram, and originally means "the way to talk".

The writing record of the generalization from the concrete material concept "five materials" to the philosophical concept "five phases" starts with *Shang Shu · Hong Fan* or *The Book of Documents · The Fundamental Principles*, which states that "The five phases: the first is water, the second is fire, the third is wood, the fourth is metal, the fifth is soil. Water is moistening and downward flowing. Fire is flaming upward. Wood is bending and straightening. Metal is transforming and changing. Soil, then, is sowing and reaping. Moistening and downward flowing generates salty [flavor]. Flaming upward generates bitter [flavor]. Bending and straightening generates sour [flavor]. Transforming and changing generates acrid [flavor]. Sowing and reaping generates sweet [flavor]." It is thus clear that the five phases do not refer to the concrete five materials any more, but to five kinds of functional attributes which are the distillations of the five materials, becoming five kinds of symbolic images or imagery symbols, thus belonging to the category of image.

In the late Warring States Period (475-221 B.C.), Lyu Buwei 吕不韦, the prime minister of the Qin Kingdom, compiled *Lü Shi Chun Qiu* or *Lyu's Spring and Autumn Annals*, which continued to use the thinking way of *Hong Fan* or *The Fundamental Principles*, affirmed that many things in the world could be attributed to the five phases according to their qualities, and related the system of five phases to flavors, sounds or tones, colors, seasons, directions, internal organs, insects and domestic animals, and grains, and universalized the attributes of the five phases as well. So, the concept of five phases in philosophical sense had formed.

Pang Pu 庞朴 (1928–) pointed out that "Almost all of the thinkers of the Pre-Qin Days talked about *wu xing* from the record of the five directions on oracle inscriptions of the Shang Dynasty (ca. 16th-11th century B.C.) to *Lü Shi Chun Qiu · Shi'Er Ji* or *Lyu's Spring and Autumn Annals · Twelve Periods* where a huge system of *wu xing* was established. The only difference lies in weight or significance and special aspects of *wu xing* in their writings."[114]

As regard to Zou Yan 邹衍 (ca. 305-240 B.C.), a philosopher of the late Warring States Period, Joseph Needham said, Zou Yan might not be the founder of the *wu xing* theory, but, undoubtedly, it was he who systematized and stabilized the thinking system that had been spread for over a century.[115]

6.2.2 Introduction of the Five Phases into Chinese Medicine

The concept of the five phases had been used in medicine as early as the Spring-Autumn and Warring States Period to explain the attributes of internal organs and relationships among them. That is to say, introduction of the philosophical five-phase theory into Chinese medicine is undoubtedly earlier than the time of *Huang Di's Inner Classic*. A quite systematic five-phase theory has already formed in the *Huang Di Nei Jing Su Wen* or *Huang Di's Inner Classic · Basic Questions*, and all of the fives in the book evolved from the five phases, such as the five *zang* organs, five flavors, five colors, five *qi*,

114 Pang Pu. 1982: 219.

115 Translated from Chinese. See: Translator: Department of History of Sciences of Shanghai Jiao Tong University; Author: Needham, Joseph. 2001: 149.

five essences, five spirits, five diseases, five excesses, five deficiencies, five methods, five grains, and so and so forth.

For example, *Jin Gui Zhen Yan Lun* or *The True Words from the Golden Chamber* states that

> "The east and the green color correspond to the liver. The liver opens into the eyes, and the essence is stored in the liver. Illness may manifest on the head. The flavor is sour, the plant is tree/wood, the animal is chicken, the grain is wheat, the planet is *Sui*/Jupiter, the number is 8, the smell is foul, the season is spring, which all pertains to the wood in *wu xing*. And the area affected is the tendons."[116]

That is to say, the direction east, the color green, the flavor sour, the plant wood/tree, the animal chicken, the grain wheat, the planet Jupiter, the number 8, the smell foul, the season spring, and the *zang* organ liver, etc. are all attributed to the wood in the five phases by the way of *Qu Xiang Bi Lei*. See Table 4.

	TONES	JUE	ZHI	GONG	SHANG	YU
NATURE	Flavors	Sour	Bitter	Sweet	Acrid	Salty
	Colors	Green	Red	Yellow	White	Black
	Transformations	Generate	Grow	Transform	Reap	Store
	Climatic factors	Wind	Heat	Dampness	Dryness	Fire
	Directions	East	South	Center	West	North
	Seasons	Spring	Summer	Late Summer	Autumn	Winter
Five Phases		Wood	Fire	Soil	Metal	Water
MAN	Zang Organs	Liver	Heart	Spleen	Lung	Kidney
	Fu Organs	Gallbladder	Small Intestine	Stomach	Large Intestine	Bladder
	Sense Organs	Eyes	Tongue	Mouth	Nose	Ears
	Tissues	Tendon	Vessel	Flesh	Skin & Hair	Bone
	Emotions	Anger	Joy	Anxiety	Sorrow	Fear
	Sounds	Shouting	Laughing	Singing	Crying	Groaning
	Movements	Grasping	Worrying	Vomiting	Coughing	Trem-bling

Table 4. Relating the Nature and Man to the Five Phases

116 The translation accords with the interpretation and commentaries by Guo Aichun, See Guo Aichun. 1999: 26.

6.2.3 How to Translate *Wu Xing* into English?

How do we translate *wu xing* into English? There are several different translations available for *Wu Xing*: the five elements, the five phases, the five agents, and the five elemental phases.

"*Wu xing*" has long been mistranslated into the five elements, which is very possibly influenced by the Greek System of the Four Elements. That is to say, translator adopts the strategy of "domestication" in order to make the translation more acceptable to the Western readers. Now let us first take a look at how the word "element" was translated into Chinese.

6.2.3.1 Element, *Yuan-Xing*, and *Yuan-Su*

The modern concept of a chemical element as a "substance that cannot be split up by any known means into something simpler" did not exist in classical Chinese natural philosophy.

When the concept of the four elements was introduced into China in the late Ming dynasty (1368–1644), the translation *yuan-xing* 元行 (original-phase) for the term "element" was influenced by the theory of *Wu Xing*. There are five *xing* (phases) in China, namely, metal, wood, water, fire, and soil, which have an interdependent cyclic relationship. In the Chinese world view, fire represents not only the real fire, but also the substances and qualities bearing characteristics of fire.

Although there were different Chinese translations for "element" in the 19th century, those terms are mostly forgotten nowadays. Only the word *yuan-su* 元素(original-element), which is derived from the Japanese language and was introduced into China after the Sino-Japanese war (1894–95), is still in use today.

As we know *Wu Xing* evolved from the "five materials", but were not five concrete materials any more, and therefore they are not five elements.

6.2.3.2 Five Phases and Four Elements

In fact, "five phases" is the most popular translation for *Wu Xing* in the literature published in the West. Ted J. Kaptchuk commented that

> "The Five Phases are not in any way ultimate constituents of matter. This misconception has long been embodied in the common mistranslation

'Five Elements' and exemplifies the problems that arise from looking at things Chinese with a Western frame of reference. The Chinese term that we translate as 'Five Phases' is *wu xing*. *Wu* is the number five, and *xing* means 'walk' or 'move', and, perhaps most pertinently, it implies a process. The *wu xing*, therefore, are five kinds of processes; hence the Five Phases, and not the Five Elements. The theory of Phases is a system of correspondences and patterns that subsume events and things, especially in relationship to their dynamics."[117]

The mistranslation "Five Elements" exemplifies the problems that arise from looking at things Chinese with a Western frame of reference. Here "a Western frame of reference" actually refers to the Greek System of the Four Elements, which was advanced by Empedocles (504-433 B.C. or 490-430 B.C.), an ancient Greek philosopher. He believed that the four elements, i.e. fire, water, soil, and air, were the basic constituents of things and objects, related the four elements to four categories like four basic properties, four humors, etc., and he also advocated that the continual change among the four elements was unceasing.[118]

Hippocratic Corpus applied the Greek System of the Four Elements to medicine, which became the system of the four humors. *Hippocratic Corpus* corresponds the four humors to the four elements (soil, air, fire, and water), the four seasons, the four specific properties (hot, cold, damp, and dry), the four stages of human age, and the four dispositions, which was used to explain the human body and pathogenesis of some diseases.[119]

---

117 Kaptchuk, Ted J. 2000: 437.

118 Teaching and Research Section of History of Foreign Philosophy, Department of Philosophy, Peking University. 1957: 73-91.

119 Translated from Chinese. Zhang Daqing, Translator; Porter, Roy, Author. 2000: 90.

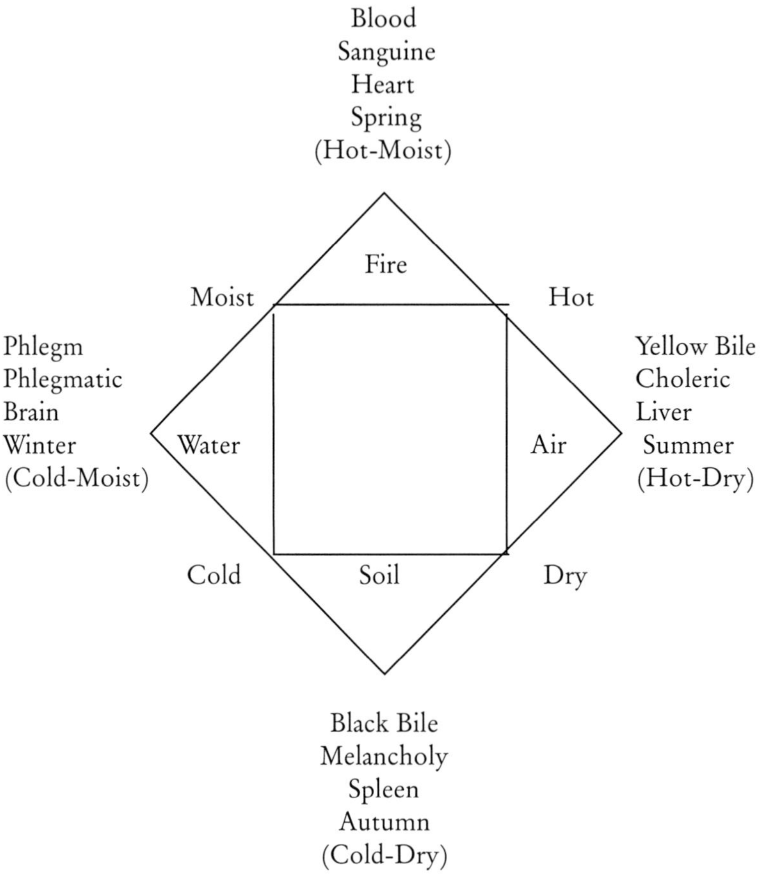

Illus. 13. The Greek System of the Four Elements

As regard to the concrete medical theory, the five-phase theory in the *Su Wen or Basic Questions* and the four-humor system in the *Hippocratic Corpus* share some similar viewpoints. But the attributes of five phases in the *Su Wen or Basic Questions* are much wider in range than that of the four-humor system in the *Hippocratic Corpus;* Integrated with *qi* and yin-yang theory, with the backing of the Visceral Manifestation and meridian-vessel theories, the five-phase theory runs through every link from physiology, pathology of the human being to diagnosis and treatment of diseases, thus forming a broad, circular, self-contained, integrated, and systematic theoretical system of Chinese medicine. While the four-humor system in the *Hippocratic Corpus* is far from bearing comparison.

6.2.3.3 Five Agents

Donald Harper, Paul U. Unschuld, and several other scholars propose to translate *wu xing* into "five agents". Unschuld comments that:

"Given the development of notions of cyclical recurrences or phases of activity of the five *xing*, a reading of 'five phases' has become popular in Western literature. In our translation we follow Harper who in his translation and discussion of the Mawangdui manuscripts adopted Marc Kalinowski's suggestion to translate *wu xing* as 'five agents'.

"The word *agent* maintains, as Harper points out, some of the material aspects of the *xing* as they are used in accounts of natural processes. A good medical example is the account of gestation in the Mawangdui medical text *Tai chan shu* 胎产书 where the bestowal of Water, Fire, Metal, Wood, and Earth/Soil on the fetus in the fourth through eight months of gestation enables blood, *qi*, muscles, bones, and skin to form."[120]

6.2.3.4 Comments on Different Translations

The *wu xing* theory, originating in China, is unique. The formation of the theory is related to the vast land of China with clear and definite five directions, clear division of the four seasons due to China's location in the North Temperate Zone, as well as rising and flourishing of the agriculture and metallurgy in the Yin-Shang Period (殷商, ca. 16th-11th century B.C.) and continual stable development afterwards. Therefore, the *wu xing* theory thrives and does not decline.

We have known that *wu xing* originates from the five materials, but are not the five materials whatsoever. The textbook of *The Basic Theories of Chinese Medicine* (5th ed.) states that "*Wu xing* refers to the movement of the wood, fire, soil, metal, and water." As regard to the content of the *wu xing* theory, it does not discuss the specific properties of the five materials in iso-

120 Unschuld, Paul U. 2003: 84.

lation, but "has by further extension come to mean that everything in the world comes into being by movement, change, and transformation of the five essential materials, i.e. wood, fire, soil, metal, and water," and "that engendering and restraining among the *wu xing* are used to expound the relationship among things."[121]

In view of the above-mentioned facts, I suggest to translate *wu xing* into five phases, five agents, or five elemental phases for "five phases" is the most popular translation in the West, and "five agents" and "five elemental phases" maintain some of the material aspects of *wu xing* and can reflect the evolution process of the term to a certain extent. Moreover, the translation "five elemental phases" is more comprehensible to the lay mind.[122]

6.2.4 Understanding the Engendering and Restraining Cycles in the Way of *Qu Xiang Bi Lei*

The engendering and restraining relationships among the five phases also come from direct observation and experiences of the phenomena among the five materials. As regards to the formation of the engendering relationship among the five phases, *Wu Xing Da Yi · Lun Xiang Sheng* or *The Great Connotations of the Five Phases· On Engendering* states that "Wood engenders fire for wood is warm in nature, fire is latent inside it and makes its way out of it and burns; Fire engenders soil for fire can burn wood, resulting in ashes, ashes can be [regarded as] a kind of soil; soil engenders metal for metal is usually found in a mountain which is composed of soil; metal engenders water for the metal can be melted into fluid, [which can be regarded as a kind of water]; water engenders wood for water can nourish wood and make it grow."

The restraining relationship among the five phases was established through observing the following natural phenomena among the five materials: water can extinguish fire, fire can melt metal, metal (such as sword and axe) can cut trees (wood), tree (wood) can take its root into soil, and dykes and dams (soil) can prevent flooding (water) from occurring.

---

121 Yin Huihe. 1984: 18.
122 Lan Fengli. 2003, 23(8): 627-28.

6.2.5 Application of Five-Phase Theory in Chinese Medicine

In Chinese medicine, the five-phase theory is mainly used to explain the physiological functions, pathological changes of the internal organs and their relationships, formulating therapeutic principles according to the engendering and restraining relationships among the internal organs, thus bearing practical significance in the clinical sense.

6.2.5.1 Five-Phase Theory and Visceral Manifestation Theory[123]

All of the knowledge related to *zang fu* organs in Chinese medicine were summarized and systematized as the theory of *Zang Xiang* or "Visceral Manifestation", which reflects the integration of the *zang-fu*'s external images and the subject's deep understanding of them, which were gained by means of metaphorizing on the basis of the idea of *Tian Ren He Yi*.

The formation of the Visceral Manifestation theory was a process of integrating knowledge on the man and classical Chinese philosophy. That is to say, it is first of all based on the ancient anatomical knowledge; then, on the attributes of the organs to the yin-yang and five phases in the way of *Qu Xiang Bi Lei* or metaphorizing guided by the idea of *Tian Ren He Yi*, and then has been proved and modified in the clinical practice.

Take the spleen as an example. The spleen is located in the middle *jiao* (the center) and below the diaphragm. According to its central position and its yellow color[124], Chinese medicine attributes the spleen to the soil in the five phases. Soil is the sowing and reaping, corresponding to the late summer in the seasons and dampness in the climate, representing the features of receiving, generating, transforming, and supporting. Therefore, the spleen's function in Chinese medicine is metaphorized as transforming the water and grain into essence, then moving and sending the essence to the whole body; thereby, the spleen is regarded as the foundation of postnatal existence, the source of the formation of *qi* and blood, is interrelated with the flesh, governs the limbs, opens into the mouth, manifests its brilliance in the lips, and so on. Finally, a spleen system is formed. The common symptoms of spleen

123 Lan Fengli. Metaphorizing: The Way to Bridge *The Book of Changes* and Chinese Medicine. In Wallner F.G., Schmisberger F., Wimmer F.M. (eds). 2010: 177-192.
124 Soil is the center of the five phases, working as the link among them.

diseases such as abdominal pain or distension, poor appetite, loose stool, diarrhea, jaundice, fatigue or weakness of the limbs, edema can be successfully relieved by treating the spleen in Chinese medicine. It is clear that the spleen in Chinese medicine does not refer to any concrete organ, maybe not the organ spleen at all (according to its central position and the yellow color, this organ may be the pancreas, which was not perceived by Chinese medicine in the ancient time), but to a functional system by applying the five-phase theory in the way of *Qu Xiang Bi Lei* guided by the idea of *Tian Ren He Yi*.

The other four organ systems have been formed in the same way. See "Table 4 Relating the Nature and Man to the Five Phases", each of the vertical columns composes a complex organ system with the attribute of five *zang* organs to the five phases as the focus and all together make up five complex organ systems.

"Wood is the bending and the straightening," having the characteristics of growing, upbearing and developing freely; while the liver thrives by orderly reaching, governs free coursing (or ensuring smooth free flow of *qi* and blood), upbearing and stirring, and is like the sprouting of "trees and plants in spring". Therefore, it is attributed to wood. Besides, the liver stores the ethereal soul, opens at the eyes, governs the sinews, its brilliance manifests in the nails, is interrelated with anger in the seven affects[125], and stands interior-exterior relationship with the gallbladder through the homing and netting connections of the meridian vessels of the two organs.[126] Thus a complex liver system, including the ethereal soul, the eyes, sinews, nails, anger, gallbladder, spring, wood, green-blue, etc., forms in this way.

"Fire is the flaming upwards," having the quality of warming, heating and rising; while the heart governs the blood and vessels, has the function of

125 Joy, anger, melancholy, anxiety, sorrow, fear and fright are the seven affects or seven emotions, which are natural human responses to the environment. Chinese medicine regards the seven affects as capable of influencing the functions of the *zang fu* organs under certain conditions, which is known as "internal damage by the seven affects". Especially vulnerable is the free coursing function of the liver. And so, the liver's function can be summarized as "prefering to function freely and disliking depression".

126 Besides, the secretion and discharge of bile is controlled and regulated by the liver's function of free coursing.

propelling *qi* and blood to warm and nourish the whole body, which is then likened to the heat of the summer, when the whole of creation thrives. Hence the heart is attributed to fire. Besides, the heart stores the spirit, opens into the tongue, its brilliance manifests in the face, is interrelated with joy in the seven affects, and stands in interior-exterior relationship with the small intestine through the homing and netting connections of the meridian vessels of the two organs. Thus, a complex heart system, including the spirit, tongue, face, joy, small intestine, summer, fire, red, etc., forms in this way.

"Metal is the working of change," having the qualities of purifying, cleaning, and reforming; while the Lungs thrive by purifying and govern downbearing. They are likened to the clear fresh air and purifying first frosts of the autumn, when the nature is withdrawing into itself. Therefore the lungs correspond to metal. In Chinese medicine, the lungs store the corporeal soul, govern *qi* and perform respiration, regulate the waterways, open at the nose, govern the skin and body hair,[127] are interrelated with melancholy in the seven affects, and stand in interior-exterior relationship with the large intestine through the homing and netting connections of the meridian vessels of the two organs. Thus a complex lung system, including the corporeal soul, *qi*, waterways, nose, skin, body hair, melancholy, large intestine, autumn, metal, white, etc., forms in this way.

"Water is the moistening and downward flowing," having the qualities of moistening, downward moving and cooling; while the Kidneys are located in the lower *jiao*, store essence and govern fluid metabolism. They are associated with the bitter cold of winter, when the nature is dormant. For this reason, the kidneys are attributed to water. Besides, the kidneys store will, are responsible for growth, development, and reproduction (or maturation), govern the bones and engender marrow, open into the ears and the two private parts: the urethra and anus, their brilliance manifests in the hair of the head, are interrelated with fear and fright in the seven affects, and stand in interior-exterior relationship with the urinary bladder through the homing and netting connections of the meridian vessels of the two organs. Thus a complex kidney system, including the will, essence (growth, development

127 It is also known as "The brilliance of the lungs manifests in the body fair." In other words, the Lungs regulate the secretion of sweat, the moistening of the skin, and resistance to the six external pernicious pathogenic factors, i.e. pathogenic wind, cold, summer-heat, damp, dryness and fire.

and maturation), water metabolism, ears, urethra and anus, head hair, fear and fright, urinary bladder, winter, water, black, etc., forms in this way.

6.2.5.2 To Explain the Inter-Organ Relationships and Prognosis

Both of the Engendering and restraining cycles have two aspects: engendering and being engendered (like that between mother and child); restraining and being restrained. The relationships of each organ to the other four of the five *zang* organs can be explained by these aspects. Let's take the liver as an example.

Liver (wood) engenders heart (fire), and is engendered by the kidneys (water); Liver (wood) restrains the spleen (soil), and is restrained by the lungs (metal). The liver relies on kidney water for nourishment, which is known as "water moistening wood"; if the kidneys fail to fulfill this function, this condition is known as "water failing to moisten wood".

The five-phase theory can also be used in disease prognosis. Generally speaking, if a condition spreads in the order of engendering cycle, i.e. the condition of disease of the mother organ involving the child organ, the prospects for a good recovery are favorable and the disease can be considered minor; If, on the contrary, a condition spreads in the opposite order of engendering cycle, i.e. the condition of disease of the child organ affecting the mother organ, the prospects are unfavorable and the disease is serious. If a condition spreads in the order of restraining cycle, the condition is more serious when over-restraining than counter-restraining.

6.2.5.3 To Determine Therapeutic Principles and Methods

Based on the five-phase theory, the general principle of treatment is "to reinforce the mother-organ in case of deficiency, and to reduce the child-organ in case of excess." Hereafter I give you some examples formulated according to the engendering cycle of the five phases:

"Banking up earth to engender metal" actually refers to the therapeutic method of fortifying the spleen to treat disorders of the lungs, which is applied in cases of lung deficiency that occur in conjunction with spleen-stomach deficiency, manifesting clinically in pale complexion, cold limbs, poor appetite, loose stool, short of breath, cough with sputum, emaciation, weak pulse, etc.

That "metal and water engender each other" actually refers to that "metal engenders water". This refers to a therapeutic method of enriching kidney yin, and complemented by nourishing lung yin, applied for lung-kidney yin deficiency, manifesting clinically in the following symptoms: enduring cough, night sweating, tidal fever, vexing heat in the chest, palms, and soles, aching and weak in the lumbar region and legs, nocturnal emission, etc.

"Enriching water to moisten wood" actually refers to the therapeutic method of nourishing kidney yin to subdue liver yang for hyperactivity of liver yang due to liver kidney yin deficiency, which presents with such symptoms as dizziness, red complexion due to rising fire, and hypertension in some cases.

In the clinical practice, the five-phase theory is applicable not only to treatment of different kinds such as medication, acupuncture, psychotherapy, but also to diagnosis, prognosis, and preventive treatment of diseases. The *Nan Jing* or *The Classic of Difficult Issues* states that "When one sees a liver disease, one should know that the liver will transmit it to the spleen. Hence one prevents such a transmission by fortifying the spleen *qi* (the 77th difficult issue)."

One point is worth to note that the meanings of water and fire are highly dependent on their contexts for they are not only two of the five phases, but also aspects of certain organs or something else.

Fire may refer to the heart or the kidney yang for the kidney yang has also been termed as "the fire of the life gate" since the rise of the life gate theory. For example, "boosting fire to engender earth" refers to a therapeutic method of warming and supplementing kidney-yang to treat spleen disorders such as clear-food diarrhea, enduring diarrhea, early morning diarrhea when caused by a spleen-kidney yang deficiency; the pathological condition of "wood fire impairing metal" does not involve three phases, actually refers to "liver fire impairing the lungs".

Water may refer to the kidneys, pathogenic water-damp, or the symptom edema. For example, "banking up earth to control water" actually refers to "fortifying the spleen and boosting *qi* to relieve edema", where the water refers to the symptom - edema.

It is worth to note that the five-phase theory is not a universal truth. It is only true under certain conditions. The five phases are used for making analogies and inferences, and sometimes broad generalization, in most cases, in the way of metaphorizing. The theory cannot fully explain the functions of the organs of the human body and the relationships among the organs alone, and just plays one of the essential roles in the formation of the *Zang Xiang* or Visceral Manifestation theory. Chinese medicine is not just based on yin-yang or/and five phases, and it is also based on a correct maybe rough understanding of man, which is composed of body and mind.

In one word, the five-phase theory enriches human's understanding of the man and nature.

> The Nature and Man are all composed by the movement and mutation of *Qi*, which makes up the underlying foundation for the cultural presupposition of Chinese medicine – *Tian Ren He Yi* or the Unity of Heaven and Humankind and the core methodology – *Qu Xiang Bi Lei* or Metaphorizing of Chinese medicine.
>
> - The Author

7 Metaphorizing: A Vital Way to Understand the Human Being

Metaphorizing is the major way of Chinese medicine to form its ontological concepts, fundamental theories, and to develop its clinical explorations. By analyzing metaphors in Chinese medicine, we become clear about implicit ontological convictions in Chinese medicine. And only by understanding the metaphors in Chinese medicine, we know that Chinese medicine is a different medical system from Western medicine which weaves natural and social phenomena together with rudimentary correct understanding of human beings as an integrity, thus revealing its methodology "*Qu Xiang Bi Lei* 取象比类 or Taking Image and Analogizing" under the guidance of "*Tian Ren He Yi* 天人合一 or The Unity of Heaven and Humankind", the core idea of classical Chinese philosophy. By this way it becomes clear that Chinese medicine must not be taken as a natural science in the Western sense, but it goes closer to geisteswissenschaften.

Here I would like to clarify this viewpoint - what Chinese medicine is based on is Chinese understanding of the live human being, compared to what Western medicine is based on is Western understanding of the dead body. For example, you can not find *Qi* and *Jing-Luo* (the meridian vessels) by dissecting dead bodies.

7.1 *Jing, Qi, Shen*: From the Nature to Man

Jing, *Qi*, *Shen* are said to be the three treasures of Chinese medicine.

7.1.1 *Jing*: From "the Selected Good Rice" in the Nature to "the Essential Part of *Qi*" in Man

The sinogram 精 *Jing*, a signific-phonetic, originally refers to the selected good rice, or polished rice, which is then extended to mean "the purest, the most refine part, the essence of things". In Chinese medicine *Jing* or essence bears three meanings: 1. the essential part of *qi*; 2. all the substances useful for the human being, e.g. food essence from diet; 3. the essential substance stored in the kidneys, also called kidney essence.

The most important creation of the Jiaxia school of the middle stage of the Warring States Period was the Theory of Essential *Qi*. The chapter of *Inner Working* of *Guan Tzu* states that "Essence is the essential part of *Qi*." It is the essential *qi* that transforms everything in the world. The chapter of *Inner Working* reads that

"The *Jing* is the essence of all things. It is with it that the Dao begins to give life. It gives life to the five grains down on the earth, and the stars up in the sky. When the Essence *Qi* drifts between the Heaven and Earth, it is called the ghost and the divine. When stored in the bosom of a particular human being, this man would become a sage."

"What I mean by the Essence is the essential part of *Qi*, with which the Dao starts to beget life."

Therefore, you see, ontologically, the Dao preceded the Essence *Qi*, which should be created by the Dao in order to beget myriad of beings.[128]

That is to say, Essence forms everything in the world, including man.

"Man comes into being by integrating the essence from the heaven and the shape from the earth. Harmony makes it happen, while disharmony fails in so-doing (The Chapter of *Inner Working* of *Guan Tzu*)."

"Man is born on the earth, hanging his life to the heaven. The union of *qi* of the heaven and earth makes up a man. Man can adapt himself to the seasons for the Heaven and Earth are his father and mother (Chapter 25 of *Nei Jing Su Wen*)."

Jing or Essence as the essential part of *Qi* is also known as Essential *Qi*. Essence, *Qi*, and blood function as the material basis for Man. Then what is *Qi* and blood?

---

128 Shen, Vincent. Dao, Qi, and Body/Mind-Huanglao Daoist Methodology of Nurturing Life. In Wallner F.G., Lan FL, Jandl M.J. (eds.). 2010: 12.

7.1.2 *Qi*: From "Cloud Air" in the Nature to "Basic Invisible Constitutent" of Man

First let us take a look at the Blood and *Qi*, two symbols of life. Confucius divided the life process into three stages: young, prime, and old. Confucius said that

> "There are three things against which a man with honour is on his guard. In his youth, when his blood and *qi* are not yet settled down, he is on guard against lust. Having reached his prime, when his blood and *qi* have become full and strong, he is on guard against strife. Having reached his old age, when his blood and *qi* is weakening, he is on guard against avarice. 君子有三戒：少之时，血气未定，戒之在色；及其壮也，血气方刚，戒之在斗；及其老也，血气既衰，戒之在得 (*The Analects of Confucius*)",

which shows that blood and *qi* were regarded as symbols of life at Confucius's time.

The sinogram for blood is 血, an ideograph, written as " " in the oracle script and " " in the Lesser Seal Script. Its lower part is a vessel, and the dot inside the vessel is a drop of the blood. Its original meaning shown by the sinogram is a blood drop from a sacrificed animal dropping down into the vessel. It thus clear that the Chinese concept of blood is a kind of vivid, direct, and visible material.

The correlation between *Qi* and blood is usually expressed by "*Qi* is the commander of blood, and blood is the mother of *qi*." That *Qi* is the commander of the blood implies that *Qi* is the dynamic force for producing and moving blood as well as keeping the blood flowing within the vessels; That blood is the mother of *qi* means that blood carries *qi* on one hand and constantly supplies *qi* with food energy on the other. Both of them are the symbols of life, a live human being. Then how did the concept of *qi* evolve in Chinese medicine?

Chinese philosophy applies the concept of *Qi* to explain the nature of existence. *Shuo Wen Jie Zi* or *The Origin of Chinese Characters · Qi Part* states that "*Qi* refers to thin, floating clouds. The sinogram 气 is a pictograph." The sinogram 气 in the oracle inscription of the Shang Dynasty (ca. 16th– 11th century B.C.) was written as " ", which resembles air current, evaporating and rising, whose image is just like cloud, will disappear very soon and become invisible. Therefore, *Qi* is invisible and formless, exists everywhere, can be gathered into a form, for instance, *Qi* can be condensed into water.

Soon afterwards, the *Qi* which surrounds and congests the man's space was abstracted into the *Qi* which bears a philosophical sense. Philosophers of the Spring Autumn and Warring States Periods (770-221 B.C.) believed that *Qi* is the basic ingredient constituting the world, and also the basic ingredient constituting the Man and that everything in the world comes into being by the movement and mutation of *Qi*, as stated in *The Book of Changes* that "Everything is transformed and generated by the enshrouding [*Qi*] of the heaven and earth. 天地氤氲，万物化生."

Later on, ancient Chinese medical experts introduced "*Qi*" into the medical field at the right moment. In the time of *Huang Di's Inner Classic*, "*Qi*" is regarded not only as the basic ingredient constituting the nature, but also as the basic ingredient constituting the Man which can be transformed into blood, essence, and body fluid, etc., and the normal functional activities of the life which is governed by "*Qi*" is known as *Shen* 神 or spirit.

Be aware, ancient Chinese philosophy regards *Qi* as the ontology of the nature, and stresses *Qi*'s material characteristics - the basic ingredient constituting the nature; while in philosophy of Chinese medicine, *Qi* is the unification of material aspect and functional activities – *Qi* is not only the basic ingredient constituting the Man, but is also used to expound the dynamic processes and functional activities of the life. The *Lei Jing* or *Classified Inner Classic* states that "All the human life depends upon *Qi*." Physiologically, *Qi* has the propelling, warming, protecting, retaining, and metabolizing functions, which keeps the life activities going in the normal process.

Thus it is clear that the concept of *Qi* in Chinese medicine was formed through a metaphorizing process by means of taking and analogizing the image of air current or vapor. That is to say, the concept of *Qi* in Chinese medicine evolved from air current or vapor in the nature to the basic invisible constituent of the nature and man, and the movement, mutation and change of *qi* result in the formation of everything in the world. *Qi* has finally become invisible and abstract, and more relates to functional activities in Chinese medicine. *Lao Tzu* states that

> "Dao begets one,
> The one begets two,
> The two begets three,
> The three begets all things in the world.

> Everything in the world bears *yin* and embraces *yang*, where the central and harmonious *qi* makes them in harmony." (Chapter 42)

Lao Tzu has more than 5,000 sinograms, but only here *Qi* is addressed.

Dao is unnamable and the way of the nature; Dao is Non-being which begets Being.

The One is the Great Ultimate or *Qi*.

The Two is Yin and Yang.

The Three is Yin, Yang and *Qi*.

Therefore, you see, ontologically, the Dao preceded the Essence *Qi*, which should be created by the Dao in order to beget myriad of beings.[129]

It's necessary to know that Yin-Yang, five phases, and eight trigrams are all the subdivisions of *Qi* of different levels from the viewpoint of *Qi*, which indicates a gradual generating and evolving process from *Qi* to Yin-Yang then to Five Phases then to Eight Trigrams. *The Book of Changes* states that "The changes have *Tai Ji* 太极 (the Supreme Ultimate, the Absolute in ancient Chinese cosmology, presented as the primary source of all created things, i.e. *Qi*), *Tai Ji* generates yin and yang, yin and yang generate the four images (i.e. the greater yang, the greater yin, the lesser yang, and the lesser yin), and the four images generate the eight trigrams."

That is to say, *Qi* can be transformed into yin and yang, yin and yang can generate and be transformed into the five phases which are composed of two pairs of yin and yang (water and fire, wood and metal) plus one middle soil. Actually, the four images and the eight trigrams indicate the five phases although the term "five phases" does not appear in this quotation: The four images can be regarded as four phases, i.e. water, fire, wood, and metal; the eight trigrams can be regarded as water (yin), fire (yang), wood (yin wood and yang wood), metal (yin metal and yang metal), and soil (yin soil and yang soil).

Therefore, the concept of *Qi* in Chinese medicine was formed through a metaphorizing process by means of taking and analogizing the image of air current or vapor. The formless *Qi* explains the structure of Chinese phi-

129 Shen, Vincent. Dao, *Qi*, and Body/Mind-Huanglao Daoist Methodology of Nurturing Life. In Wallner F.G., Lan FL, Jandl M.J. (eds.). 2010: 12.

losophy, and *Qi* has the corresponding place of the Western ontology, and is also the foundation of the model of *Qi*, Yin-Yang, and Five Phases.[130]

7.1.3 *Shen*: From "Lightening" in the Nature to "Spirit" in Man

The concept SHEN reminds me a poem – *Auguries of Innocence* by William Blake (1757-1827):

> "To see a world in a grain of sand,
> And a heaven in a wild flower,
> Hold infinity in the palm of your hand,
> And eternity in an hour."

I think SHEN is the very "grain of sand", "the wild flower", "the infinity", and "the eternity" in Chinese culture and Chinese medicine. Actually, *Shen* is a half religious and half scientific concept in Chinese culture, and bears many meanings. For example, *Dictionary of Commonly Used Characters in Archaic Chinese* explains *Shen* as "god or supernatural being; the law in the nature; spirit; magic, superb, excellent."[131] So first, let's start understanding *Shen* based on its etymology.

The nature has been constantly changing in most of the time with certain regular rules such as the alternate change of the four seasons and the corresponding changes in the nature: growing, developing, transforming, harvesting, and storing. Generally speaking, people can live a calm and peaceful life under such conditions. But there are still sometimes radical changes in the nature such as thunder, lightening, violent storm, sudden downpour, flooding, earthquake, and so on, which are characterized by a sudden onset, unpredictable changing, and being very powerful. Facing such radical changes in the nature, ancient Chinese people were deeply shocked, felt helpless, but held in awe and veneration toward such mysterious and unpredictable phenomena.

The Book of Changes reads that "The Supreme Being (Di, 帝) came out from Zhen (震 Thunder, East);" "The myriads of beings (in the nature)

130 Lan Fengli. Intercultural Philosophy and Chinese Medicine: Reflections of Philosophy of Chinese Medicine in Chinese Language. In Wallner F.G., Lan FL, Jandl M.J. (eds.). 2011: 14-33.
131 *Dictionary of Commonly Used Characters in Archaic Chinese* [Z]. 1998: 254.

came out from Zhen (震 Thunder, East);" "Arouse with thunderclap, and moisten with wind and rain;" "The great virtue of the heaven and earth is to give birth;" "SHEN is to create the myriads of beings (in the nature)." *Huang Di's Inner Classic· Basic Questions* states that "Thunder Qi connects with the heart"[132] and that "Heart stores *Shen*"[133] for both thunder and heart are attributed to fire.

The sinogram for SHEN 神 has undergone the following evolution process:

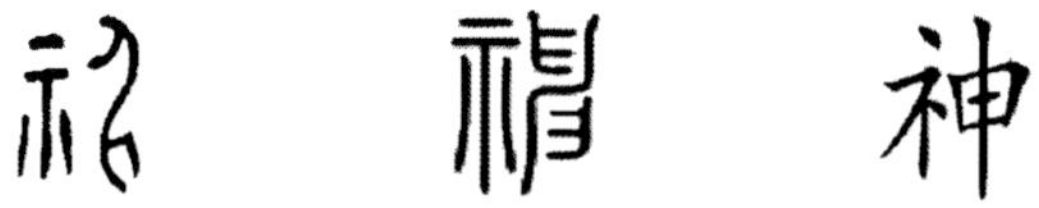

Illus. 14. "SHEN 神" from Bronze, Lesser Seal to Regular Script

The sinogram 神, an associative compound, is composed of two parts: "示" and "申". The ancient form of the right part "申" is the image of lightning in the sky, and is actually the ancient writing form of "電"(the upper is the rain radical 雨, the lower is 电, indicating the meaning); the ancient Chinese people named lightning as "SHEN 申" for they believed that the lightning was so changeable, unpredictable, invincible, knew no bounds, and therefore mysterious, and was governed by or the embodiment of "SHEN or Gods". *Shuo Wen Jie Zi* or *The Origin of Chinese Characters* explains that "申 refers to 神." The left part "示", also an associative compound, is made up of "二" (the ancient form of "上" , means "upper" or "heaven"), and the three falls ("小") , representing the sun, moon and stars. The ancient form of "示" was written as "T", representing the image of a sacrificial altar. The part "示" is a radical, and the meanings of the sinograms with "示" are usually related to offering sacrifices to gods or ancestors, or to rites. *Shuo Wen Jie Zi* or *The Origin of Chinese Characters* explains "示" as "The heaven hangs down images to show man good or ill luck, following 二. The three falls stand for the

---

132 See chapter 5 "Great Discourse on Images Corresponding to Yin and Yang from Macrocosm to Microcosm" (*Yin Yang Ying Xiang Da Lun*, 阴阳应象大论).

133 See chapter 23 "Elucidating the Five Qi" (*Xuan Ming Wu Qi*, 宣明五气).

sun, moon and stars. Observing the images in the sky[134] to detect the current changes. 示 indicates SHEN's things. All with 示 part follow such a connotation." Thus, we can figure out the ancient Chinese people's mysterious feeling about the future world and their great reverence for the gods.

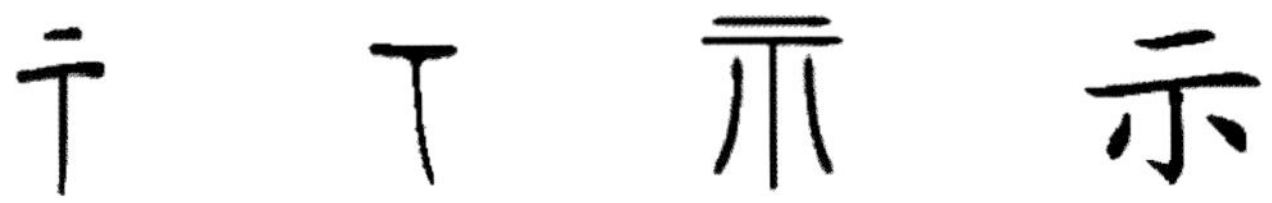

Illus. 15. "SHI 示 (礻)" from Oracle, Bronze, Lesser Seal to Regular Script

Shuo Wen Jie Zi or *The Origin of Chinese Characters* interprets SHEN as "Tian (Heaven) SHEN who induces all things of creation." Xu Xuan 徐铉 (916-991)[135] interprets "SHEN 申 as induce 引", and further explains that "The heaven governs downbearing qi to induce all things of creation". Here you can also see how difficult to translate or interpret archaic quotations from classical Chinese texts: The SHEN in the compound TIAN SHEN 天神 of this quotation may imply both "lightening" and "god".

Yang Bojun 杨伯峻 (1909-1992) explained SHEN in *Zuo's Spring Autumn Annals* as bearing two specific meanings:[136]

One refers to the spirits of all things on the earth including the heaven, earth, mountains, rivers, and so and so forth, e.g. "The people are the governor of SHEN (the spirits);"

The other refers to the spirits of famous men or of those who had performed exceptionally meritorious services after they died, e.g. "In former times, Yao[137] killed Gun[138] in the Yushan[139] mountain, and Gun's SHEN

---

134 天文 is usually translated into astronomy, but I think here it is better translated into the images in the sky.

135 The most important Northern Song scholars on the study of *Shuo Wen Jie Zi* or *The Origin of Chinese Characters* were the Xu brothers – Xu Xuàn 徐鉉 (916-991) and Xu Kǎi 徐鍇 (920-974).

136 Yang Bojun, Xu Ti. 1985: 559.

137 Yao 尧 was a Chinese ruler, one of the Three Sovereigns (Fu Xi 伏羲, Nu Wa 女娲, and Shen Nong 神农) and the Five Emperors (Huang Di 黄帝, Zhuan Xu 颛顼, Di Ku 帝喾, Yao 尧, and Shun 舜), which were mythological rulers and culture heroes of China during the period from ca. 2852 B.C. to 2205 B.C., the time preceding the Xia

(Spirit) transformed into a yellow bear, which went into a deep pool of the mountain."

The Book of Changes states that "The unpredictable changes of Yin-Yang are named SHEN." Here SHEN refers to the unpredictable, mysterious and wonderful changes.

To sum up, SHEN originally refers to the lightening in the nature, and then was first metaphorized to mean the God who created the world, and then was extended to mean the spirits of the nature, the spirits of dead famous or great men (gods and ghosts), and the unpredictable wonderful changes.

Here is worth to mention "*Gui* 鬼", which is explained in *Shuo Wen Jie Zi* or *The Origin of Chinese Characters* as 'what the people return to is named *Gui*, following the part of human and metaphorizing the image of the head of the dead'. Duan Yucai 段玉裁 (1735-1875)[140] further explains that SHEN is yang while GUI is yin. *Gui* originally refers to the spirits of the dead, and is usually translated into ghost. Actually ghost is not a satisfied translation for it is still different from *Gui* in Chinese culture, and here ghost is used only in a metaphorical way.

In the chapter on *Moving Essence and Changing Qi* of *Huang Di's Inner Classic · Basic Questions,* it reads that "A patient with SHEN is apt to recover from illness, while a patient losing SHEN has a poor prognosis." Then what is it meant by SHEN in Chinese medicine?

A Concise Dictionary of Chinese Medicine interprets SHEN as "a collective term for life activities of man in a broad sense" and "thinking and awareness activities in a narrow sense;"[141]

The Basic Theories of Chinese Medicine, the national textbook of the fifth edition on fundamental theories for higher education of Chinese medi-

---

Dynasty.

138 Gun 鲧 was Yu's father. Yu the Great 大禹, the legendary founder of the Xia Dynasty (ca. 2100-1600 B.C.), is best remembered for teaching the people flood control techniques to tame China's rivers and lakes.

139 Yushan 羽山 refers to the northwest of the Donghai County, Jiangsu Province of nowadays (see Page 274 of *Dictionary of Zuo's Spring Autumn Annals*).

140 Duan Yùcái 段玉裁 (1735-1815), due to the quality of his research in *Shuo Wen Jie Zi* or *The Origin of Chinese Characters*, stands above all the other scholars in this field of study. His annotated edition of *Shuo Wen Jie Zi* or *The Origin of Chinese Characters* is the most commonly used one today.

141 Li Jingwei, Ou Yongxin, Yu Ying'ao, et al. 2001: 775.

cine in China, reads that "SHEN bears 3 meanings in the Chinese medical theory: the first, the transformations, changes, and functions of the materials in the nature; the second, all of the activities of man's life; the third, thinking and awareness of man."[142]

To maintain a wellbeing of body and spirit" 形与神俱 is the very point to preserve, cultivate and promote health, which reads in the first chapter of *Basic Questions* that "The people of the remote antiquity practiced Dao by following the rules of yin-yang, harmonizing themselves with the nature by performing some exercises such as *Dao-Yin*,[143] having a balanced diet, arising and retiring at regular hours, avoiding overstressing their body and mind, therefore they maintained a wellbeing of body and spirit, and lived over one hundred years which was beyond their natural life span." Besides, *Shen*'s condition also affects man's healthy conditions, as the 62nd chapter of *Basic Questions* reads that "Spirit (*Shen*) in excess results in continuous laughing; while Spirit (*Shen*) in deficiency leads to being grief."

As regards to the relationship between the body and spirit, there are two famous metaphors in classical philosophical texts. One is the metaphor of candle and its flame, in which candle metaphorizes the body and its flame the spirit.[144] The flame (the spirit) will immediately disappear as long as the candle (the body) burns out and does not exist, which shows that the spirit exists on the body. The other is the metaphor of a sword and its sharpness, which was put forward by Fan Zhen (范缜, ca. 450-515)[145]. He said, "The body is the substantial foundation of the spirit, and the spirit is the function of the body. ... The relationship between the spirit and its substantial foundation is just like that between the sword and its sharpness; the relationship between the body and its function is just like that between the sword and its sharpness. However, there is neither sword without its sharpness nor

142 Yin Huihe. 1984: 3.

143 *Dao-Yin* 导引 refers to an exercise combining stretching, massaging, and breathing to promote the flow of *qi*.

144 See *Xin Lun · Xing Shen* 《新论 · 形神》 by Huan Tan 桓谭 (23 B.C.- 50 A.D.), the first treatise on body and spirit in the history of Chinese philosophy.

145 Fan Zhen 范缜 (ca. 450-515) was a Chinese philosopher of the Southern Dynasty, remembered today for his treatise *Shén Miè Lùn* (《神灭论》, "*On the Annihilation of the Spirit*").

sharpness without the sword. As there is no sharpness without a blade, it is impossible for a spirit to exist without its body. "

It thus clear that the concept *Shen* evolved from the lightening in the Nature to the spirit in Man – first "Lightening in the nature", then "Heaven God who created the world", then "Unpredictable, marvelous, wonderful changes in the nature", and then "Spirit in Man".

To sum up, the concepts of *Jing*, *Qi*, and *Shen*, the three treasures of Chinese medicine, are all formed by the way of *Qu Xiang Bi Lei* or Taking Image and Analogizing or the metaphorizing process from the Nature to Man:

Qi: originally from the "cloud air or vapor" in the nature, then to "the invisible basic substance that forms the nature and man and produces everything in the world through its movements, mutations and changes";

Jing or Essence: originally from "the selected good rice" in the nature, then to "the purest, the most refine part, essence of things", and then to "the essential part of *Qi*";

Shen: originally from "lightening" in the nature, then to "Heaven God who created the world", then to "unpredictable, marvelous, wonderful changes in the nature", and then to "Spirit in Man"; *Shen* can also be understood as the liveliness derived from Essence and *Qi*.

7.2 The Visceral Manifestation: Weaving Yin-Yang, Five Phases, and Social Phenomena with Basic Understanding of Internal Organs Together

All of the knowledge related to *zang fu* organs was systematized as the visceral manifestation theory. *Zang Fu* 藏府, now written as 脏腑 in Chinese, is a collective term for the internal organs and a pair of specific concepts in Chinese medicine, which are metaphors formed in the way of observing, taking images from and analogizing the social storing system of the remote antiquity.

7.2.1 *Zang Fu* 藏府: Metaphorizing the Social Storing System of the Remote Antiquity

7.2.1.1 *Zang* 藏: Storing but Not Discharging

The sinogram "脏 *Zang*" underwent such an evolution process "臧-藏-臟-脏". 脏 *Zang* was originally written as "臧" before the Han Dynasty (206 B.C. – 220 A.D.), such as in *Han Shu·Yi Wen Zhi* or *Treatise on Literature* of *The History of the Former Han Dynasty* where all the sinograms of "藏" were written as "臧". Later on, "臟" was made to be used as a specific sinogram for man's *zang* organs by adding the flesh moon 月 part to "藏". "脏" is the simplified writing form of "臟".

As regards to the meaning of "藏", Chinese medical books usually interpret it as follows: "藏 zang4，藏 zang2 也", which means "藏 zang4 is used to store."[146] "*Shuo Wen Jie Zi* or *The Origin of Chinese Characters* with Annotations from Duan Yucai" states that "藏 *Zang*" is the place to store valuable and precious things, i.e. "storehouse".

The sinogram "藏" bears two pronunciations, one is "cang2", mainly used as a verb，means to "hide 隐藏", "to collect and store up 收藏", "to save and preserve 储藏" or "to store 储藏"; the other is "zang4"， originally refers to "a place to store valuable and precious things", i.e. "precious deposits 宝藏", "treasure house 宝库", which is the original meaning of "脏 *zang*" in the compound words "内脏 the internal organs".

Shi Ji·Lao Zi Zhuan or *The Historical Records·Biography of Lao Tzu* states that Lao Tzu was "the official to guard the treasure house of the Zhou Dynasty (ca. 1100-256 B.C.)". One annotation interprets "the official to guard the treasure house" as "the official to guard the treasure house for storing valuable documents and files". Such a specialized establishment for storing imperial mandates, files, gold, jades and other precious things had been handed down to later generations. For example, *Zhong Zang Fu* 中藏府, also know as *Zhong Zang* 中藏, was set up in the Han Dynasty (206 B.C. –

146 Note: The number after the pinyin indicates the tone of the pronunciation of the character.

220 A.D) with officials known as *Ling* 令 and *Cheng* 丞 to be in charge of documents and precious things.

Therefore, we see that the prototype of *zang* 藏 is a kind of storehouse established by kings of the remote antiquity for storing precious documents, files, imperial mandates, imperial jade seal, and other valuable things. All the things inside the storehouse "藏" are extremely precious or invaluable, which are generally stored inside and not taken out. The five *zang* organs "五藏" in Chinese medicine function to store the essential *qi* and not discharge it, which resembles the function of zang "藏", therefore, "藏" is used to name man's five *zang* organs "五脏（藏）" and state their common physiological function by the way of *Qu Xiang Bi Lei*.

7.2.1.2 *Fu* 府: Discharging but Not Storing

Fu 腑 was originally written as "府" in the ancient times. The part "flesh moon 月" was supplemented to "府" afterwards to make a specific sinogram "腑" for expressing man's *fu* organs.

In the ancient literature, "府" at least bears the following meanings:

1. the place to store money, goods, or documents. *Shuo Wen Jie Zi* or *The Origin of Chinese Characters* interprets the original meaning of *Fu* 府 as "the place to store documents".

2. the official being in charge of money, goods, and documents. *The Rites of Zhou [Dynasty]* (*Zhou Li ·Tian Guan ·Zai Fu* 《周礼·天官·宰夫》) states that "The fifth is *Fu*, who has official contract to administer the storehouse."

3. the place of gathering something. *Zuo's Spring and Autumn Annals · The 27th Year of Xigong's Reign* states that "*The Book of Songs* and *The Book of Documents* are the *Fu* of *Yi*, the place of gathering meanings."

4. a general name for a feudal official or local authorities. *The Rites of Zhou [Dynasty]* (*Zhou Li ·Tian Guan ·Da Zai* 《周礼·天官·大宰》) states that "Eight methods are used to govern the feudal officials." One annotation interprets *Fu* as "the places where all the officials reside."

5. high officials' or noble lords' residences.

Actually, the earliest meaning of "*fu* 府" is a storing system established by kings of the remote antiquity to govern six kinds of money and goods. *The Book of Documents* (*Shang Shu · Da Yu Mo* 《尚书 · 大禹谟》) states that "The earth is even, the heaven is ready-made, and the six *Fu* and three kinds of things are all in order, which will be relied on by all the later generations to live." Kong Yingda's[147] annotation reads that "*Fu* is the place to store money." *Yu Pian· Guang Part* 《玉篇·广部》[148] reads that "*Fu* is the place to store goods". What kinds of goods were stored in the *Fu*? Six kinds of money or goods, i.e. water, fire, metal, soil, wood, and grain, were stored in the "*Fu*", which were often consumed in the daily life and indispensable to ancients' life. The six kinds of money or goods to consume were administered by six officials of six departments respectively, and the institutions where the officials reside are also known as six *Fu*.

The Rites of Zhou [Dynasty] (*Zhou Li · Qu Li* 《周礼·曲礼》) states that "The son of Heaven's six *Fu* are set up to administer soil, wood, water, grass, utensils, and goods." It can be seen that the specific names of the six *Fu* in the Zhou Dynasty (ca. 1100-256 B.C.) slightly changed, but their functions and official system remained the same.

Six kinds of money or goods were to be constantly consumed, which of course needed corresponding fresh supplies. How to supply them? They should be supplied by collecting and gathering them from the common people. As a matter of fact, "six *Fu*" were also the tax bureau of the remote antiquity, the officials of the six *Fu* were a general name of "six tax officials" of the king's official system of that time, as what was recorded in the annotation on six *Fu* of the *The Rites of Zhou [Dynasty]* (*Zhou Li · Qu Li*) that "(six) *Fu* governs the storing of the tax of six kinds of things" in the remote antiquity.

It is thus clear that the six *Fu* administered by the six corresponding officials stored six kinds of necessities for everyday life, which were consumed and supplied everyday, so coming in and out were their characteristics. While "藏 *Zang*" was characterized by only coming in without coming out.

To sum up, "府 *Fu*" was a kind of storehouse established by kings of the remote antiquity to hold six necessities for everyday life, known as "six materials"; the institutions were also known as six "*Fu*", governing collecting or levying tax, therefore, the official names administering the six *Fu* also had

147 Kong Yingda 孔颖达 (574-648), a famous Confucian scholar and an expert in Confucian classics of the Sui-Tang Dynasties.

148 *Yu Pian* 《玉篇》, a dictionary arranged according to forms and structures of sinograms compiled by Gu Yewang 顾野王 (519-581) in 543.

the sinogram "府 *Fu*". The "六府 six *Fu*" were characterized by constantly coming in and out of the money or goods, resembling the function of man's "六腑(府) six *fu* organs" which receive, transform, move water and grain and discharge the waste out of the body but not to store, therefore, "府 *fu*" is used to name man's "六腑(府) six *fu* organs" and state their common physiological function by the way of *Qu Xiang Bi Lei*.

It can be seen that the establishment of "臧 *zang*" and "府 *fu*" started in the Xia Dynasty (ca. 2100 – ca.1600), was gradually perfected till Shang and Zhou Dynasties (ca. 1600 – 256 B.C.) according to the record in *The Book of Documents* (*Shang Shu Da Yu Mo* 《尚书·大禹谟》). It can be inferred that the origin and formation of the Chinese medical theory were really time-honored.

To Sum up, the sinogram 脏 *Zang* underwent such an evolution process "臧—-藏—臟—脏". "Zang 藏" originally refers to "a place to store precious things or treasure house". *Shuo Wen Jie Zi* or *The Origin of Chinese Characters* reads that "藏 zang4 is used to store (藏 cang2)", which was annotated by Duan Yucai that "*Zang* 藏" is the place to store valuable and precious things, i.e. "storehouse". In the remote antiquity, *Zang* 藏 is a specialized establishment for storing imperial mandates, files, gold, jades and other precious things, and all the things inside the storehouse "*Zang* 藏" were extremely precious or invaluable, which were generally stored inside and not taken out. Such "*Zang* 藏" was taken and analogized the five organs in the body which are said to store the essential *qi* but not discharge it – Heart, Liver, Spleen, Lungs, and Kidneys.

Fu 腑 was originally written as "府". The earliest meaning of "*fu* 府" is a storing system established by kings of the remote antiquity to govern six kinds of money and goods, known as "Six Materials", i.e. water, fire, metal, soil, wood, and grain. What were stored in the "*Fu*" were often consumed and of course needed corresponding fresh supplies and indispensable to ancients' life. Therefore the Six *Fu* were taken and analogized the organs in the body which are said to receive, transform, move water and grain and discharge the waste out of the body but not to store – Gallbladder, Stomach, Large Intestine, Small Intestine, Bladder, and Triple *Jiao*.

7.2.1.3 *Zang* 藏 or *Fu* 府: Who Decided?

Who decided which organ was attributed to *Zang* or *Fu* is still unclear. *Huang Di Nei Jing Su Wen · Yin-Yang Ying Xiang Da Lun* or *Huang Di's Inner Classic ·Basic Questions · Great Discourse on Images Corresponding to Yin-Yang* states in the name of Huang Di that

"I have heard that in the remote antiquity, the sages talked about and theorized the human body by differentiating *zang* from *fu*, understanding the distribution and function of the vessels, giving the names to the acupuncture points ..."

Huang Di Nei Jing Su Wen · Wu Zang Bie Lun or *Huang Di's Inner Classic ·Basic Questions · Further Discourse on the Five Zang Organs* states also in the name of Huang Di that

"I have heard from persons educated in medicine the different classifications of the *zang* and *fu* organs. Some regard the brain and marrow, the intestines and stomach as *zang* organs; others regard these organs as *fu*. People all disagree."

The two quotations indicate that the ancient Chinese had formulated the meanings of "藏府 *zang fu*", but developed into different schools as regards to the specific classification or differentiation of them.

7.2.1.4 Triple *Jiao:* Having a Name but No Shape?

Triple *Jiao,* the collective term for the upper, middle, and lower *Jiao*, is the sixth *fu* organ, a specific and unique organ in Chinese medicine. *The Nan Jing* or *The Classic of Difficult Issues* proposes that Triple *Jiao* "has a name but no shape", which evoked disagreement on its physical shape, location, and meaning among physicians of the later generations.

Triple *Jiao* first appeared in "*Basic Questions·Discourse on the True Words in the Golden Cabinet*", which reads that "As regards to yin and yang of the *zang-fu* or depots and palaces, *zang* or depots are yin while *fu* or palaces are yang. Thus the liver, heart, spleen, lungs, and kidneys are yin while the gallbladder, stomach, large intestine, small intestine, bladder, and triple *Jiao* are yang." But, its shape and location are not shown in this quotation.

7.2.1.4.1 Explanations of the "Tripe *Jiao*" from Different Schools

What does "triple *jiao*" really mean and what is the term explanation of it? Physicians over the ages hold different views of "triple *jiao*", some explain it with physical forms, while others explain it by its functions. Ren Yingqiu 任应秋（1914-1984）in *Theories of Schools of Chinese Medicine* 《中医各家学说》 summarized the explanations of "triple *jiao*" from physicians over the ages from Three Kingdoms (220-265), Jin dynasty (265-420) to People's Republic of China (1949–) in five categories:

The first school holds that the "triple *jiao*" has no shape, represented by Sun Yikui (孙一奎，1522-1619). In his viewpoint, "triple *jiao*" has its meridian vessel but has no *fu* or palace, and it is the function of the bladder and the sea of *qi* of the chest center (Dan Zhong, 膻中); And so it has a name but no shape.

The second school regards the "triple *jiao*" as a cavity, represented by Yu Tuan (虞抟, 1438-1517) and Zhang Jiebin (张介宾, 1563-1640). For example, Zhang Jiebin held that the "triple *jiao*" is one of the six *fu* or palaces, residing "outside the *zang-fu* or depots and palaces but inside the body, embracing all the *zang* or depots, and being the largest *fu* or palace like a cavity."

The third school takes the stomach as the "triple *jiao*", represented by Luo Mei (罗美, dates unknown), a famous doctor in Kangxi's Reign (1661-1722) of the Qing Dynasty (1644-1911). In his viewpoint, the "triple *jiao*" is the division for the stomach – "Therefore, we know that triple *Jiao* is the division for the stomach according to its upper and lower rough outlines. The location of the triple *Jiao* is the same as that of Yangming or Yang Brightness (i.e. stomach). What the triple *Jiao* governs is just what the Yangming or Yang Brightness (i.e. stomach) gives."

The fourth school takes the "triple *jiao*" as a fat membrane, represented by Tang Rongchuan (唐容川, 1846-1897). In his viewpoint, the sinogram 焦 ("jiao") is interchangeable with 膲 ("jiao"), and 膲 ("jiao") is an internal fleshy organ. That is to say, the membrane of the body is the "triple *jiao*". He said, "Triple *Jiao* is the membrane of the body, connecting the stomach, intestines with the bladder," "linking *banyou* or the leaf fat with *jiguanyou* or the cockscomb fat, attaching to the small intestine, and stretching out to become interstices of the lumbar and abdomen."

The fifth school regards the "triple *jiao*" as three sections of the body, represented by Yang Xuncao [杨玄操, dates unknown, a doctor in Tang Dynasty (618-907)] and Li Gao (李杲, 1180-1251). In this viewpoint, the "triple *jiao*" is explained as the upper, middle and lower sections of the body - Heart and lung disease is called "the upper *Jiao* disease"; Spleen and stomach disease is named "the middle *Jiao* disease"; Parturition, menstrual disorders and abnormal vaginal discharge, impotence and sterility as well as weakness and aching of the lumbar and the legs are considered as "the lower *Jiao* disease".

The statement that the triple *Jiao* has a shape was first proposed by Chen Wuze (陈无择, 1131-1189) in his monograph entitled *A Unified Treatise on Diseases, Symptoms, and Remedies According to the Three Causes*" 《三因极一病证方论》. He held that the triple *Jiao* is a piece of membrane: "Triple *Jiao* is a fat membrane as large as a hand, just being the opposite of the bladder."

Qian Bingqiang 钱秉强 simulated a method of archaeology prevailing in the world today and figured out that the original meaning of "triple *jiao*" referred to the portal vein-oriented veins in thoracic and abdominal cavity through animal-dissecting tests.

Referring to the physiological knowledge of Western medicine, most of modern scholars seek for anatomical organs, tissues or systems corresponding to the "triple *jiao*" according to its functions, such as the Lymphatic system hypothesis proposed by Zhang Taiyan (章太炎, 1869-1936), Lu Yuanlei (陆渊雷, 1894-1955) and the research team for Chinese and Western Medicine of the Jiangyin Health Bureau, Jiangsu Province, pancreas hypothesis by Zhao Dihua 赵棣华 and the hypothesis of the body fluid equilibrium system by Xia Han 夏涵, etc.

The proposed organ, tissue or system may explain some of the functions of the "triple jiao". For example, liquid and humor metabolism explains its role in regulating the waterways but leaves out its qi transforming function - "Governing all kinds of qi", which is also impossible to cover that the "triple jiao" is divisible but inseparable with all the other zang-fu or depots and palaces. Therefore, many scholars point out that the "triple jiao" is reasoned, concluded and analyzed to be a theory of a combination of intuition and reasoning based on clinical symptoms, physiological phenomena and observation of exposed corpses. Regardless of the differences between the Chinese and Western medical systems, the farfetched equation of "triple jiao" with certain organs, tissues or systems perceived by Western medicine would inevitably lead to controversies and disagreements. Such understanding is very insightful. Such easy equations and comparisons are wrong from the beginning when concerning the great differences in cultural backgrounds, philosophical foundations (such as epistemology, methodology), and theoretical systems between Chinese and Western medicine.

"Triple jiao", in essence, is the place and passage for generation and transformation of essence, qi, and body fluid. It is not like the other zang-fu or depots and palaces, but the others cannot independently perform their biochemical activities without it; it is not like the other tissues but they have its presence, otherwise the body's basic biochemical activities can not commence.

Such "external fu or palace" or "solitary fu or palace" can only be explored through multi-system, multi-tissue and multi-level connections. It has the implication of a functional "unit", but is not a fictitious non-existent abstraction. As one of the six fu or palaces, "triple jiao" certainly has its material basis. The "形 xing" in the statement of Nan Jing or The Classic of Difficult Issues that "The triple jiao has a name but no xing" means "xing zhuang 形状 or shape", not "xing zhi 形质 or material basis", which implies that "triple jiao" has its name but does not bear a certain shape. A Japanese scholar 玄医 held that "The gathering of the space among the flesh and blood, among the zang and fu or the depots and palaces is the triple jiao." Triple Jiao connects the upper and reaches the lower, covers and includes the interior and the exterior, distributes essential qi and fluid to the whole body, and penetrates into the zang-fu or the depots and palaces, meridian vessels, organs and tissues. Thereby, some scholars support that such understanding is the true meaning of the triple jiao.

7.2.1.4.2 Understanding the "Tripe Jiao" Based on Etymology of the Sinogram "焦 Jiao"

There are three versions of interpreting the sinogram "jiao":

1. The sinogram "焦 Jiao" follows fire, is interchangeable with "燋 jiao" which means roast with fire. This implies that the triple Jiao plays a role in digesting and decomposing water and grain.

2. The sinogram "焦 Jiao" is interchangeable with "膲 jiao", which is believed to be one of the fleshy organs of the body, such as the membrane. Miraculous Pivot · Dew of the Year 《灵枢 · 岁露》 states that "毛发残，膲理薄，烟垢落", which can be translated into "One will lose his/her hair of

the body and head, his/her texture of the muscles will be sparse, and the sebum will exfoliate to be like smoky dust."

Zhang Zhicong (张志聪, 1616-1774) annotated that "The sinogram 理 *li* refers to the texture of the muscles, the place which the triple *jiao* communicates and meets. That's why it is named 膲理 *jiaoli*." [149] *Miraculous Pivot · On Great Confusion* 《灵枢·大惑论》states that: "邪气留于上膲，上膲闭而不通", which can be translated into "Evil *qi* congests the upper *jiao*, leading to the obstruction of the upper *jiao*."

3. *Five Methods of Integrating Chinese Medicine with Western Medicine* 《医学汇通五种》 by Tang Rongchuan（唐容川, 1846-1897） holds that "焦 *jiao*" was written as " [illegible] *jiao*" in ancient times; that the sinogram " [illegible] *jiao*" follows "采 *cai*" which means "strata or layers can be identified", follows "韋 (韦) *wei*" which means hides of cattle because the triple *jiao* looks like it, and follows "焦 *jiao*" because it (the triple *jiao*) has wrinkles like the skin burnt by fire; and that parts of the sinogram "采 *cai*" and "韋 (韦) *wei*" are omitted, leaving only "焦 *jiao*" which is not correctly understood by later generations.

We can find the sinogram [illegible] but cannot find the sinogram [illegible] in *Shuo Wen Jie Zi* or *The Origin of Chinese Characters*. Tang Rongchuan mistook [illegible] with [illegible] probably because the seal scripts of "米 *mi*" and "采 *cai*" were so similar to each other. The sinogram " [illegible]" refers to something contracting because " [illegible]" follows "米 *mi*" and pronounced as "焦 *jiao*", originally means collecting grains by gathering and contracting. Accordingly we can see that " [illegible]" is a soft leather-like constricted substance contracting from "all sides" to the central. In the human body, it is a membranous organ wrapping the *zang-fu* or the depots and palaces, and is one of the six *fu* or palaces. It is widely distributed in the body cavity with variable shape and closely linked with the wrapped internal organs (the *zang-fu* or the depots and palaces), so the generations fail to recognize its shape.[150]

I believe that the concept formation of the "triple *jiao*" is certainly based on some anatomical knowledge and has a certain material basis. The

149 Wang Xiaolong. 2001: 507.
150 Wang Hongtu. 1997: 197.

second and third explanations of "焦 *jiao*" in ancient medical classics are quite reasonable.

7.2.1.4.3 English translation of "*San Jiao*"

The "*Standard Acupuncture Nomenclature* (Part 1 and 2)" approved and issued by the World Health Organization in 1991 recommends "triple energizer" as the standardized English translation of "三焦 *San Jiao*". However, a considerable number of authors and translators, especially Western scholars, refuse to use this term. Among them, some use the *pinyin* transliteration "*san jiao*", some use "triple burner", and some use "triple warmer" or "triple heater", and "Triple burner" is the most popular one. The English translations of "上焦 *shang jiao*", "中焦 *zhong jiao*", and "下焦 *xia jiao*" all depend on the translation of "焦 *jiao*".

The Introduction of "*WHO International Standard Terminologies on Traditional Medicine in the Pacific Region*" (Why the word "Terminology" is used here in plural form?) issued in 2007 explains the principles of the English translation of the nomenclature, which are as follows: Accurate reflection of the original concept of Chinese terms; No creation of new English words; Avoidance of *Pinyin* (Romanized Chinese) use; Consistency with WHO's *Standard Acupuncture Nomenclature*.[151]

Obviously, the World Health Organization can not follow the four principles simultaneously when selecting the standardized translation of "三焦", but it makes appropriate adjustments based on the current use of the translation. It uses "triple energizers" as the standardized translation of "三焦", which is consistent with the "*Standard Acupuncture Nomenclature*" (1991), and in the following "Definition/Description" also mentions "triple burners": "triple burners: a collective term for the three portions of the body cavity, through which the visceral *qi* is transformed, *also widely known as triple burners.*"[152] What is puzzling is that why "energizers" and "burners" are in plural form behind "triple" in the nomenclature approved and issued by World Health Organization?

151 WHO. 2007: 4.
152 WHO. 2007: 23.

According to the term explanation of "三焦", the current English translations of "三焦" all fail to accurately reflect the meanings of the term. "Triple energizer" puts particular emphasis on *San Jiao*'s function of "governing all kinds of *qi*" as *qi* is usually regarded as a kind of "energy". The translation "Triple burner" results from the misunderstanding of "焦", just as what Prof. Xie Zhufan (谢竹藩, 1924–) said that "As a common word, this character (焦) does mean 'burnt' or 'charred', but as a medical term, it means 'passage or space within the body.' This definition is well explained in some specialized Chinese dictionaries like *Concise Dictionary of Characters in Chinese Medicine* 《简明中医字典》 published by Guizhou People's Publishing House in 1985."[153]

Translations like "triple burner", "triple warmer" and "triple heater" are all related to heat or fire, reflecting translators' understanding of "焦 jiao": following fire, being interchangeable with "燋 jiao", thus meaning roast with fire, which implies that the triple Jiao plays a role in digesting and decomposing water and grain.

I am very doubtful about one of the translation principles proposed by the World Health Organization – "Avoidance of *Pinyin* (Romanized Chinese) use". Transliteration has been used in the translation practice for over one thousand years. Xuan Zang (玄奘, 602-664), a famous translator of Buddhist scriptures of the Tang Dynasty (618-907), systematically summed up five principles for applying transliteration in the Preface of *Fanyi Mingyi Ji* 《翻译名义集·序》, namely "Five reasons for no translation":

1. "For secrets": Sutra passphrase should be transliterated;

2. "For polysemies": Polysemies in the Buddhist scriptures should be transliterated;

3. "For concepts without equivalents in the target language": Concepts without equivalents in the target language (Chinese) should be transliterated;

4. "For following ancient transliteration": The ancient transliteration established by the people through long practice should be kept in use;

5. "For respecting the original work, e.g., the transliteration "般若 bō rě" for a concept in Buddhist scriptures shows respect to the original while

153 Xie Zhufan. 2003: 41.

its translation "wisdom" sounds unimportant and superficial.: Using transliteration to avoid losing the true meaning of the original.

Such principles are of great significance to keep the original meaning and effect, to fill semantic vacancies caused by cultural and linguistic differences and to introduce foreign words.[154] The practice of translating Chinese medical texts into a Western language shows that the "Five reasons for no translation (i.e. transliteration)" tally fully with the actual situation of the translation of Chinese medicine. For example, the concept "气 *qi*" apparently bears many meanings, no matter "energy", "influence" or "atmosphere" is all unable to convey all its meanings, and so it should be *pinyin* transliterated as "*qi*".

The practice of translating Chinese medical texts into a Western language shows that use of *pinyin* transliteration is gradually becoming more widely used. Words formed through *Pinyin* transliteration such as "*yin*", "*yang*", "*qi*", "*Dao(Tao)*", etc. have long been accepted by English vocabulary system.

According to etymology of the Sinogram "Jiao 焦 ", as one of the six *fu* or palaces, "triple *jiao*" certainly has its material b asis. Based on the term explanations of "triple *jiao*" and its available translations, I believe that *Pinyin* transliteration, i.e., "*san jiao*" or "triple *jiao*", is the best translation of "三焦" in order to avoid ambiguity and confusion.

7.2.2 The Visceral Manifestation: Weaving Social Phenomena with Basic

Understanding of Internal Organs Together. – How did the visceral manifestation theory in Chinese medicine evolve and form?

7.2.2.1 Anatomical Knowledge of the Body

First, the visceral manifestation theory is based on a correct anatomical knowledge of the body. *Huang Di's Inner Classic · Miraculous Pivot · Rivers and Vessels* reads that

"Regard the body of an eight *chi* (feet) man, when alive, take his measurement, feel his pulses; when dead, dissect his body and regard the strength

154 Chen Hongwei. 1998: 7.

of his *zang* organs, the size of his *fu* organs, the volume of the trunk cavity and the organs within it, then the length of the vessels, the clarity of the blood and the state of the *qi* … All are shown to conform to a standard."

I think that is the basic requirement for medical practitioners of that time. Actually there are some more accurate anatomical records in *Huang Di's Inner Classic.* For example, the ratio of the esophagus and the intestinal canal of human beings was 1.6 *chi*: 55.8 *chi*, i.e. 1: 34.87, which is very close to 1:34 in the modern anatomy.[155]

Anatomical knowledge was the foundation to construct the theoretical system of Chinese medicine. The procedure of dissecting the body is just like to open a treasure house, from which the concepts of exterior-interior and *Zang-Fu* came out, and the physical structure level – skin, vessel, flesh, sinew, and bone was understood. Then the further anatomical practice showed shapes or structures of internal organs, helped build the concept of Triple *Jiao* and its relative theory, learned relationship among internal organs, and discovered the partial physiological functions of internal organs.

For example, the sinogram for *heart* evolved from a direct vision of the organ, which underwent from  in the oracle script through  in the bronze script and  in the lesser seal script to 心 in the regular script; others like the sinogram  in the lesser seal script and 肺 in the regular script for the *lungs*, and the sinogram  in the bronze script,  in the lesser seal script, and 胃 in the regular script for the *stomach*, etc. all embody the direct vision of the internal organs.

Physiological functions of the organs were also discovered partly by dissecting dead bodies, for example:

1. The heart governs blood and vessels; the vessels are the residence of the blood;

2. The lungs govern *qi*, perform respiration, open at the nose, relate to all the vessels, help the heart to move the blood;

3. The kidneys govern water metabolism;

4. The major physiological functions of the stomach, the small intestine, and the large intestine: The stomach governs food intake and decomposition, then sends the decomposed food down to the small intestine, where it is separated into the clear and the turbid; Then the clear is absorbed and dis-

155 Wang Hongtu. 2004: 25.

tributed through the body, while the turbid is further passed down to the large intestine, through which it becomes the waste and is discharged from the body through the anus.

All of the above mentioned take the anatomical knowledge as their background and foundation. Bacause of the limitation of anatomical knowledge, *Huang Di's Inner Classic* interpretes the life phenomena and constructs its own system by integrating the philosophical theories of essential *qi*, yin-yang, and five phases with the accumulation of practical knowledge together with the limited anatomical knowledge.

7.2.2.2 The Attributes of the Organs to the Yin-Yang and Five Phases by the Way of Metaphorizing Guided by the idea of *Tian Ren He Yi*

The five *zang* organs were attributed to the five phases at least partly according to their colors in ancients' eyes, which gained from observing the organs after dissecting dead bodies:

Heart – red – fire,
Liver – brown (blue-green) – wood,
Spleen – yellow – soil,
Lungs – pink to grey (white) – metal[156],
Kidneys – dark red (black) – water.

Thereby, their physiological functions, pathological changes, and their relationships were inferred through analogizing the five phases' characteristics and the engendering and restricting relationships among them.

7.2.2.3 Long-term Observation on Physiological and Pathological Phenomena

For example, if people wear too less or the weather is too cold, people may catch a cold, and then may present with the following symptoms such as nasal obstruction, running nose, sneezing, and coughing. Long-term observation of this series of phenomena resulted in the understanding of the close relationship among the skin, nose and lungs – Lungs govern the skin and the hair of the body, and open at the nose.

---

156 Nowadays, many people's lungs tend to be black because of smoking and/or air pollution.

7.2.2.4 The Theory Being Modified and Proved in the Long-term Clinical Practice

Repeated medical practice explained and proved some physiological functions from the aspects of pathological phenomena and therapeutic effects. For example, many eye diseases were cured by treating the liver, so "the liver opening into the eyes" was concluded as a theory; many kidney-supplementing agents promoted the healing of fractures, thereby that "the kidney essential *qi* has the function of promoting the growth of bone" was drawn out, which resulted in the theory that "the kidneys govern bones and engender marrow."[157]

7.2.2.5 Why Did Anatomy Decline in Chinese Medicine?[158]

Why does Chinese medicine not need anatomy anymore for a better understanding of *zang fu* organs? Actually, this question can be transformed into the question "why the concepts and theory of *Zang Fu* organs of Chinese medicine have evolved from anatomical organs to functional entities." You can get some idea from the Table 5

Based on the genesis of the Visceral Manifestation Theory, I would like to advance the following viewpoints:

1. The main reason that medical practitioners lost motive force of dissecting dead bodies to know the morphological structure of the human body was not the restriction from the Confucian or feudal ethical codes, but the influences of Chinese thinking ways – *Si Wai Zhuai Nei* 司外揣内 or Inspecting the exterior to predict the interior, *Qu Xiang Bi Lei* 取象比类 or Taking image and analogizing, and *Yi Xiang Ce Zang* 以象测藏 or Speculating pathological changes of internal organs by observing the external manifestations of life guided by *Tian Ren He Yi* 天人合一 or The Unity of Heaven and Humankind;

2. The ontology of Chinese culture decides the holistic, dynamic, functional, interacting and interrelating thinking to be the core thinking of Chi-

157 Yin Huihe. 1984: 28.

158 Lan Fengli. Why Anatomy Declined in Chinese Medicine: The Concepts and Theory of Zang Fu Organs. CMIR, London, 2009.

nese medicine, which does not need reductionist ideology to understand the human being;

3. Chinese medicine is a practical, clinical medical system, which pays much more attention to practical knowledge which aims to prevent and cure illnesses, not the basic anatomical knowledge which only aims to understand the human body;

4. The integration of *Qi*, Yin-Yang, and Five-Phase theories into Visceral Manifestation Theory systematizes the open and complicated system of human being, successfully explains almost all of the physiological functions and pathological changes of the organs;

5. Repeated clinical observations and practices have proved that the transformation of the concepts and theory of *Zang Fu* organs of Chinese medicine from anatomical organs to functional entities is successful.

Heart	*Hippocratic Corpus*[159]	*Huang Di Nei Jing*[160]
General Under-standing	Has two atriums and two ven-tricles;	The organ as a Monarch, from which spirit originates; the root of life, the seat of the spirit; the greater yang within yang;
Main Func-tions	The right atrium provides lungs with blood, accepts air from lungs, exchanges air;	Rules the body's blood and vessels; opens into the tongue; it's brilliance mani-fests in the face;
Relations to Others	There is only air, no blood in the left atrium;	South, summer, hot & fire, bitter, red, *zheng*, elation,

159 Note: Here the contents from *Hippocratic Corpus* are translated into English from the Chinese translation.

160 *Huang Di Nei Jing* came out at about the same time as *Hippocratic Corpus* about 2,000 years ago. As Unschuld said in "Prefatory Remarks" of "HUANG Di NEI JING SU WEN: Nature, Knowledge, Imagery in an Ancient Chinese Medical Text" (University of California Press, 2003: IX) that it "plays a role in Chinese medical history comparable to that of the Hippocratic writings in ancient Europe. Progress and significant paradigm changes have reduced Hippocrates to the honored originators of a tradition that has become obsolete. In contrast, many practitioners of Chinese medicine still consider the *Su Wen* a valuable source of theoretical inspiration and practical knowledge in modern clinical settings. "

	the left atrium is the location of intrinsic heat.	laughing, and the Heart, etc. are all attributed to fire in the five elemental phases; the heart (fire) engenders the spleen (earth).
Outcome	A Morphological Heart Organ: Focuses on the morphological structure of the heart, thus providing direction, possibilities and leaving space for the further study on its anatomical structure and corresponding physiological functions.	A Heart Complex System: Separates "Heart" from the organ "Heart" in anatomical sense, integrates "Heart" with the theories of Yin-Yang and Five Phases, social phenomena (Monarch), natural phenomena (season, direction, climate, flavor, color), and other aspects of man (spirit, joy, tongue, face, spleen) into "A Heart Complex System
Analysis	Guides Western medicine to develop on the philosophical foundation of reductionism, mechanism and dichotomy, thus embodying the analytical thinking	Establishes the Visceral Manifestation theory, embodying the holistic approach "Four Seasons - Five *Zang* Organs – Yin-Yang" guided by "The Unity of Heaven and Humankind".
Conclusion	Western Medicine continuously refreshes itself because of the application of advanced scientific technology and instruments (tools).	Chinese medicine has formed a self-contained fruitful paradigm, so can be enriched and developed in the same framework - *Qu Xiang Bi Lei* guided by *Tian Ren He Yi* established about 2,000 years ago, survive up till today.

Table 5. Different Views of Heart in *Hippocratic Corpus* and *Huang Di Nei Jing*[161]

161 Lan Fengli. Intercultural Philosophy and Chinese Medicine: Reflections of Philosophy of Chinese Medicine in Chinese Language. In Wallner F. G., Lan Fengli, Jandl M.J (eds.). 2011: 14-34.

Take "*Pi* 脾" or the spleen for another example.

Pi or spleen in Chinese medicine is located in the Middle *Jiao* and below the diaphragm; it is attributed to Soil in the five phases, which is sowing and reaping, thus representing the features of receiving, generating, transforming, and supporting; by metaphorizing the soil's characteristics it governs movement and transformation of water and grain (food), i.e. transforms the water and grain into essence, then moves and sends the essence to the whole body, and thus is regarded as the source of the formation of *qi* and blood, and the foundation of postnatal existence; it controls blood, governs the flesh and the limbs, opens into the mouth, manifests its brilliance in the lips, is interrelated with anxiety in the emotions and saliva in the fluids, and stands in exterior-interior relationship with the stomach, etc.; in the nature, it is related to the late summer in the season, and dampness in the climate, etc.[162] It is thus clear that *Pi* or spleen in Chinese medicine is responsible for digesting food, and is extremely important and indispensable to a man. Abdominal pain or distension, poor appetite, loose stool, diarrhear, jaundice, fatigue or weakness of the limbs, edema, etc. are common symptoms of the spleen disease, which can be relieved or cured by treating the spleen.

While Western medicine understands the spleen as the largest lymphatic organ, which is located in the top part of the abdominal cavity behind the stomach and below the diaphragm; it appears to act to remove dead blood cells and fight infection, but its functions are not fully understood and an adult can live normally after his spleen has been removed; etc.[163]

You see Chinese understanding of the spleen is so different from Western understanding of the spleen. What's the underlying reason? The underlying reason is that they are based on different cultural presuppositions.

Chinese understanding of the spleen is based on the specific cultural foundation of classical Chinese science, e.g. the philosophical theories of yin-yang and five phases, the methodology of *Qu Xiang Bi Lei* or Taking Image and Analogizing guided by the idea of *Tian Ren He Yi* or The Unity of Heaven and Humankind, etc. and thus finally forming *a spleen complex system* which involves Nature and Man but centers the spleen.

---

162 Yin Huihe. 1984: 34-36.
163 Collin, P.H. 2001: 550.

While Western understanding of the spleen is based on the cultural foundation of Western science, e.g. the analytic approach based on reductionist ideology, mechanism, dichotomy, the methodology of deduction and induction, the methods of anatomy and experiments, etc.

Successful practice of Chinese medicine and Western medicine demonstrates that each of the both understandings about the spleen is true under its specific cultural presuppositions.

7.3 The Vessel Theory: From Rivers in the Nature to Vessels in Man

What is *Jing-Luo* system? Several translations are available for *Jing-Luo* system 經絡系統: "Meridian System" is the standard translation approved by WHO, but the word "Meridian" only indicates a two-dimensional grid while *Jing-Luo* system is supposed to carry *qi* and blood, and thus must be a three-dimensional system; "Channel System" is the most popular translation in the English literature on Chinese medicine, but the word "Channel" is polysemous; I think "Vessel System", a translation shown in *Huang Di Nei Jing Su Wen* by Paul U. Unschuld in 2003 is the best if we take into account the origin and development of the concepts of *Mai* 脈 and *Jing-Luo* 經絡.

Based on some anatomical knowledge on *Mai* (脈, vessel) and medical practice esp. the application of acupuncture, moxibustion, *tuina*, and *qigong*, the concepts of *Jing-Luo* 經絡 are actually metaphors formed in the way of observing, taking images of and analogizing the water flow in the rivers under the earth and the longitudinal lines of the textiles, which are embodied in their writing forms. The chapter *Water & Earth* of *Guan Tzu* states that "Water is the *qi* and blood of the earth, running on (under) the earth just like *qi* and blood flowing in the vessels."

The sinograms 脈 and 衇 are two common original complex forms of 脉. Its lesser seal script is  . This sinogram is a signifc-phonetic compound: the left part is the signific component 月 (flesh moon) or 血 (blood), indicating that *mai* 脈 functions to carry and move blood and is a part of the body; And the right part is the phonetic, indicating both pronunciation and meaning at the same time. In the medical books unearthed from Mawangdui Han Tomb, most of *mai* 脈 were written as "温". "水" is the variant form of " 氵 ", "目" the variant form of "flesh moon 月", "皿" the variant form of "blood 血". The structure of the sinogram has clearly illustrated that the ancients analogized or metaphorized water flow with blood flow.[164] It is thus clear that "*mai*" of the early days referred to blood vessels, so "*mai* 脉" is also known as "blood vessel 血脈", as stated in *Huang Di Nei Jing Su Wen · Mai Yao Jing Wei Lun* or *Huang Di's Inner Classic ·Basic Questions ·Discourse on Subtleties and Essentials of Vessels* that "The vessels 脈 are the residence of the blood." Be aware, *Qi* does not show up in this quotation.

The concepts "*jing*" and "*luo*" appeared later than "*mai* or vessel". *Jing* and *luo* are further divisions of "*mai* or vessel", i.e. "*jing*" vessel and "*luo*" vessel, which was first recorded in the *Huang Di Nei Jing Ling Shu Mai Du* or *Huang Di's Inner Classic·Miraculous Pivot · On Vessels*: "*Jing* vessels reside in the interior; their branches running transversely are known as *luo* vessels; the branches of *luo* vessels are known as grandchild vessels."

The sinograms "經 *jing*" and "絡 *luo*" share the same silk part "糸", which is originally used in the textiles.

The concept "*jing-mai* 經脈" is a metaphor formed in the way of *Qu Xiang Bi Lei* or taking images and analogizing. The right part of "經" is "巠", indicating both pronunciation and meaning, which is interpreted in *Shuo Wen Jie Zi* or *The Origin of Chinese Characters* as "water vessels, following <<< (川), pictographic, indicating rivers, under the 一; 一, refers to the earth." That is to say, "巠" refers to the water vessels running under the earth. *Jing* 經 is explained in *Shuo Wen Jie Zi* or *The Origin of Chinese Characters* as "the longitudinal lines of the textiles or warps." The reason that "*jing* 經" is used to name the main stems of the vessels is closely related to the origin of the sinogram "*jing* 經", which contains two images and reflects the similarities between the longitudinal lines of the textiles or warps, the rivers running under the earth and the running routes of the main stems of the vessels.

Another part of "*luo* 絡" is "各", indicating both pronunciation and meaning, which is interpreted in *Shuo Wen Jie Zi* or *The Origin of Chinese Characters* as "divergent views being different". Another interpretation of "*luo* 絡" is that "It originally meant unreeled silk, hemp, or cotton fiber, and from its association with stringy fibers came to be used in Chinese medicine

164 Li Ding. 1998: 2-3.

as a noun that means network and as a verb that means to net."[165] Anyway, *luo* 絡 is used to name divergent branches of the vessels.

Huang Di Nei Jing Ling Shu Ben Zang or *Huang Di's Inner Classic · Miraculous Pivot · On Viscera* states that "*Jing* vessels 經脈 function to move *qi* and blood, nourish yin and yang, moisten tendons and bones, and lubricate joints." Compared to the statement that "The vessels 脈 are the residence of the blood," quite a lot new contents were supplemented to *jing* vessels, among which the most remarkable point is that the function of moving *blood* was extended to moving *qi* and *blood*.

"*Xue mai* 血脈", "*jing* 經" and "*luo* 絡" appear together in the *Han Shu·Yi Wen Zhi* or *Treatise on Literature* of *The History of The Former Han Dynasty*, "Medical classics explore the origins of *blood vessels* 血脈, *jing-luo* 經絡, bone marrow, yin-yang, exterior and interior in order to treat various diseases from the root," where seemingly differentiated blood vessels from *jing-luo.*

Jing-luo 經絡 functions to carry and move *qi* and blood in the body. *Guan Tzu · Water & Earth* states that "Water is the *qi* and blood of the earth, running on the earth which is just like *qi* and blood flowing in the vessels." Judged from the cognizing order, the flow of *qi* and blood in man is analogized and inferred from the natural phenomenon of water flow in the rivers under the earth. The extensions from "vessel 脈" to "*jing-luo* 經絡" and from "blood" to "*qi* and blood" are also closely related to the application of acupuncture, moxibustion, *tuina*, *qigong*, etc, which explore the phenomenon of *qi* and blood flowing in the body, thus enriching the understanding on the "vessels".

To sum up, the concepts and theory of *jing-luo* were formed first on the basis of some anatomical knowledge on "vessels 脈"; then by the way of *Qu Xiang Bi Lei*, i.e. observing and taking images of the water flow in the rivers on/under the earth and the longitudinal lines of textiles or warps, then analogizing, enlightened by the idea of *Tian Ren He Yi*; and then have been proved and modified in the medical practice esp. the application of acupuncture, moxibustion, *tuina*, and *qigong*. That is to say, *jing-luo* or the vessels are metaphors, referring to the circular or round pathways of the living system.

165 Wiseman Nigel and Zhang Yuhuan. 2003: 174.

Therefore, I believe that it will take forever to find any three-dimensional structure of *jing-luo* 經絡 through dissecting dead human bodies. *Jing-luo* 經絡 system or the vessel system is more like a functional concept reflecting a certain image, which is embodied in their writing forms. As stated in the *Huang Di Nei Jing Su Wen·Li He Zhen Xie Lun* or *Huang Di's Inner Classic · Basic Questions · Discourse on Leaving and Uniting of True Qi and Evil Qi* that "The sages formulated principles, which must conform to the heaven and earth. Therefore, the heaven has 365 degrees and 28 constellations, the earth has 12 *jing* rivers, and man has 12 *jing* vessels."

Here we can conclude that metaphorizing or *Qu Xiang Bi Lei* is a vital way to understand the human being for the concepts of Essence, *Qi*, *Shen*, the Visceral Manifestation theory, and the Vessel Theory were all formed by the way of *Qu Xiang Bi Lei* or Taking Image and Analogizing, the metaphorizing process, guided by the idea of *Tian Ren He Yi* or the Unity of Heaven and Humankind.

The numbers start at one, end with ten, and complete with three.

- *Shi Ji. Lyu Shu* or *Historical Records. Calendar*

8 Number Metaphors for Constructing the Theoretical System of Chinese Medicine

The numbers in Chinese medicine embody philosophy of numbers in Chinese culture.

8.1 Numbers in Chinese Medicine

Numbers are everywhere in Chinese medicine, for example:

- One: *Tian Ren He Yi* 天人合一: Literally means "Heaven and Humankind Uniting into One", while my translation is "the Unity of Heaven and Humankind"; and One pillow for pulse taking;
- Two: Yin and Yang;
- Three Yin & Three Yang: Taiyin, Shaoyin, Jueyin & Taiyang, Yangming, Shaoyang;
- Three Materials: three resources of Chinese materia medica - herbs, minerals, and animal parts;
- Three Grades: three grades of Chinese material medica – Top, Medium, and Low Grade Medicinals;
- Three treasures: Essence, *Qi*, and Spirit – man as one unity with three dimensions;
- Three *Jiao*: also known as "triple energizer" or "triple burner", a collective term for the three portions of the body cavity, i.e. Upper, Middle and Lower *Jiao*, through which *qi* and fluids are transmitted;
- Three pathogenic categorizations: All of the disease-causing factors can be classified into three – internal, external, non-external & non-internal pathogens;
- Four *Qi*: four properties of Chinese medicinal substances – cold, hot, warm, and cool;
- Four examinations: inspection, listening & smelling, inquiry (history-taking), and palpation (including pulse taking) – four diagnostic methods of examining a patient and collecting information for making a diagnosis;

- Five flavors: five flavors of Chinese medicinal substances – sour, bitter, sweet, acrid, and salty;
- Five *zang* organs: heart, liver, spleen, lungs, and kidneys;
- Six *fu* organs: gallbladder, stomach, large intestine, small intestine, bladder, Triple energizer;
- Six *Qi*: six climatic influences, i.e. wind, cold, summer-heat, dampness, dryness and fire, the normal climatic conditions in the nature;
- Six excesses: the six pathogenic excessive or untimely climatic influences as exopathogenic factors – pathogenic wind, cold, summer-heat, dampness, dryness and fire; `
- Six meridians: Taiyang, Yangming, Shaoyang, Taiyin, Shaoyin, and Jueyin;
- Seven emotions: also known as "seven affects" - Joy, anger, melancholy, anxiety, grief, fear, and fright;
- Eight therapeutic methods: sweating, vomiting, precipitating (mainly refers to "purgation"), warming, clearing, harmonizing, supplementing, dispersing;
- Eight principal patterns: yin and yang, exterior and interior, cold and heat, deficiency and excess patterns;
- Eight extraordinary vessels: governing, controlling, girdling, thoroughfare, yin heel, yang heel, yin link, yang link vessels;
- Twelve regular meridian-vessels: the main passages for *qi* and blood, namely Lung Meridian of Hand Taiyin (LU), Large Intestine Meridian of Hand Yangming (LI), Stomach Meridian of Foot Yangming (ST), Spleen Meridian of Foot Taiyin (SP), Heart Meridian of Hand Shaoyin (HT), Small Intestine Meridian of Hand Taiyang (SI), Bladder Meridian of Foot Taiyang (BL), Kidney Meridian of Foot Shaoyin (KI), Pericardium Meridian of Hand Jueyin (PC), Triple *Jiao* Meridian of Hand Shaoyang (TJ), Gallbladder Meridian of Foot Shaoyang (GB), and Liver Meridian of Foot Jueyin (LR);

  ...

See Chapter 2 for the interpretation of One and three. Here, let us take a look at some other commonly emcountered important numbers – five, six, and twelve.

8.2 Five *Zang* Organs and Six *Fu* Organs

The Book of Changes states that "Heaven is one, earth is two; heaven is three, earth is four; heaven is five, earth is six; heaven is seven, earth is eight; heaven is nine, earth is ten. There are five heavenly numbers, and there are also five earthly numbers. When they are distributed among the five places, each finds its complement. The sum of the heavenly numbers is twenty-five, and that of the earthly numbers is thirty. The sum total of heavenly numbers and earthly numbers is fifty-five. It is this which results in the changes and transformations and moves demons and gods."

That is to say, in the numbers from one to ten, the odd are heavenly numbers, while the even are earthly numbers. Six is a heavenly number, while five is an earthly number. Therefore, the heaven has six climatic influences, i.e. wind, cold, summer-heat, dampness, dryness, and fire, and man has six *fu* organs, which pertain to Yang; The earth has five phases, i.e. wood, fire, soil, metal, and water, and man has five *zang* organs, which pertain to Yin.

Six to five, why? I have consulted ancient Chinese classics and have got some related quotations for your information.

Guo Yu. Zhou Yu or *Records of States. Records of Zhou* reads that "The heaven is six and the earth is five, which are the rules of the numbers."

Zuo Zhuan. Zhao Gong Yuan Nian or *Zuo's Spring and Autumn Annals. The 1st Year of Zhao Gong's Reign* reads that "The heaven has six climatic influences, which go down to give birth to five flavors, to present with five colors, and to manifest in five tones."

Han Shu. Lyu Li Zhi or *History of the Former Han Dynasty. Treatise on Calendar* reads that "The heaven is six and the earth is five, which are the rules of the numbers. The heaven has six climatic influences, which go down to give birth to five flavors. The five plus the six is the number in between the heaven and earth. ... The eleven terminates the way of the heaven and earth."

In ancient Chinese people's eyes, the evolution of the *zang fu* organs was a kind of group development following the rule of the nature. *Nan Jing Ji Zhu* or *A Collection of Annotations on The Classic of Difficult Issues*[166]

166 *Nan Jing Ji Zhu* 《难经集注》 or *A Collection of Annotations on The Classic of Difficult Issues*: the extant earliest collection of annotations on *The Classic of Difficult*

reads that "The reason that the *zang* organs are five and *fu* organs are six is that the five *zang* organs respond to the five phases on the earth, and the six *fu* organs echo the six climatic influences upon the heaven, among which the triple *jiao* is the premier fire and is attributed to Hand Lesser Yang. Therefore, only *fu* organs are six."

All of the knowledge related to *zang fu* organs was systematized as the Visceral Manifestation Theory. *Zang Fu* 藏府, now written as 脏腑 in Chinese, are metaphors formed in the way of observing, taking images from and analogizing the social storing system of the remote antiquity. Five *zang* organs 五藏 store the essential *qi* but not drain, like *zang* 藏 or depots which stored the invaluable treasures and were not allowed to take out; Six *fu* organs 六府 transform the water and grain (food) but not store, like *fu* 府 or six palaces which stored six kinds of goods and were daily consumed and supplemented with.

Zuo Zhuan. Wen Gong Qi Nian or *Zuo's Spring & Autumn Annals. The 7th Year of Wen Gong's Reign* reads that "Water, fire, metal, wood, soil, and grain are termed six *Fu*." An annotation reads that "Six is the number of man's *fu* organs."

Why is that - the heaven six and the earth five? The answer would be that culture depends on natural and social environments, and that science depends on culture.

8.3 Regular Meridians: From Eleven to Twelve

There were only 11 vessels recorded in *The Moxibustion Classic of 11 Vessels of Arms & Feet* and *The Moxibustion Classic of 11 Vessels of Yin & Yang*, two monographs on moxibustion unearthed from Mawangdui Han Tomb. But as we know, there have been 12 regular meridians since the time of *Ling Shu* or *Miraculous Pivot.* Then which one is missing?

In the above mentioned two monographs, there were only two hand yin meridian vessels, and one was missing for the heart in Chinese medicine is said to be "the governor of the five *zang* and six *fu* organs ... Evils are not permitted to invade the heart;" and then that "the pericardium protects the

---

Issues from Lu Guang 吕广 of the Three Kingdoms (220-265), Yang Xuancao 杨玄操 of the Tang Dynasty (618-907), and Ding Deyong 丁德用, et al of the Song Dynasty (960-1279) by Wang Jiusi 王九思 in 1505 of the Ming Dynasty (1384-1644). It has 5 volumes and 13 chapters.

heart by taking the invading evils instead (*Ling Shu. Xie Ke* or *Miraculous Pivot. Evils Visited*)."

Later on, one heart meridian vessel became divided into two, i.e. Heart Meridian of Hand Shaoyin (HT) and Pericardium Meridian of Hand Jueyin (PC). And then the six pairs of meridian vessels - one *zang* and one *fu*, one yin and one yang; three yin and three yang, six hand medians and six foot meridians, were recorded in the *Ling Shu. Jing Mai* or *Miraculous Pivot. Meridian Vessels,* thus forming the so-called the Twelve Regular Meridians.

In Chinese culture, the number twelve was a specific and the greatest number of the heaven. For example, the Ten Heavenly Stems have been used as serial numbers and also in combination with the Twelve Earthly Branches to designate years, months, days, and hours since oracle scripts of the Yin-Shang Dynasty (ca. 17th – 11th Century B.C.).

Shi Ji. Lyu Shu or *Historical Records. Calendar* reads that "The numbers start at one, end with ten, and complete with three." *Shuo Wen Jie Zi* or *The Origin of Chinese Characters* reads that "*Shi* 十 or Ten completes the numbers. The horizontal stroke '一' indicates East-West; the vertical '丨' indicates South-North, and then the sinogram 十 possesses the four directions and the center." Kong Yingda 孔颖达 (574-648) annotated that "Ten is the extreme of the numbers." Such understanding may result from that the counting of man's fingers ends with ten.

In ancient Greece, Pythagoras (580? – 500? B.C.) school also attached great importance to the number Ten. As we know from *The Book of Changes* that from one to ten, the odd numbers "one, three, five, seven, and nine" are heavenly numbers, while the even numbers "two, four, six, eight, and ten" are earthly numbers, so the number Ten is the largest earthly number.

In classical Chinese culture, the number "ten" represent the mysterious perfect, and many, numerous. For example, "*Shi Quan Shi Mei* 十全十美", an Chinese idiom, literally means "ten completenesses and ten beauties", actually means "be perfect in every aspect", "flawless and perfection", "be done to perfection"; "*Shi Mu Suo Shi, Shi Shou Suo Zhi* 十目所视，十手所指", another Chinese idiom originally from *Li Ji. Da Xue* or *The Book of Rites. The Great Learning*, literally means "ten eyes watching, and fingers of ten hands pointing", actually means "with many eyes watching and many fngers pointing – One cannot do wrong without being seen; Nothing could be done without public supervision."

The Twelve Earthly Branches are usually used to echo the twelve months. *Shi Ji. Lu Shu* or *The Historical Records. Calendar* names the Ten Heavenly Stems and the Twelve Earthly Branches as "Ten mothers and twelve sons". *Huai Nai Tzu. Tian Wen Xun* reads that "The numbers start from *Jia* 甲 and Zi 子, in which mother and son are matching to each other." *Bai Hu Tong* 白虎通[167] reads that "The heavenly stems such as *Jia* 甲 and *Yi* 乙 are the trunk (stem), while the earthly branches such as *Zi* 子 and *Chou* 丑 are the branches." Actually the number twelve reflects the classical Chinese thinking of *Tian Ren He Yi* 天人合一 or The Unity of Heaven and Humankind, such as the twelve months in a year, the twleve two-hour periods in a day – Midnight (PM 23:00 – AM 1:00), Rooster Crowing (AM 1:00-3:00), Daybreak (AM 3:00-5:00), Sunrise (AM 5:00-7:00), Eating Time (AM 7:00-9:00), Midmorning (AM 9:00-11:00), Midday (AM 11:00 – PM 1:00), Sun Westing (PM 1:00-3:00), Late Afternoon (PM 3:00-5:00), Sunset (PM 5:00-7:00), Dusk (PM 7:00-9:00), Man Sleep (PM 9:00-11:00), which takes the movement of the sun to show the time order, and the twelve animals used to symbolize the year in which a person is born, etc.

Huai Nan Tzu. Patterns of Heave reads that "The heaven has the four seasons to regulate the twelve months; the man has the four limbs to make the twelve joints." And *Ling Shu. Wu Luan* reads that "The twelve vessels are supposed to respond to the twelve months."

Therefore we see that numbers in Chinese culture are far beyond the numbers. Numbers reflect the world view of ancient Chinese people. Numbers in Chinese medicine show that understanding of Man is based on the understanding of the nature, that Man and Heaven unit and resemble each other, and that man mirrors the heaven.

---

167 *Bai Hu Tong* 《白虎通》 was compiled during the reign of Han Zhang Di 漢章帝 (58-88 A.D.). The work started in the year 79 A.D. when he summoned his officers to hold a conference. The results were recorded and compiled by Ban Gu 班固 (32-92), a famous scholar. This becomes standard answers to questions about the study of *Jing Xue* 經學 or study of Confucian classics. It is interesting that this book even includes a section on sex education.

"To truly modernize Chinese medicine, we must first demystify these theories."

(Wang Ming-wei)[168]

9 Metaphorizing: A Vital Way to Understand and Modernize Chinese Herbal Medicine

The formulation of most of the books on Chinese materia medica has been almost fixed in the writing pattern of "General Introduction" and "Classified Medicinals" arranged according to their chief actions with "Properties, Flavors, Meridians Entered, Actions, Cautions & Contraindications" since the era of *Shennong's Classic of Materia Medica*[169], but few explain or illustrate whys and hows. Chinese herbal medicine, just like Chinese medicine, has evolved under the guidance of *Tian Ren He Yi* 天人合一 or The Unity of Heaven and Humankind through *Qu Xiang Bi Lei* 取象比類 or Taking Image and Analogizing, which refers to the Metaphorizing Process in Chinese Herbal Medicine.

9.1 Differences between *Ben Cao* and *Yao*

It is well known that Chinese medicine uses mixtures of different medicinal substances formulated according to a certain strategy in a holistic approach to disease. Here first of all, I would like to discuss the differences between *Ben Cao* (Materia Medica，本草) and *Yao* (Medicine, 藥).

Ben Cao (Materia Medica，本草) and *Yao* (Medicine, 藥) have been taken as the same since the teaching mode of Chinese medicine has transformed into the modernized or Westernized or professional one at the early of the 20th century. That is to say, *Yao* is a modernized term of *Ben Cao.* Actually, they do not refer to the same thing.

168 Qiu, Jane. April 2007: 590-591.
169 Ling Yikui. 1984: 1.

Ben Cao, the materia medica, is a collective term for all of the individual substances with healing properties, i.e. the medicinal substances or the medicinals, including herbs, minerals and animal parts. *Ben Cao* is divided into three grades in the *Shennong's Classic of Materia Medica*:

- Top-grade medicinal is non-toxic, possesses a rejuvenating effect and can be taken frequently and for a long period of time without causing any harm;
- Medium-grade medicinal has no or only slight toxic effect and is effective in treating diseases or supplementing deficiencies;
- Low-grade medicinal is effective in expelling pathogens, but is toxic and should not be taken for a long period of time.

Yao 药, with its original sinogram as 藥, is explained to be "harmony of different medicinal substances", and is used to "treat illnesses" (the sinogram is 疒 with 樂 inside it, a variant form of *liao* 療, the simplified writing form is 疗), i.e. restoring the harmonious state to the individual. The two sinograms of the original forms share the same part 樂 (the simplified form is 乐, means music, and is explained to be "harmony of different tones" in *Shuo Wen Jie Zi* or *The Origin of Chinese Characters*). Thus, it is clear that *Yao* 藥 refers to the medicine ready to be taken for treating illnesses, which is usually composed of more than one medicinal substance formulated according to the strategies of *Jun Chen Zuo Shi* or Chief, Associate, Assistant and Guide medicinals, i.e. formula. I think Chinese herbal medicine is composed of the two parts: *Ben Cao* (Materia Medica，本草) – discussion of individual medicinals and *Yao* (Medicine made from a Formula, 藥) – Formulas and Strategies.

9.2 Properties, Flavors, and Meridian Entry

Theory of Chinese materia medica comes from metaphorizing qi, yin-yang and five phases. Everything in the world, including Man and Chinese Materia Medica, comes into being by the movement and mutation of *Qi*, which begets Yin-Yang, and the five phases (two pairs of yin and yang, i.e. water and fire & wood and metal, plus one middle soil).

The Four Properties (*si qi*, 四气) result from metaphorizing the Yin-Yang of the Heaven, varying according to the four seasons – Warm and

Hot, the Yang of the Heaven; Cool and Cold, the Yin of the Heaven. In specific, properties of a medicinal come from metaphorizing its living environment, growing seasons and rules, collecting time, and/or medicinal part (including its shape, color, etc.), etc.

The Five Flavors (*wu wei*, 五味) result from metaphorizing the Yin-Yang of the Earth, varying according to the five phases – Acrid, Sweet, and Bland, the Yang of the Earth; Sour, Bitter, and Salty, the Yin of the Earth. It is well known that flavors of many medicinals are far away from their real tastes.

The Meridian Entry (*gui jing*, 歸經) results from attributing the medicinal's properties and flavors to Man's *zang-fu* organs according to the theories of Yin-Yang, Five Phases and Meridian Vessels.

9.3 Metaphorizing: A Vital Way for Genesis of Actions of Materia Medica

Tian Ren He Yi or The Unity of Heaven and Humankind is the cultural presupposition for metaphorizings of Chinese materia medica, and metaphorizing is the way to understand actionns of Chinese medicinals, which of course have been confirmed and proved in the clinical practice.

Actions of a Chinese medicinal are from metaphorizing its property, or its flavor, or its color, or its shape, or its quality, or its disposition, or its growing time, or its growing place, or its pronunciation, etc. which is used to harmonize the *zang-fu* organs and restore Yin-Yang balance to the individual with its predominating actions. Briefly speaking, actions of Chinese medicinals are chiefly based on the principle of "*Like attracts like.*"

Metaphorizing Its Property: Cool or cold medicinals have the actions of clearing heat, draining fire, cooling blood and reducing toxicity, etc; while warm or hot medicinals have the actions of warming the interior, dispersing cold, supplementing fire, reinforcing yang, warming the meridians and freeing the network vessels, restoring yang from collapse, etc.

Metaphorizing Its Flavour: Generally speaking, acrid medicinals can disperse and promote the flow of *qi* and blood; sweet can tonify, moderate, and harmonize; sour can astringe; bitter can drain fire and dry dampness; salty can soften the hardness and free the bowels; bland can promote urination, etc.

Metaphorizing Its Colour: Such a viewpoint has been systematized and theorized by the aid of the five-phase theory since the Han dynasty (206

B.C. – 220 A.D.). *Essentials of Materia Medica*[170] (*Ben Cao Bei Yao. Yao Xing Zong Yi*) states that medicinals of green-blue with sour flavor pertains to wood, all enter the Liver and Gallbladder Meridians. – The liver stands interior-exterior relationship with the gallbladder, the gallbladder is *Jia* wood, the liver is *Yi* wood; medicinals of red with bitter flavor pertains to fire, all enter the Heart and Small Intestine Meridians. – The heart stands interior-exterior relationship with the small intestine, the small intestine is *Bing* fire, the heart is *Ding* fire; medicinals of yellow with sweet flavor pertains to earth, all enter the Spleen and Stomach Meridians. – The spleen stands interior-exterior relationship with the stomach, the stomach is *Wu* earth, the spleen is *Ji* earth; medicinals of white with acrid flavor pertains to metal, all enter the Lung and Large Intestine Meridians. – The lungs stand interior-exterior relationship with the large intestine, the large intestine is *Geng* metal, the lungs is *Xin* metal; and that medicinals of black with salty flavor pertains to water, all enter the Kidney and the Bladder Meridians. – The kidney stands interior-exterior relationship with the bladder, the bladder is *Ren* water, the kidney is *Gui* water.[171]

For example: There are five colours of beans to enter the five *zang* organs respectively. Black bean, black in color, its shape is like that of the kidneys, the grain of the kidneys, so can tonify the kidneys; Red bean, red in color, the grain of the heart, with downbearing property, can free the small intestine and has the function of diuresis; the white hyacinth bean, white and yellowish, the grain of the spleen, can regulate the spleen and warm the stomach. The following are some other examples illustrated with pictures.

170 *Ben Cao Bei Yao*《本草备要》, or *Essentials of Materia Medica*: a clinical manual of materia medica and a door to Chinese medicine with 8 volumes and published in 1694 by Wang Ang 汪昂 (1615-1695).

171 *Jia, Yi, Bing, Ding, Wu, Ji, Geng, Xin, Ren, Gui*: the ten heavenly stems.

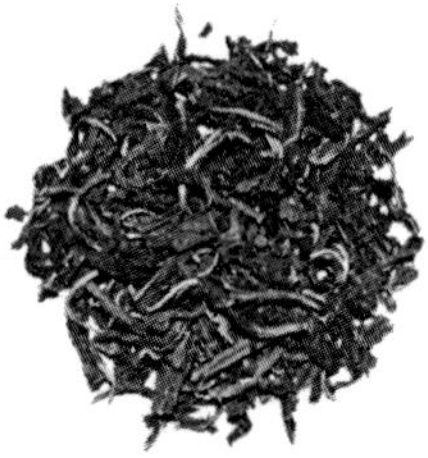

Fig. 1. *Sang Ye*

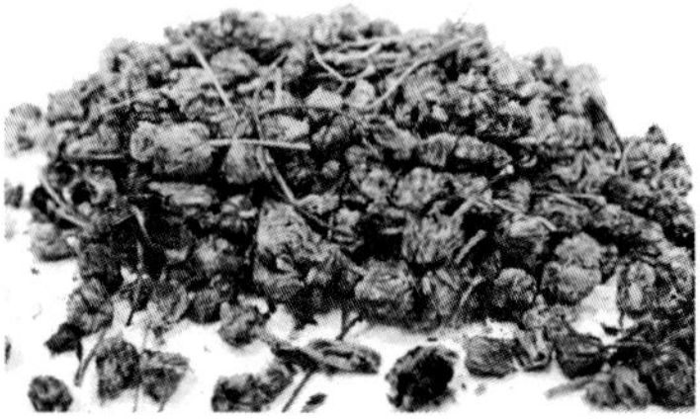

Fig. 2. *Ju Hua*

The greenish, whitish, yellowish medicinals are usually said to enter the phase of *qi*, used to treat exterior pattern, such as mulberry leaf (Folium Mori, *Sang Ye*; Fig. 1) and chrysanthemum (Flos Chrysanthemi, *Ju Hua*; Fig. 2)

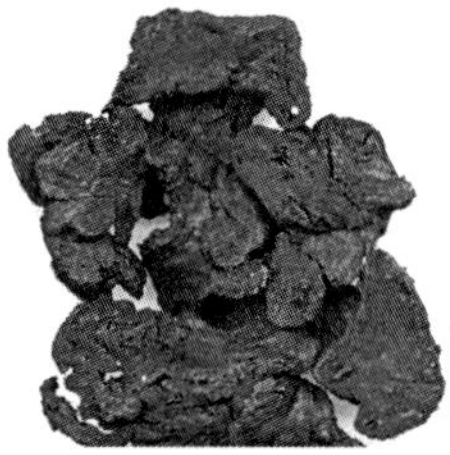

Fig. 3. *Di Huang*

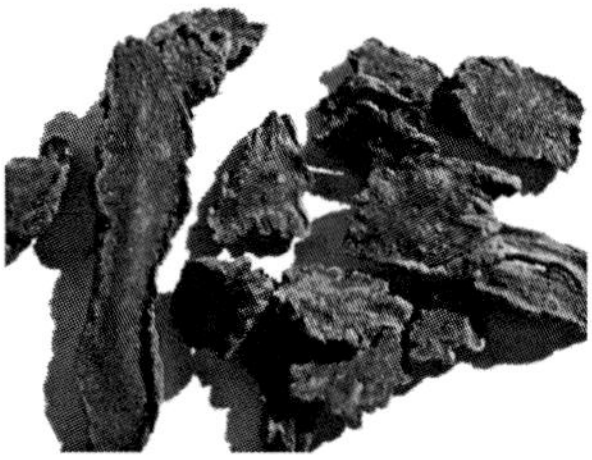

Fig. 4. *Xuan Shen*

The reddish, blackish, dark yellow medicinals are usually said to enter the phase of blood, used to treat interior pattern, such as rehmannia (Radix Rehmanniae, *Di Huang*; Fig.3) and scrophularia (Radix Scrophulariae, *Xuan Shen*; Fig.4).

Besides, green-blue, red, yellow, white and black medicinals are attributed to different *zang-fu* organs according to the five-phase theory. For example:

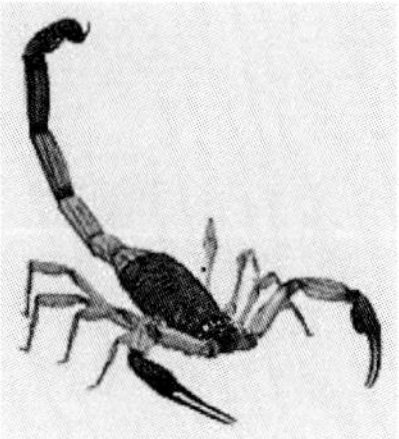

Scorpion (Buthus, *Quan Xie*, Fig. 5), whose body colour is *green-blue*, is said to enter the *Liver* Meridian, and is therefore used to treat *wind disease*, such as convulsion, spasm, stubborn *bi* syndrome, e.g. arthritis, etc.

Fig. 5. *Quan Xie*

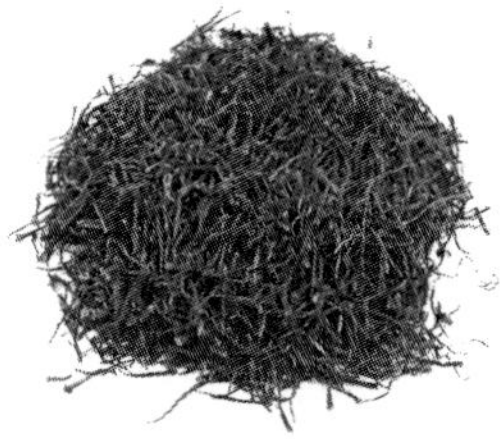

Fig. 6. *Hong Hua*

Carthamus (Flos Carthami, *Hong Hua*, Fig. 6), whose colour is *red*, is said to enter the *Heart and Liver* Meridians, and therefore is used to promote the flow of blood, remove blood stasis, and free menstruation for the *blood* is from the heart and is stored in the liver.

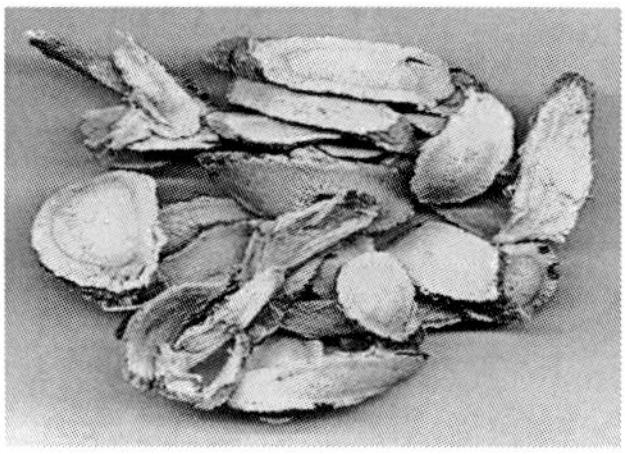

Fig. 7. *Huang Qi*

Astragalus (Radix Astragali, *Huang Qi*, Fig. 7), whose colour is *yellow* and whose flavour is *sweet*, is said to enter the *Spleen* Meridian, and is therefore very effective in *tonifying the Spleen and benefiting Qi*.

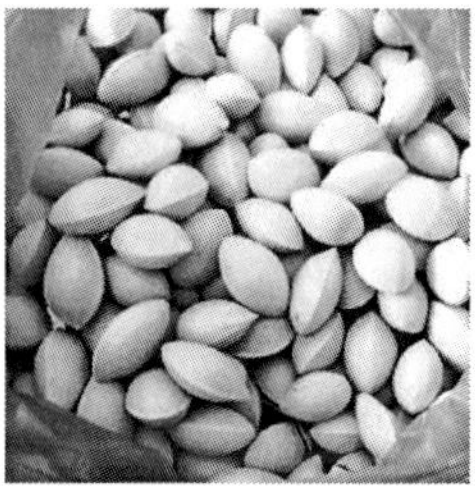

Fig. 8. *Yin Xing*

Gingko (*Yin Xing*, Fig. 8), whose colour is *white*, is said to enter the *Lung* Meridian, and is therefore used to supplement the Lung *Qi* and arrest coughing.

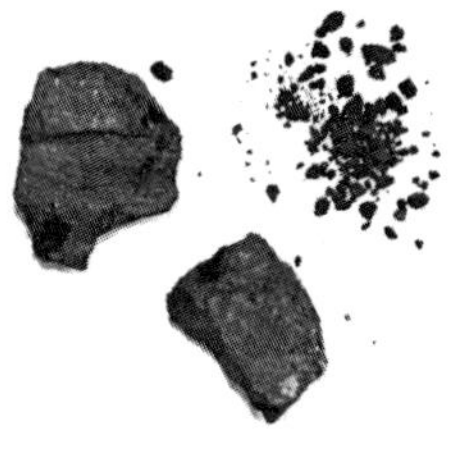

Fig. 9. *Ci Shi*

Magnetite (*Ci Shi*, Fig. 9), whose colour is *black* and *heavy* in quality, is said to enter the *Kidney* Meridian, and is therefore used to tonify the Kidney and subdue yang, arrest panting, deafness and tinnitus caused by Kidney deficiency, downbear the reverse upward flow of *Qi*.

Some medicinals with more than one colour or even five colours can be used to treat various diseases. For example, Jujube is formed from small white flower to fruit of first green, then white and yellow, then red after being ripe, then blackish after being picked up and dried under the sun, bearing the colours and qualities of the five phases, and therefore can nourish the Spleen and Stomach, free and open the nine orifices, benefit the twelve meridians, supplement *qi*, engender fluid, tonify the blood, supplement deficiencies of all kinds, harmonize all of the other medicinals, etc. (Zhang Zhicong, *Ben Cao Chong Yuan* or *The Origin of Materia Medica*[172]. *Ben Jing Shang Pin* or Top Grade Medicinals of *Shennong's Classic of Materia Medica*)

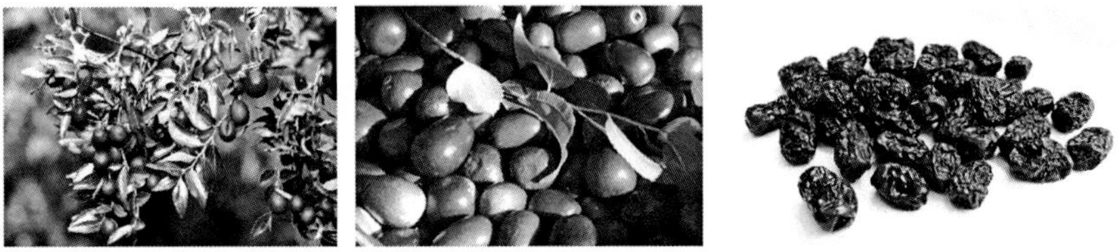

Fig. 10. Jujube (Chinese Date, *Da Zao*)

Metaphorizing Its Shape: The typical example is ginseng. The Chinese name is *Ren Shen* 人参, of which *Ren* 人 means human being. *The Origin of Materia Medica.* Top Grade Medicinals of *Shennong's Classic of Materia Medica* (*Ben Cao Chong Yuan. Ben Jing Shang Pin*) by Zhang Zhicong states that the root of ginseng is like the shape of the human being with head, face, and the four limbs. It receives the brilliance of the Heaven and the vastness and richness of the Earth, and forms into the shape of the human being after a long time, thus having the quality of the Heaven, Earth, and human being. Therefore, it is mainly indicated in supplementing or tonifying the human being.

172 *Ben Cao Chong Yuan* 《本草崇原》 or *The Origin of Materia Medica:* a monograph on materia medica, which annotates *Shennong's Classic of Materia Medica,* by Zhang Zhicong 张志聪 (1616-1674). Based on the five circuit phases, six climatic factors, and waxing and waning between yin and yang, Zhang Zhicong founded the *Yao Qi* 药气 theory to expound actions of medicinals in details, which starts from the formation of properties and flavors, attributes of yin-yang and five-phases as well as shapes and colors of medicinals, and correlates the machanism of curing an illness. His approach deeply influenced such medical experts as Xu Dachun 徐大椿 (1693-1771) and Chen Xiuyuan 陈修园 (1753-1823).

Besides, Ginseng mainly grows in the damp shadow places of forests in the North-East of China, can survive in one of the world coldest places, and is therefore very effective in restoring yang from collapse and contraindicated in excessive heat patterns, such as the famous Pure Ginseng Decoction (*Du Shen Tang*).

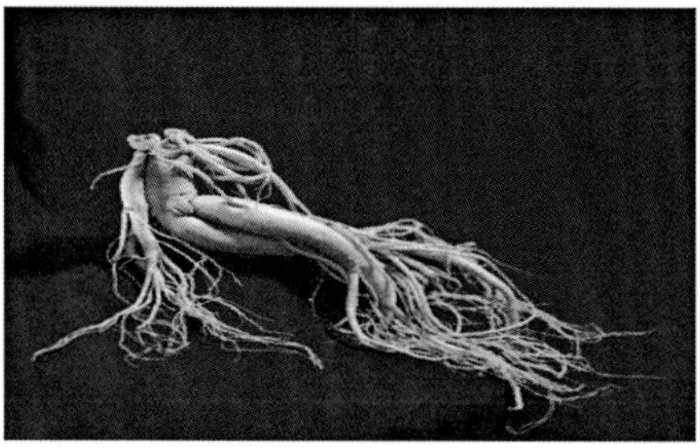

Fig. 11. Ginseng

Metaphorizing Its Disposition: Generally speaking, flower is usually on the tip of a branch, and therefore can expel the pathogenic factors on the head and eyes; the leaves distribute around a plant in different directions, and therefore can disperse; stem and branch can treat diseases of the limbs; seed conceives a new life, and therefore can tonify the Kidneys, strengthen sexuality, help conceiving a fetus, and treat sterility (male) and/or infertility (female); hollow medicinals or with holes can free the flow of *qi* and free the network vessels; medicinals rich in fluid can increase humour; vine can free the network vessels; and so and so forth. Take krait for example.

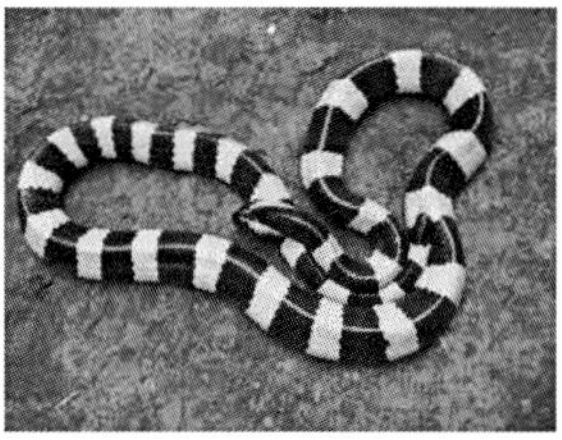

Fig. 12. Krait

"The snake can treat all kinds of wind diseases. ... The wind moves swiftly and is changeable. The snake also moves swiftly and exuviates (casts off or sheds) many times in its life. Therefore, it can track wind deep into the bone, stabilize convulsions (caused by wind), and is an important medicinal for wind blockage disease, convulsions, leprosy, tinea, serious sores and ulcers for it can move through the bowels and viscera inside, run through the skin outside, can reach nowhere in the body." (Li Shizhen, *Ben Cao Gang Mu* or *The Compendium of Materia Medica*)

Metaphorizing its pronunciation[173]: Take seeds as an example. "*The seed* (籽) *can produce semen* （子）." Seed conceives a new life. *Shen Nong's Classic of Materia Medica* reads that *Wu Wei Zi* (schisandra, Schisandrae Fructus) can benefit or supplement the male's semen; *Ben Cao Jing Ji Zhu* or *A Collection of Annotations on Classic of Materia Medica* states that *Gou Qi Zi* (lycium berry, Lycii Fructus) can tonify essential *qi*, strengthen sexuality; *Yao Xing Lun* or *On Properties of Medicinals* records that *Tu Si Zi* (cuscuta, Cuscutae Semen) can benefit essence or semen and supplement marrow, and that *Fu Pen Zi* (rubus, Rubi Fructus) is indicated in deficiency or depletion of kidney essence for the male and infertility for the female; *Ben Cao Hui Yan* or *A Collection of Words on Materia Medica* states that *Che Qian Zi* (plantago seed, Plantaginis Semen) can strengthen sexuality and help conceiving a fetus; and so and so forth.

A version of textbook "*Chinese Herbal Medicine*" published in the 1950's states that "Most of the medicinals rich in seed are said to enter the kidney," and we know that the kidneys are responsible for growth, development and reproduction (maturation) in Chinese medicine. There are some formulae which are mainly composed of different seeds, such as Seven-Seed Powder recorded in the *Bei Ji Qian Jin Yao Fang* or *Invaluable Prescriptions for Emergencies* mainly for male's sterility due to deficiency of essential *qi*, Five-Seed Progeny Pill recorded in *Yi Xue Ru Men* or *Introduction to Medicine* as "the No.1 prescription for conceiving a fetus of all times", and Pill of

173 There are three important methods to explain a sinogram in ancient Chinese texts: "discerning meaning by interpreting and analyzing its structure", "discerning meaning in the light of pronunciation", and "discerning meaning in its contexts". It is worth to note that "structure" here refers to that of sinograms in the Oracle, Bronze, or Lesser Seal Script such as the approach in *Shuo Wen Jie Zi* or *The Origin of Chinese Characters*, not that in Simplied Lesser Seal or Regular Script; that "pronunciation" refers to that of sinograms of the Zhou, Qin, and Han Dynasties (ca. 11th Century B.C. – A.D. 220), which are generally known as pronunciation of the ancient times; All of the three methods should be used in a rigorous way, esp. the second one "discerning meaning in the light of pronunciation", and observe the principle that "Single evidence is untenable". Actually "discerning meaning in the light of pronunciation" is also a specific Chinese cultural phenomenon. Take *Hu Lu* 葫芦 or the bottle gourd as an example. Its pronunciation sounds like *Fu Lu* 福禄 or blessing and emolument, so it has long been regarded as a traditional symbol for blessing and emolument among Chinese people.

Five-Seed and Whole Deer recorded in *Chi Shui Xuan Zhu* or *The Black Bead in the Red Water* for sterility and infertility due to yang deficiency.

To sum up, all of the Chinese medicinals come into being and shape from the *Qi* of the Heaven and Earth, have different actions, and therefore can treat different illnesses, which can be inferred from metaphorizing their *qi* (property), flavour, colour, shape, quality, etc. through *Qu Xiang Bi Lei* outlined in the framework of *Tian Ren He Yi*.

9.4 Metaphorizing: A Vital Way to Understand Medicine made from a Formula/Prescription[174] (*Yao*)

It is a great qualitative leap of the development of Chinese herbal medicine from the use of a single medicinal to a compound formula, in which therapeutic interactions among different medicinals are strengthened, and toxicity or side effect is reduced through coordinating actions of different medicinals. To diagnose a disease, identify the pattern and establish a treating principle is the premise of formulating a formula/prescription, which is generally composed of Chief, Associate, Assistant and Guide medicinals, a holistic approach to disease treatment of harmonizing different aspects of the patient:

- *Sovereign [Chief]:* provides the principal therapeutic action;
- *Minister [Associate]*: helps strengthen the principal action;
- *Adjuvant [Assistant]*: relieves secondary symptoms or tempers the action of the Chief when the latter is too potent;
- *Courier [Guide]*: directs action to the affected Meridian or site.

9.5 Metaphorizing: A Vital Way to Modernize Chinese Herbal Medicine

Previous attempts to modernize Chinese herbal medicine have focused on isolating active ingredients from herbal remedies and screening them one at a time, which accords with the Western way of thinking, i.e. analytical or abstract thinking. And such an approach has led to a handful of new treatments,

174 I use "formula" for one with a fixed name and a fixed group of component medicinals with fixed dosages, and "prescription" for one prescribed by a practitioner aimed at a specific patient in his/her specific condition.

such as artemisinin for treating malaria and the decongestant ephedrine, "but there has been no goldrush of approved drugs." The Western way of thinking can be an ideal complement to the Chinese way of thinking, and the corresponding research outcome provides valuable references for both researchers and practitioners. But I think the Chinese way of thinking should be of more significance in guiding the studies on modernizing Chinese herbal medicine.

The 1st Example – Tripterygium Wilfrodis (*Lei Gong Teng*, 雷公藤)[175]: Li Leishi 黎磊石 discovered for the first time the therapeutic effect of Tripterygium Wilfrodis in treating various chronic nephritis, lupus nephritis, and purpuric nephritis, and spread it to the whole country through metaphorizing Tripterygium Wilfrodis's immunosuppressive action in taking effect in treating nephritis and allergic dermatological diseases. Later on he proved the effect of an ingredient isolated from this herb in acute rejection after renal transplantation, and clarified Tripterygium Wilfrodis's immunosuppressive action in an all round way.

The 2nd Example – Realgar-Indigo Naturalis Formula (RIF, *Fu Fang Qing Dai Wan*, 复方青黛丸)[176]: The main components of RIF are realgar (*xiong huang*, 雄黄), *Indigo naturalis* (*qing dai*, 青黛) and *Salvia miltiorrhiza* (*dan shen*, 丹参) with tetraarsenic tetrasulfide (A), indirubin (I), and tanshinone IIA (T) as their major active ingredients respectively. The research group took the active ingredients as the representatives of the three medicinals (a kind of metaphorizing) to study the synergy in the treatment of a murine APL model *in vivo* and in the induction of APL cell differentiation *in vitro*. Their data also indicate A as the principal component of the formula, whereas T and I serve as adjuvant ingredients. They therefore suggest that dissecting the mode of action of clinically effective formulae at the molecular, cellular, and organism levels may be a good strategy in exploring the value of traditional medicine. This case has been regarded as a successful case of researching compound formulas of Chinese medicine. Therefore, the strategy of composing a formula (Chief, Associate, Assistant and Guide medicinals) will be a valuable strategy in discovering or synthesizing new drugs.[177]

175 Li Leishi. 1998, 18 (12):707.

176 Wang Lan, Zhou Guangbiao, Liu Ping, et al. 2008, Vol. 125 (12): 4826-4831.

177 Qiu, Jane. 2007 (6): 506-507.

To sum up, I think metaphorizing is a vital way to understand, to research, and to modernize Chinese herbal medicine, and will be also a valuable strategy in discovering or synthesizing new drugs.

He who has health, has hope; and he who has hope has everything.

- Arabian Saying

If you are not in tune with the universe, there is sickness in the heart and mind.

-Navajo Saying

The principle of *Bian Zheng Lun Zhi* 辨证(証)论治 or "Pattern Identification and Treatment" advanced by Ren Yingqiu results not only from political influences of Mao Zedong Thought and "dialectics" in philosophy, but also an overall development of the former methodologies of treatment in Chinese medicine. Individualized treatment, one of the greatest advantages of Chinese medicine, needs that disease diagnosing, pattern identifying, and symptom considering function together.

- The Author

10 Metaphorizing: A Vital Way to Understand the Concept of Health and Disease

Diverse cultures have diverse worldviews, which accounts for the differences in how people of different cultural and ethnic backgrounds shape their views of health and well-being in both the physical and spiritual realm. Dualistic (or dichotomy) or holistic worldviews and mechanistic or non-mechanistic worldviews also account for cultural perceptions of everything from the concepts of health, well-being and illness (or disease), the causes (or origins) of illnesses, to prevention and treatment of the illnesses.

There are two major cultures in this world, i.e. European (or Western) and Chinese (or Eastern) cultures, which are distinguished by a variety of identifiers: dualistic (or dichotomy) versus holistic worldviews, reductionism versus holism, reason versus intuition, objectivity versus subjectivity, or being scientific versus being philosophical, and so and so forth. Chinese medicine is deeply rooted in its culture, and this part will show you how Chinese people conceive the concepts of health, well-being, disease, and treatment of diseases with pictures and images in the way of *Qu Xiang Bi Lei* or Metaphorizing.

10.1 The Concept of Health in Chinese Culture: The Playing of A Piece of Mild, Smooth Symphony in the Nature

Based on investigation of the etymologies of some sinograms - *Jian* 健, *Kang* 康, *Ping* 平, *Yue* 樂, *Yao* 薬 and *He* 和 and related discussions from *Huang Di Nei Jing*,we can conclude that the state of being healthy in Chinese culture is dynamic harmonious functioning of all the component parts of a being (composed of body and mind) with the nature, just like the playing of a piece of mild, smooth symphony in the nature.

10.1.1 Introduction: Definition of Health by WHO

It is well known that the compound *Jian Kang* 健康 has always been taken as the Chinese equivalent for the words "health" and "healthy", both of which are of Germanic origins with their etymology as "hale" (free from disease or infirmity), "whole", or "related to whole".[178,179] Obviously, that "Health is a state of complete physical, mental, and social well-being and not merely the absence of disease or infirmity", the most famous and enduring definition of "Health" given by the World Health Organization (WHO)[180] in 1946, accords with the etymology of the word "health" and its original meaning very well. But this definition is severely criticized for it has been subject to controversy, in particular as being lack operational value and because of the problem created by use of the word "complete"[181, 182] although

178 *Oxford Dictionary of English*, 2nd Edition, Oxford University Press, 1998, 1999, 2001, 2003, 2005.

179 *Webster's Encyclopedic Dictionary of the English Language*, New Revised Edition, 1994.

180 www.who.int/bulletin/archives/80(12)981.pdf *WHO definition of Health*, Preamble to the Constitution of the World Health Organization as adopted by the International Health Conference, New York, 19–22 June 1946; signed on 22 July 1946 by the representatives of 61 States (Official Records of the World Health Organization, no. 2, p. 100) and entered into force on 7 April 1948.

181 Callahan D. "The WHO definition of 'health'."*The Hastings Center Studies*, 1(3), 1973 - http://www.jstor.org/pss/3527467

182 Jadad AR, O'Grady L. "How should health be defined?" *BMJ* 2008; 337:a2900 - http://www.bmj.com/cgi/content/full/337/dec10_1/a2900

the word "complete" is synonymous with the word "whole", the etymology of "health".

Then, how should we define "health"? Hereafter are several other famous definitions about health:

Health "is a fundamental human right (The Declaration of Alma-Ata, 1978)."

Health is also "a resource for everyday life, not the objective of living. Health is a positive concept emphasizing social and personal resources, as well as physical capacities (The WHO's *Ottawa Charter for Health Promotion*, 1986)."

Health is the level of functional or metabolic efficiency of a living being. In humans, it is the general condition of a person's mind, body and spirit, usually meaning to be free from illness, injury, or pain (as in "*good health*" or "*healthy*") (Merriam-Webster, 2011; wikipedia, 2012.).[183,184]

How does Chinese culture understand health? Are these definitions also identical with Chinese understanding of health? Spector's answer reads that "Chinese medicine teaches that health is a state of spiritual and physical harmony with the nature."[185] Our answer will be based on the analysis of some sinograms- *Jian* 健, *Kang* 康, *Ping* 平, *Yue* 樂, *Yao* 藥 and *He* 和, and related discussions from *Huang Di Nei Jing*.

10.1.2 Jian 健: (of Human) "Energetic, Vigorous, Powerful, and Strong"

The sinogram"健 Jian", a signific-phonetic and an associative compound, is composed of two parts: 亻 and 建. The right part "建 Jian" means "to build, to found, to create, to establish, to construct", implying that the underlying capacity and energy being strong and powerful. In fact, most of the sinograms carrying "建 Jian" relate to "strong, powerful, energetic", for example:

腱: being composed of the signific flesh moon 月(indicating "of or related to a body part"), and Jian 建, referring to strong and tough sinews or tendons;

---

183 Merriam-Webster.*Dictionary* – "*Health*", accessed 21 April 2011.
184 http://en.wikipedia.org/wiki/Health, accessed 8 July 2012.
185 Spector, R.E. 2004: 212.

犍: being composed of the signific cattle 牛 and Jian 建, referring to powerful bullock;

键: being composed of the signific metal 钅 and Jian 建, referring to firm metal keys which are used to fix doors or axles.

健: being composed of the signific human 亻 and Jian 建, referring to (of human) "energetic, vigorous, powerful, and strong".

Shuo Wen Jie Zi or *The Origin of Chinese Character* interprets "健 Jian" as "Kang 伉", which means "to pair", "to counter-balance", "tall and big", "powerful", "to undertake", and "to resist". It is worth to note that the Chinese compound "*Jian Kang* 健康" shows up very late until the 20th century, but the pronunciations of the two sinograms are very similar to "健伉 Jian Kang", which are used to mutually interpret each other in *Shuo Wen Jie Zi* or *The Origin of Chinese Characters.*

Zeng Yun 增韻 interprets "健 Jian" as "strong and powerful".

The Book of Change interprets the image of the first hexagram "*Qian* or *The Creative*" as "The movement of heaven is *Jian* or Full of Power, and thus the man with honor makes himself strong and untiring."

It is worth to note that the sinogram"健 Jian" does not show up in *Huang Di Nei Jing* (*Huang Di's Inner Classic*) nor *Nan Jing* (*The Classic of Difficult Issues*), nor *Shang Han Lun* (*On Cold-Induced Diseases*). In *Jin Gui Yao Lue* or *The Synopsis of the Golden Chamber*, the sinogram"健 Jian" shows up only once:

時病差未健，食生菜，手足必腫。

This clause can be translated into:

"Eating raw vegetables during the recovering period from an epidemic will cause the extremities to swell."

In *Shen Nong Ben Cao Jing* or *The Shennong's Classic of MateriaMedica*, the sinogram"健 Jian" shows up altogether 11 times, among which it appears 9 times with "Fei 肥" as "FeiJian 肥健", which means "to make sb. gain weight and become strong"; it is followed by "Xing 行" twice as "Jian Xing 健行", which means "to walk with vigorous strides".

10.1.3 Kang 康: The Playing of A Musical Bell

See Illus. 16 for the evolution of the sinogram"康 Kang", an ideograph. The first one 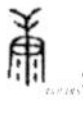, is the bronze script of the modern writing: the four spots in the sinogram signify music emitted by shaking a bell, indicating the playing of a musical bell,[186] but were mistaken as "Mi 米 or Rice" in the lesser seal script . It is well known that *Shuo Wen JieZi* or *The Origin of Chinese Characters* explains sinograms based on the analysis of their writing forms of the lesser seal script. That is why *Shuo Wen Jie Zi* mistakes it as the original sinogram of "糠", which means "chaff", "bran". Now let us take a look at how *Er Ya* or *Approaching to the Standard* explains this sinogram.

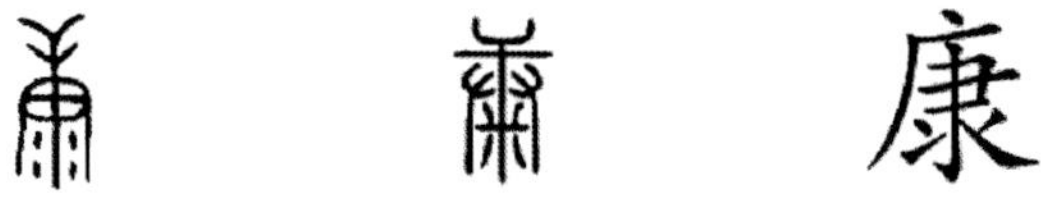

Illus. 16. "*Kang* 康" from Bronze, Lesser Seal to Regular Script

10.1.3.1 Kang 康: "樂"or Music, Happiness, and Harmony

Shi Gu or *Explaining the Old [Words]*, the first chapter of *ErYa* or *Approaching to the Standard,* explains it as "樂", which is written as in *Xiao Zhuan* or the lesser seal script, a pictograph indicating a kind of drum. *Shuo Wen Jie Zi* or *The Origin of Chinese Characters* explains it as "the general term for five tones and eight sounds". Actually its original meaning is known as *Yue*or music, harmony of different tones and sounds, which usually brings *Le* or happiness to the listeners and was used as *Yao* or medical treatment to relieve people's sufferings.

In fact, in ancient times, *Yue* or music, *Le* or happiness and*Yao* or medical treatment are three pronunciations and three correspondent meanings born with the sonogram "樂". And then the concept "*He* 和" must be mentioned here.

"*He* 和" is usually translated into "harmony" in the Western world, which shows a simplified and reduced understanding of this concept by the Westerners. This concept, as shown by its original form 龢, bears two aspects of meaning: the first is different, the second is harmonious. That is to say, being both different and harmonious can be termed "*He* 和".

186 Gu Yankui. 2008; 2010: 1297.

It is really indeed the case that the simplified Chinese characters (the popular style of writing now in China) have also reduced the cultural connotations implied in their original forms. "*He* 和" is the simplified form of the sinogram 龢. As stated in *Shuo Wen Jie Zi or The Origin of Chinese Characters*, its original form is composed of two parts: the left part is a pictographic part symbolizing a musical instrument made of bamboo with three holes used to harmonize different tones, and the right part 禾 is the phonetic part, indicating its pronunciation "He"; Its original meaning refers to harmony of different music tones.

The development of Chinese characters shows that harmony of different foods is known as 𤮺,[187] that harmony of different tones is known as 樂 (music), and that harmony of different medicinal herbs is known as 藥 (medicine), which was originally written as 樂 (music) – obviously, music therapy is one of the earliest therapies in the remote antiquity, which was gradually replaced by "Yao 藥" (herbal medicine) afterwards. One of the variant forms of the sinogram 療 (treat) also has the 樂 part, which shows that restoring harmony is the goal of all the Chinese medical treatments.

It is well known that Chinese medicine uses mixtures of different medicinal substances formulated according to a certain strategy in a holistic approach to diseases, i.e. *Yao* or Medicine 藥, which is different from *Ben Cao* or Materia Medica 本草. *Ben Cao*, the material medica, refers to all of the individual medicinal substances with healing[188]properties, i.e. the medicinal substances or the medicinals, including herbs, minerals and animal parts. While *Yao,*藥, with its original sinogram as 樂 (music) - harmony of different tones, is explained to be "harmony of different medicinal substances", and is used to "treat illnesses" (the sinogram is 疒 with 樂 inside it, a variant form of 療, the simplified sinogram is 疗), i.e. restoring the harmonious state to the individual. Thus, it is clear that *Yao* 藥 refers to the

187 The upper part means to harmonize; the lower part 甘, means sweet, which is applied to harmonize the other tastes i.e. sour, bitter, acrid, and salty. See *The Origin of Chinese Characters · Gan part* 《说文解字 · 甘部》.

188 The word "heal" shares the same etymology with the words "health" and "hale" (*Oxford Dictionary of English; Webster's Encyclopedic Dictionary of the English Language*).

medicine ready to be taken for treating illnesses, which is composed of two or more medicinal substances formulated according to the strategies of *Jun Chen Zuo Shi* or Chief, Associate, Assistant and Guide medicinals, i.e. formula.

Obviously, explaining "康 Kang" as "樂" associates so many sinograms and so much information together, and indicates that "health and harmony", the ultimate aim human beings have been untiringly pursuing, are of the same origin and form a direct line of succession in Chinese culture. Actually, "Kang Le 康乐" has become a common compound, which means "health and happiness" or "healthy and happy".

10.1.3.2 Kang 康:
"An 安" or "Free From Any Danger", "Calm", "Safe", and "Peaceful"

Besides, *Shi Gu* or *Explaining the Old [Words]*, the first chapter of *ErYa* or *Approaching to the Standard,* also explains it as "安 An", an associative compound being composed of "Mian 宀, a deep room" and "Nü 女, a virgin ", reflecting the image of "a maiden staying in a deep room", indicating that the original meaning of the sinogram is "free from any danger", "calm", "safe", and "peaceful", etc. Actually, "An Kang 安康" has also become a common compound, which is translated into "good health"; and a popular English translation for "Zhu Nin An Kang 祝您安康" is "Wishing you the best of health"[189].

10.1.3.3 Kang 康: An Unobstructed Road Leading to Five Directions

Shi Gong or Explaining Dwellings, the fifth chapter of Er Ya or Approaching to the Standard states that

> "What unobstructedly leads to one direction is called *Dao Lu* 道路 or Road;
> "What unobstructedly leads to two directions is called *Qi Pang* 歧旁 or Fork;

189 Wu Guanghua. 2010.

"What unobstructedly leads to three directions is called *Ju Pang* 剧旁 (In a road is the point at which it divides into three branches to three directions);
"What unobstructedly leads to four directions is called *Qu* 衢 or Crossroads;
"What unobstructedly leads to five directions is called *Kang* 康 or an unobstructed road leading to five directions;
"What unobstructedly leads to six directions is called *Zhuang* 庄 or an unobstructed road leading to six directions;
"What unobstructedly leads to seven directions is called *Ju Can* 剧骖 or an unobstructed road leading to seven directions;
"What unobstructedly leads to eight directions is called *Chong Qi* 崇期 or an unobstructed road leading to eight directions;
"What unobstructedly leads to nine directions is called *Kui* 逵（馗）or an unobstructed road leading to nine directions".

"*Kang Zhuang Da Dao* 康庄大道", a common Chinese compound, actually refers to "wide free road which leads to anywhere."

Explaining "康 Kang" as "an unobstructed road leading to five directions"is of vital importance to understand the concept of health in Chinese culture. According to the meridian theory in Chinese medicine, that *Qi* flows smoothly and vigorously in the meridians is a prerequisite to a healthy person; and a person will surely suffer a kind of illness if one or more of his meridians are obstructed to some extent.

The sinogram"康 Kang" only shows up several times in the "Seven Comprehensive Discourses on Theory of Five Periods and Six Qi" of the *Su Wen* or *Basic Questions*, which are generally considered to be supplemented by later generations, but does not appear in either *Ling Shu* (*Miraculous Pivot*) or *Nan Jing* (*The Classic of Difficult Issues*) or *Shen Nong Ben Cao Jing* (*Shennong's Classic of Materia Medica*) or *Shang Han Lun* (*On Cold-induced Diseases*) or *Jin Gui Yao Lue* (*Synopsis of the Golden Chamber*).

Then how does *Huang Di Nei Jing* or *Huangdi's Inner Classic* understand health? Let us now take a look at "Ping 平".

10.1.4 Ping 平:
Melody Being Mild and Balanced, Breathing Being Gentle and Leisurely

The sinogram"Ping 平", written as  in the bronze script and  in the lesser seal script, is an associative compound. In its bronze script, it follows

亏 (于), which means "melody being mild and leisurely", and 八, which means "to divide equally". Its original meaning is "melody being mild and balanced, breathing being gentle and leisurely". "The tone being mild and slow" - what is explained for this sinogram in *Shuo Wen Jie Zi or The Origin of Chinese Characters* is actually its extended meaning.[190]

Huang Di Nei Jing or *Huangdi's Inner Classic* calls "a person free from any illness" as "Ping Ren 平人"or "a healthy person". Based on the current materials, this compound shows up first in *Nei Jing*. There are two discourses on "*Ping Ren* 平人" in *Huang Di Nei Jing* or *Huangdi's Inner Classic:* one is "*Ping Ren Qi Xiang Lun* or *Discourse on Pulse Conditions in a Healthy Person*", the 18th chapter of *Su Wen* or *Basic Questions*; and the other is "*Ping Ren Ju Gu* or *Fasting in a Healthy Person*", the 32nd chapter of *Ling Shu* or *Miraculous Pivot,* which talks about that the digestive system of a healthy person must function normally to maintain the normal functioning of life. Hereafter are some discussions on "*Ping Ren* 平人"or "a healthy person" from *Huang Di Nei Jing.*

10.1.4.1 *Su Wen* or *Basic Questions*: The Pulse Image of a Healthy Person

The pulsation of a healthy person, according to the 18th chapter of *Su Wen* or *Basic Questions, Ping Ren Qi Xiang Lun* or *Discourse on Pulse Conditions in a Healthy Person,* should arrive five times during one breathing period and the normal pulse should have stomach *qi*. It states that[191]

> Huang Di asked, "What is the pulse image of a healthy person like?"
> Qi Bo answered, "The pulse of a healthy person beats rhythmically five times in one breathing period - twice in one exhalation, another twice in one inhalation, and once more during the interchange between the inhalation and the exhalation. One exhalation and one inhalation make up one breathing period, i.e. one respiration. A healthy person refers to a person free from any illness."
> ...

190 Gu Yankui. 2008; 2010: 148.

191 The translation here is from the author, which accords with GuoAichun's interpretation. See Guo Aichun. 1999: 105-106.

"The source of the normal pulse of a healthy person is the stomach, and so the stomach *qi* is the normal *qi* of the pulse of a healthy person."[192]

Besides, the nine indicators of a healthy person's pulses should be concert, and his yin and yang should be balanced. The 62nd chapter of *Su Wen* or *Basic Questions, Tiao Jing Lun* or *Discourse on Regulating the Meridians,* states that

"The yin and yang meridians possess *shu* or stream points, where transportation and convergence of *qi* and blood occur. Blood and *qi* of a yang meridian will transport to the yin meridians. The yin meridians then fill and nourish the body. When yin and yang are balanced, the body becomes robust. The nine indicaors of the body's pulses will also be concert. This occurs in a healthy person."

10.1.4.2 *Ling Shu* or *Miraculous Pivot:* Six Features of A Healthy Person

The 9th chapter of *Ling Shu* or *Miraculous Pivot*, *Zhong Shi* or *Beginning and Ending*, identifies that "a healthy person" should have the following six features:

1. Being free from any illness;
2. The *Cunkou* pulse at wrist and *Renying* pulse at neck suit the changes of the four seasons;
3. The pulses at *Cunkou* (wrist) and *Renying* (neck) should be concert (e.g. in frequency and amplitude);
4. The pulses of the other parts of the body should be neither blocked nor agitated;
5. The temperature of the trunk and the extremities should be more or less the same, which indicates that the extremities are warm and the body temperature is normal – a manifestation of free smooth flow of *qi* and blood in the vessels and yin and yang in a balanced state;

---

192 The normal pulse of a healthy person is said to have stomach, spirit and root, also known as three features of a normal pulse. Having stomach [*qi*] refers to the pulse being neither floating nor sunken, neither rapid nor slow, but clam and mild with regular beats; The image of a pulse with spirit is identical with that with stomach *qi*; The pulse with root refers to the *Chi* portion of the pulse being powerful when heavily pressed for *Chi* portion indicates the condition of the kidneys, which are generally regarded as the root of the being in Chinese medicine.

6. The physical form (flesh) outside the body and blood and *qi* inside the body should be mutually appropriate.

Here it is worth to stress the 2nd feature –"The *Cunkou* pulse at wrist and *Renying* pulse at neck suit the changes of the four seasons," which indicates that the harmony in between the man and the nature is essential for a healthy person. As the *Huang Di's Inner Classic· Basic Questions* states in the chapter 25 "*Discourse on Protecting Life and Preserving Physical Appearance*" that "Man is born on the earth, hanging his life to the heaven. The union of Heaven *qi* and Earth *qi* make up a man. Man can adapt himself to the seasons for the Heaven and Earth are his parents."

If a person has the above mentioned six features, he or she must be healthy. Here we can see whether a person is healthy or not is mainly determined by his or her pulses, which accords very well with the explaining of "康 Kang" as "an unobstructed road leading to five directions"–"free smooth of *qi* and blood in the vessels."

10.1.5 Conclusion: The Concept of Health in Chinese Culture

Based on the above analysis, we can conclude that "being healthy" in Chinese culture signifies "(of human) being energetic, harmonious, mild, balanced, happy, peaceful in the world", indicating a state of free smooth flow of *qi* and blood in the vessels, which might be achieved in the remote antiquity by musical and medicinal treatments. Hence, we would like to say that the state of being healthy in Chinese culture is dynamic harmonious functioning of all the component parts of a being (composed of body and mind) with the nature, just like the playing of a piece of mild, smooth symphony in the nature, which accords with the etymologies of some sinograms mentioned in this part very well.

10.2 Etymology-based Understanding of the Concept of Disease in Chinese Culture: "Lack of Ease" and Pictorial Thinking

Based on investigation of etymologies of some sinograms - "*Chuang* 疒", "*Ji* 疾", and "*Bing* 病", and of the words "disease" and "disorder", it can be concluded that Western and Chinese cultures conceive the concept of disease in a similar way at the first beginning, and that Chinese understanding of disease is derived from "lack of ease" to all diseases, which reflects a pictorial thinking compared to Western conceptual thinking developed later along with the rise of application of Western science and technology in the Western medicine. In Chinese culture, diseases are usually caused by the agents which are usually not considered as causes of disease in the Western culture.

10.2.1 Introduction: Three Health Belief Systems

Despite the diversity in worldviews, a paradigm in which all health belief systems can be divided into three major categories: scientific/biomedical, magico-religious, and holistic, each with its own corresponding system of health beliefs.[193]Among the three health belief systems, the magico-religious system is quite primitive, and exists in almost all the cultures in their infancy periods. This system derives from a worldview in which the world is seen as an arena in which supernatural forces predominate.[194] The ill person is a victim of punishment rendered by the supernatural agent. Treatment involves achieving positive association with spirits, deities, and so forth.[195] While the other two systems represent two mature medical knowledge systems originated from Western and Eastern cultural perspective respectively.

The Western scientific or biomedical system is derived from the dualistic (or dichotomy) and mechanistic worldview in a reductionistic, allopathic approach, and is the dominant health belief system in the West, including Europe, America, and some other parts of the world. Actually, this system is also the dominant medical system in China if the flow of funds is considered although the government of China has proposed to equate Chinese medicine with Western medicine since 1949.

Under this paradigm, life is controlled by a series of physical and biochemical processes that can be studied and manipulated by humans. Human

193 Andrews, M.M. The Influence of Cultural and Health Belief Systems on Health Care Practices. In Andrews M.M, Boyle J.S. (eds). *Transcultural Concepts in Nursing Care*[C]. 4th ed. Philadelphia: Lippincott Williams and Wilkins, 2003: 75.
194 *Ibid.*
195 Angelucci, P. Notes from the Field: Cultural Diversity: Health Belief Systems. *Nursing Management*, 1995, 26 (8): 8.

health is understood in terms of physical and chemical processes;[196] and disease is understood as ascertained abnormalities in the sense of human biology, which can be determined by physical, chemical and/or other specific examinations. This system focuses on identifying causative agents of disease by applying modern scientific and technological methods, making diagnosis according to the objective data gained through tests, examinations, and machines, and thus offering a so-called scientific explanation of disease, and finally conquering disease by battling the onslaught of microorganisms and diseased cells, destroying or removing the causative agents (e.g. with antibiotics), repairing, removing, or even replacing the affected body part with a new one if it cannot be repaired (e.g. the development of surgery and organ transplantation), or controlling the affected body system (e.g. with inhibitors, modulators). And besides, "Prevention of disease involves avoiding pathogens, agents, or activities known to cause abnormalities."[197] To sum up, the Western scientific or biomedical system is an applied medical system based on modern Western science.

The Eastern holistic system is derived from a worldview – *Tian Ren He Yi* 天人合一 or the Unity of Heaven and Humankind for they are supposed to be composed of the same ingredient – *qi* in the same way, which bridges and closes the incompatibilities in between Man and Heaven (Nature). Therefore, health is a dynamic harmonious functioning of all the component parts of a being (composed of body and mind) with the nature. Holistic approach to the human being is non-mechanistic and explains illness or disease as a result of imbalance or disharmony between yin and yang in the being or between Man and nature, e.g. Chinese medicine explains illnesses as a result of impersonal conditions such as wind, cold, summer-heat, dampness, dryness, and fire.

Then how does Chinese culture conceive the concept of disease, and interpret the origins of disease?

---

196 Andrews, M.M. The Influence of Cultural and Health Belief Systems on Health Care Practices. In Andrews M.M., Boyle J.S. (eds). *Transcultural Concepts in Nursing Care*[C]. 4th ed. Philadelphia: Lippincott Williams and Wilkins, 2003: 76.
197 Angelucci, P. Notes from the Field: Cultural Diversity: Health Belief Systems. *Nursing Management*, 1995, 26 (8): 8.

10.2.2 The Concept of Disease in Chinese Culture: From "Lack of Ease" to All the Diseases

Chinese understanding of disease originates from a kind of direct feeling in the remote antiquity. Most of the disease names recorded in the oracle inscriptions were named according to abnormal physiological function of a certain body part, e.g. *Chuang Shou* 疒首 or disordered head, *Chuang Er* 疒耳 or disordered ear, *Chuang Kou* 疒口 or disordered mouth, *Chuang Chi* 疒齿 or disordered tooth/teeth, *Chuang Bi* 疒自（鼻） or disordered nose, etc.

Disease-related sinograms recorded in the *Shuo Wen Jie Zi* or *The Origin of Chinese Characters* involve internal, external, gynecological, pediatric, ENT, and epidemic diseases, etc., and vivid explanations of these sinograms embody a unique Chinese understanding of diseases. *The Disease Part* of *The Origin of Chinese Characters* 《说文解字 · 疒部》 explains 102 disease-related sinograms[198], among which three denote "disease", i.e., "Chuang 疒", "Ji 疾", and "Bing 病".

10.2.2.1 "Chuang 疒": A Patient or a Pregnant Woman Lying on the Bed for Recuperating or Resting

Now let us start with the signific sinogram for disease –"Chuang 疒". "疒", was written as in early oracle inscriptions, resembling a man with sweating (a sweating man indicates a patient) lying on the bed (a bed with its legs towards right); later, it was written as , resembling a pregnant woman lying on the bed ; and then written as in late oracle inscriptions, which was simplified into a man lying on the bed (the bed since then with its legs towards left). Thus it is clear that the original meaning of "Chuang 疒" is a patient or a pregnant woman lying on the bed for recuperating or resting.

, its writing form in seal scripts, was further simplified by adding an indicating symbol on the bed , indicating "lying on the bed". Afterwards, "疒" has been only used as a signific to symbolize suffering or being ill, and almost all disease-related sinograms have this part as their signific.

198 Originally by [Han] Xu Shen, Annotated by [Qing] Duan Yucai. 1988: 348-353.

Another oracle script writing form of this sinogram was composed of three similar parts, but the bed  was at the left part with its legs towards left. See *Detailed Interpretation of Chinese Characters: Origin and Evolution of 1,000 Sinograms* by Zuo Min'an or *Dictionary of Etymologies of Chinese Characters* by Gu Yankui.

① ② ③ ④

Illus. 17. "*Chuang* 疒" from Oracle, Bronze, Lesser Seal to Regular Script[199]

The Disease Part of *The Origin of Chinese Characters* 《说文解字 · 疒部》 reads that "疒，倚也。人有疾病，象倚箸之形," which can be translated into "疒, leaning on or against. When a man has an illness or a disease, his image is just like the image of leaning on or against something;" that "Ji 疾, illness;" and that "Bing 病, serious illness."

In English language, as we all know, the word "disease" (dis- + ease), usually explained with the word "disorder" (dis- + order), is used to express various kinds of illnesses or "Ji Bing 疾病". "Disease" came to be a word of Middle English in the sense of "lack of ease; inconvenience" from Old French "desaise" – "lack of ease" from "des-" (expressing reversal) + "aise" (ease); "Disorder", a word of the late 15th century, is also of French origin – "desordener", ultimately based on Latin "ordinare" – ordain.[200] This is quite interesting for the etymologies of English words "disease", "disorder", and of the sinogram "Chuang 疒" show that Western and Chinese cultures conceive the concept of disease in a similar way at the very beginning. Thereby, the original meaning of "Chuang 疒" can be summed up as the same as the original meaning of the word "disease" – "Lack of Ease".

As regards to "Ji Bing 疾病" or diseases, modern scholars classify them into three concepts: 1. Disease, a medical term, refers to ascertained abnormalities in the sense of human biology, which can be determined by physical,

199 Zuo Min'an. 2005: 368.

200 *Oxford Dictionary of English* [Z], 2nd Edition, Oxford University Press, 1998, 1999, 2001, 2003, 2005.

chemical and/or other specific examinations; 2, Illness, refers to a person's self feeling and self judgment. For example, a person believes he or she is ill[201] when he or she feels uncomfortable. Under some conditions, an illness can be diagnosed as a kind of "disease" after medical checkup; but in much more cases, an illness is not a disease in the medical sense but just a kind of psychological or social imbalance; 3. Sickness[202], is a kind of description for a person's social status – that is, others (or the society) know or admit this person being in an unhealthy state. Most of the so-called "Ji Bing 疾病" or diseases are actually "illnesses".[203]

While "Ji Bing 疾病" in Chinese medicine also bears three different meanings: 1. Disease, refers to a pathological process with certain manifestations. The occurrence, development, changes, and manifestations of a disease go along a certain specific law, such as epilepsy, leprosy, and cholera; 2. Symptom, refers to either a subjective feeling of the patient or an abnormal change discerned by physician's examinations. In this case, the disease is usually named after the patient's chief complaint/suffering such as headache, palpitation, insomnia, vomiting, diarrhea, etc, or a visible image of the disease such as ox hide lichen – an episodic skin disease characterized by thickening and hardening of the skin that gives it the appearance of the skin of an ox's neck, crane's-knee wind – a disease marked by a painful suppurative swelling of the knee associated with emaciation of the lower legs, etc; 3. The major pathogenesis of the disease, such as wind disease, blockage disease.

Based on the proposition that Chinese medicine is another complete medical system dependent on Chinese culture, "Ji Bing 疾病" in Chinese medicine, in most of cases, should be illness or disease in its original mean-

---

201 As regards to the etymology of the word "ill", Webster's Encyclopedic Dictionary of the English Language (Revised ed., 1994) reads: "Middle English ill(e) < Scand; cf. Icel illr ill, bad"; The Online Etymology Dictionary reads: "c. 1200, 'morally evil' (other 13c. senses were 'malevolent, hurtful, unfortunate, difficult'), from O.N. *illr* 'ill, bad,' of unknown origin. Not related to *evil*. Main modern sense of 'sick, unhealthy, unwell' is first recorded mid-15c., probably related to O.N. idiom 'it is bad to me.' Slang inverted sense of 'very good, cool' is 1980s. As a noun, 'something evil,' from mid-13c." (http://www.etymonline.com/index.php?term=ill)

202 The etymology of the word "sick" is described as "Old English *sēoc* 'affected by illness', of Germanic origin; related to Dutch *ziek* and German *siech*".

203 Translated into English from Chinese. See H. P. Chalfant. 1987: 14.

ing – lack of ease, not disease in the sense of modern Western medicine which can be determined by physical, chemical and/or other specific examinations.

10.2.2.2 "Ji 疾" and "Bing 病": From "Being Hurt by an Arrow" to All Diseases

The sinogram "Ji 疾" is an associative compound and a pictophonetic as well. Its oracle writing form follows man and arrow, resembling the image of a man's right armpit being hit by an arrow. Its writing form in the bronze inscription, still keeps this image. It is thus clear that the original meaning of "Ji 疾" is "being hit/hurt by an arrow". Being hurt by an arrow is, of course, a kind of disease, and so it evolved into in the lesser seal script, in which the part man [204] transformed into the signific for disease – 疒; later it evolved into 疾 in the regular script, and has been kept in use until now. Here below shows the evolution of the writing form of this sinogram.

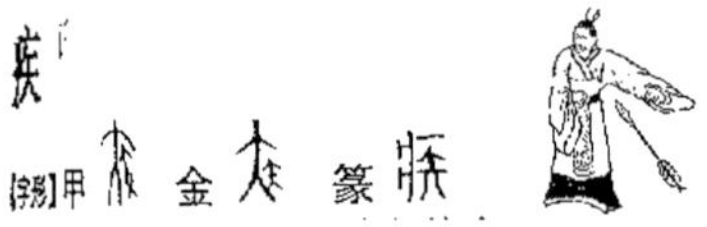

Illus. 18. "*Ji* 疾" from Oracle, Bronze, Seal Script to Its Original Pictograph[205]

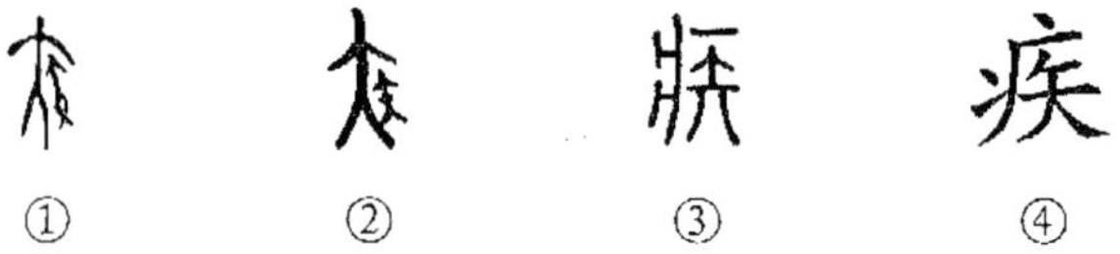

Illus. 19. "*Ji* 疾" from Oracle, Bronze, Lesser Seal, to Regular Script[206]

---

204 You may understand this as the bronze script writing form of 大 (means "Great"). In fact, the sinogram 大 (Great) really resembles the image of man for "Heaven is Great, Earth is Great, Man is also Great; Man abides by Earth, Earth abides by Heaven, Heaven abides by Tao, and Tao abides by the nature". Therefore, undoubtedly, this writing form stands for the image of a man.

205 Gu Yankui. 2008; 2010: 1109.

"Being hurt by an arrow" indicates a mild disease due to external injury. Duan Yucai 段玉裁 (1735-1815) annotated that "An arrow can hurt man; [When an arrow hits and hurts a man,] the arrow should be removed extremely quickly; therefore, it follows the arrow – ." So, it also indicates an acute disease.

Here we can see a good example of pictorial thinking in understanding diseases in the Chinese way. The pictorial thinking has the advantage over the Western conceptual thinking that it is to make diseases more imaginable. This is also one condition for the individualized treatment because it makes the speaking between the patient and the physician more intimate.

Generally speaking, a mild disease, an acute disease, or a disease in its early stage or in the exterior is called "Ji 疾"; while a serious "Ji 疾" is called "Bing 病". For example, 病入膏肓, Bing Ru Gaohuang[207], a Chinese idiom, literally means "Bing 病 or The disease has progressed into the cardio-diaphragmatic interspace," which actually indicates that "The disease is beyond cure."

The Biography of Bian Que[208] *and Cang Gong*[209] from *The Historical Records* also tells the difference between "Ji 疾" and "Bing 病" – "Ji 疾" could be relieved but "Bing 病" was incurable. It reads that:

Bian Que passed through the Qi Kingdom, and Marquis Huan of the Qi (Qi Huan Hou) treated him as his guest. When going to the court to visit the Marquis, Bian Que said upon seeing him: "Your Excellency, you have *Ji* or an illness in the skin structures. If it is not be cured now it will go

206 Zuo Min'an. 2005: 368.

207 Gaohuang 膏肓, refers to the region below the heart and above the diaphragm, situated deeply in the body in Chinese medicine. Therefore it is translated into "cardio-diaphragmatic interspace".

208 Bian Que, surnamed Qin and named Yueren, was a famous physician of the Warring States Period (475-221 B.C.). The people of his time honored him with the name of a lucky bird "Bian Que" to praise his excellence in medical skills and medical morality. He was said to be the founder of the pulse study of Chinese medicine and the first physician to apply the four examinations – inspection, listening and smelling, inquiry, and palpation, to diagnose disease. He was especially good at diagnosing and treating internal, external, gynecological, and ENT diseases. His both works – *Inner Classic* and *Outer Classic*, had been lost long before.

209 Cang Gong (205 B.C.? –?), surnamed Chun and named Yuyi, was also a famous physician of his time. *Shi Ji* records 25 medical case reports from him, known as "Zhen Ji 诊籍" or diagnosing records, the extant earliest medical records in China.

deeper." Marquis Huan replied: "I don't have any *Ji* or illness." After Bian Que had left, Marquis Huan said to those around him: "Physicians are fond of gains, and so they prefer to treat those who are not ill for the purpose of achieving a success!"

Five days later, Bian Que revisited the Marquis, and said to him: "Your *Ji* or illness has gone deeper to the blood vessels. If it is not be cured now it may go deeper." Marquis Huan replied: "I don't have any *Ji* or illness." After Bian Que had left, Marquis Huan became unhappy.

Another five days later, Bian Que revisited the Marquis again, and told him: "Your Excellency, Your *Ji* or illness has gone deeper to the region of your intestines and stomach. If it is not be cured now it will go deeper." Marquis Huan did not respond. After Bian Que had left, Marquis Huan became unhappy.

Another five days later, Bian Que revisited the Marquis for the fourth time, but he immediately ran away as long as he looked at him from a distance. Marquis Huan sent someone to ask him for the reason, and Bian Que told him: "When *Ji* or an illness is located in the skin structures, it can be reached and thus be cured by hot bathing and hot compressing; when being in the blood vessels, it can be reached and thus be cured by needles and stones; when being in the intestines and stomach, it can be reached and thus be cured by medicinal wine; but when being in the morrow of the bones, even *Si Ming* or Life God can not do anything any longer! Now, the Marquis's disease is in the marrow of the bones. Therefore, I preferred not to ask for an audience with the Marquis."

Another five days later, Marquis Huan's body became *Bing* or diseased, and sent someone out to summon Bian Que. But Bian Que had already fled. Subsequently, Marquis Huan died.

We can see from this story that Marquis Huan's *Ji* of different levels could be cured by different means according to their locations, but died of *Bing*, which penetrated through the skin, the blood vessels, the intestines and stomach, and finally progressed to the marrow of the bones.

To sum up, "Ji 疾" refers to illness or mild disease, while "Bing 病" refers to serious disease. But nowadays, the meanings of both sinograms tend to be the same, and the two sinograms always show up together as a compound to mean "disease".

10.2.3 Origins of Disease in Chinese Culture

As we have mentioned at the introduction part of the part, the Western scientific or biomedical system regards disease as being caused by abnormalities in the structure and function of the body systems in biological concerns, which are "more 'real' and significant in contrast to psychological and sociological explanations of illness"[210]; magico-religious approach believes that disease is caused by supernatural factors, such as God's approval or disapproval of one's behavior.

While in Eastern (or Chinese) holistic culture, man and nature unit and resemble each other, which indicates that man is just like a microcosm that follows macrocosmic laws and is continually informed and influenced by macrocosmic influences. In the chapter "Comprehensive Discourse on Regulating Spirit in Accordance with the Four Seasons" of *Huang Di's Inner Classic. Basic Questions*, it reads that

> "Yin-yang and the four seasons, they constitute the end and the beginning of the myriad beings [in the world], and are the foundation of death and life.
> Opposing them will result in catastrophes and harm life.
> Following them will prevent severe diseases from emerging.
> This is called 'Achieving Dao'."

The Eastern holistic approach to the origins of disease proposes that there are natural laws that govern myriad things and beings in the world, i.e. the fundamental principles of the yin-yang theory, namely

> All the things and beings in the world have two facets: a Yin aspect and a Yang aspect;
> Any Yin or Yang aspect can be always further divided into Yin and Yang;
> Yin and Yang are rooted in each other, and mutually create each other;
> Yin and Yang counterbalance each other; and
> Yin and Yang transform into each other under certain conditions.

Actually you can get all these principles of the yin-yang theory from reading the Yin-Yang Diaphragm or *Tai Ji Tu* 太极图. As *Huang Di's Inner Classic. Basic Questions · Comprehensive Discourse on Images Corresponding to Yin-Yang* states that

---

210 Luckman J. 1999: 47.

> "Yin and yang, they are
> the Way of Heaven and Earth,
> the fundamental principles governing the myriad beings,
> mother and father to all the changes and transformations,
> the origin and beginning of generating and killing, and
> the palace of man's spirit."

10.2.3.1 Imbalance or Disharmony between Yin and Yang: The General Origin for All the Diseases

For a person to be healthy, he or she must remain in harmony with laws of the nature and willingly adjust and adapt to changes in their environments.[211] As the *Huang Di's Inner Classic. Basic Questions* states in the chapter 25 "*Discourse on Protecting Life and Preserving Physical Appearance*" that

> "Man is born on the earth, hanging his life to the heaven.
> The union of Heaven qi and Earth qi make up a man.
> Man can adapt himself to the seasons for Heaven and Earth are his parents."

In Chinese culture, man and the nature are not separated from each other, man does not control or conquer or remake the nature, but man lives in harmony with himself and with the nature. Therefore, imbalance or disharmony between yin and yang of the man or between man and the nature accounts for the general origin of all the diseases.

10.2.3.2 Different Classification of Concrete Origins of Disease

Common Chinese people often talk reasons of their illnesses as results of "being attacked by wind/cold/dampness", or of "the fire flaming upward". Actually, origins of disease in Chinese culture are various and generally not considered as causes in the mainstream Western scientific biomedical system. In order to explain the nature and characteristics of the origins of disease, ancient Chinese medical experts tried to group them into three major categories, i.e. internal, external, and non-internal & non-external.

---

211 Luckmann J. 1999: 49.

10.2.3.2.1 External Origins: Six Excesses and Pestilential Qi

1. Abnormal weather conditions, known as six excesses, also known as six exogenous pathogenic factors, six climatic pathogenic factors, or six external pernicious influences, refer to the six climatic conditions in excess as pathogenic factors – pathogenic wind, cold, summer-heat, dampness, dryness, and fire. Under normal conditions, they are actually six normal climatic variations of the nature, and are therefore also called "six natural factors". And when do the six natural factors become six external pernicious influences?

Generally speaking, when the climatic variations are too unusual, or when the occurrence of the six natural factors is too excessive or insufficient or unreasonable, or when the climatic variations are too rapid and violent, and more important when the healthy *qi* of the being is too weak to adapt to the climatic variations of the nature, these impersonal factors will cause diseases, which are known as the so-called externally contracted diseases such as cold-induced diseases, sun stroke, etc.. The common symptoms of diseases caused by the six external pernicious influences include aversion to the particular influence (e.g. cold, wind), fever, chills, body aches, general malaise (discomfort), which are actually the result of the healthy *qi* esp. the guard *qi* attempting to expel the influence.

2. Epidemic or pestilential factors, causes a virulent contagious or fulminating infectious (in the air) diseases such as plague, cholera, diphtheria, mumps, SARS, etc.

10.2.3.2.2 Internal Origins: Seven Affects

Emotional distresses, known as seven emotions or seven affects, refer to joy, anger, melancholy, anxiety, grief, fear, and fright. The differences between melancholy and grief, fear and fright appear to be of degree. The seven emotions appear in healthy individuals, and are normal reactions of the being to external environments. And when do the seven emotions become seven affects, or the seven emotional pathogenic factors? When an emotion is either excessive or insufficient over a long period of time, or when it arises very suddenly with great force, it can generate imbalance and illness, which is termed as "internal damage due to seven affects". That is to say, internal disharmony can generate unbalanced states, and leading to the so-called psychosomatic diseases such as depression, insomnia, etc.

10.2.3.2.3 Non-Internal & Non-External Origins: The Way of Life

1. Improper diets or dietary irregularities, will affect the physiological functions of the spleen and stomach, eventually resulting in various diseases. Soil is sowing and reaping. The spleen and stomach function together to take in, decompose, move, and transform food into essence, and thus providing the material basis for the being and working as the foundation for the postnatal existence. And therefore, the spleen and stomach are metaphorized to soil in the five phases. Li Dongyuan 李东垣 (1180-1251) stressed the role of the spleen and stomach for the being, and proposed that "Internal damage of the spleen and stomach will result in the occurrence of various diseases," and thus established the Soil-Supplementing School, one of "the Four Great Medical Schools in the Jin-Yuan Dynasties (1115-1368)".

2. Physical overstrain or lack of physical exercise, particularly over a long period of time, may cause diseases. As *Huang Di's Inner Classic. Basic Questions* states that "Physical overstrain consumes *qi;*" and that "Seeing for a long time impairs the blood; lying in bed for a long time impairs *qi*; sitting for a long time impairs the muscles; standing for a long time impairs the bones; and walking for a long time impairs the sinews."

3. Overindulgence in sex, may consume kidney essence, resulting in sexual disorders such as hyposexuality, impotence, premature ejaculation, general weakness, listlessness, dizziness, and tinnitus. Kidneys are regarded as being responsible for growth, development, maturation and reproduction for they store the essence, i.e. Kidney Essence, which functions as the root and foundation for reproduction and sexuality.

Besides, traumatic injuries, physical cuts, insects or animal bites, parasites, etc. have also been regarded as origins of non-internal & non-external category, which result in different diseases.

To sum up, in Chinese culture, diseases are usually caused by the agents which are usually not considered as causes of disease in the Western culture. As Kaptchuk points out that "The idea of causality in Chinese medicine is ultimately a means for identifying and qualifying the important relationship between environment, emotional character, personal lifestyle, and health and illness."[212] And the treatments in Chinese medicine all aim to restore the

212 Kaptchuk, T. J. 2000: 165-166.

balance between yin and yang to each individual in their specific natural, social and individual conditions.

10.3 The Nomenclature, Cultural Connotations, and Translation of Disease Names in Chinese Medicine

The name of a disease in Chinese medicine is generally named after its origin, chief symptom, pathogenesis, affected area, or the combination of the above four aspects. The underlying cultural connotations of disease names in Chinese medicine can be summarized into 2 points: one is self-feeling, and the other is relationship centering metaphorizing. As regards to how to translate the disease names in Chinese medicine, I hold that adopting natural equivalents can be used to translate most of the disease names named after symptoms; that literal translation should be the major approach for translating most of the specific disease names so as to preserve systematicness, independence, and integrity of the theoretical system of Chinese medicine; that paraphrase can be used to translate some disease names when their meanings can be identified according to the *Shuo Wen Jie Zi* or *The Origin of Chinese Characters*, *Yu Pian*, and/or *Zhu Bing Yuan Hou Lun* or *Treatise on Origins and Symptoms of Diseases*; and that a combination of Pinyin transliteration + paraphrase can be used to express some disease names in certain contexts after referring to related dictionaries.

10.3.1 The Nomenclature of Disease Names in Chinese Medicine

Disease names in Chinese medicine involve diseases of almost all clinical branches, including internal, external, gynecological, pediatric, ENT departments, etc., the sources of which are also many and varied, including various "symptoms", "patterns", and "diseases". The nomenclature of disease names in Chinese medicine can be classified into the following five categories:

1. Named after the chief symptom, e.g., coughing, vomiting, diarrhea, constipation, *Jue* 厥 or syncope,[213] *Wei* 痿 or atrophy-flaccidity[214], etc;

---

213 *Jue* 厥 or syncope refers to a morbid state characterized by temporary loss of consciousness with cold limbs resulting from disordered flow of *qi* and blood.

2. Named after the chief origin, e.g., *Shang Han* 伤寒 or cold-induced disease, *Shang Shu* 伤暑 or summerheat-induced disease, *Zhong Feng* 中风 or wind stroke, etc;

3. Named after the chief pathogenesis, e.g. *Bi* 痹 or blockage,[215] etc;

4. Named after the chief affecting body part, e.g., headache, abdominal pain, lower back pain, etc;

5. Named after a combination of the chief origin, symptom, pathogenesis, and diseased body part, e.g., *Han Jue* 寒厥 or cold syncope, *Re Jue* 热厥 or heat syncope, *Qi Jue* 气厥 or *qi* syncope, Jue Xin Tong 厥心痛 or *heartache with cold limbs*, *Xin Feng* 心风 or Heart Wind, *Gan Feng* 肝风 or Liver Wind, *Pi Feng* 脾风 or Spleen Wind, *Shen Feng* 肾风 or Kidney Wind, *Da Chang Ke* 大肠咳 or Large Intestinal Coughing, etc.

10.3.2 Self-Feeling and Metaphorizing: The Underlying Cultural Connotations of Disease Names in Chinese Medicine

Ancient Chinese understanding of disease reflects the medical level of that time in a certain sense. Chinese understanding of disease originates from a kind of direct feeling in the remote antiquity. Most of the disease names recorded in the oracle inscriptions were named according to abnormal physiological function of a certain body part, e.g. *Chuang Shou* 疒首 or disordered head, *Chuang Er* 疒耳 or disordered ear, *Chuang Kou* 疒口 or disordered mouth, *Chuang Chi* 疒齿 or disordered tooth/teeth, *Chuang Bi* 疒自（鼻）or disordered nose, etc. As we have discussed before, Chinese conceive the concept of disease in a pictorial way - "lack of ease" as *The Disease Part* of *The Origin of Chinese Characters* 《说文解字 · 疒部》 reads that "疒，倚也。人有疾病，象倚箸之形," which can be translated into "疒, leaning on or against. When a man has an illness or a disease, his image is just like the image of leaning on or against something."

Diseases involved in Chinese medicine actually include the concepts of disease, disorder, illness (ailment), and sickness in English. Besides, a

214 *Wei* 痿 or atrophy-flaccidity refers to a morbid state characterized by flaccidity paralysis with muscular atrophy of a limb.

215 *Bi* 痹 or blockage refers to a diseased state characterized by invasion of the pathogenic factors that cause stagnation of *qi* and blood and blockage of the meridian vessels.

"symptom", the English equivalent for "Zheng 症", "change in the way the body works or change in the body's appearance, which shows a disease or disorder is present and is noticed by the patient himself,"[216] such as vomiting, coughing, and headache, is also a concept of disease in Chinese medicine if it happens to be the chief complaint or the major suffering of the patient.

Generally speaking, disease in Chinese medicine bears three different meanings:

1. Disease, refers to a pathological process with certain manifestations. The occurrence, development, changes, and manifestations of a disease go along a certain specific law, such as epilepsy, leprosy, and cholera, etc.

2. Symptom, refers to either a subjective feeling of the patient or an abnormal change discerned by physician's examinations. In this case, the disease is usually named after the patient's chief complaint/suffering such as headache, palpitation, insomnia, vomiting, diarrhea, etc, or a visible image of the disease such as ox hide lichen – an episodic skin disease characterized by thickening and hardening of the skin that gives it the appearance of the skin of an ox's neck, crane's-knee wind – a disease marked by a painful suppurative swelling of the knee associated with emaciation of the lower leg, etc.

3. The major pathogenesis of the disease, such as wind disease, blockage disease. Take wind disease as an example. Wind is air in motion. It usually comes and goes abruptly, makes things move, sway the branches of trees, and blows harder at the tops of mountains than at the bottoms. Thereby, symptoms or diseases metaphorizing the features of wind are believed to be caused by wind, and are known as wind symptom or disease:

a) Symptoms or diseases with sudden onset and quick disappearance, e.g., mild cases of upper respiratory infection or allergic rhinitis with only sneezing and running nose, urticaria ("wind-rash") and angioneurotic edema;

b) Diseases with lesions that move from one place to another, e.g., rheumatic arthritis with migratory joint pains ("wind-arthritis"), and cutaneous pruritus with no fixed location;

c) Diseases marked by tremors, twitching, convulsions, or vertigo, apoplexy with sudden onset of hemiplegia ("wind-stroke"), and facial paralysis.

---

216 See Collin, P.H. 2001: 574. If a symptom is noticed only by the doctor, it is a sign ("Zheng 征" in Chinese).

Among the above conditions, some are known as exogenous wind caused by exogenous pathogenic wind from outside the human body in any season, which may invade the upper respiratory tract as in allergic rhinitis, the skin as in urticaria and cutaneous pruritus, and the meridians as in migratory arthritis and Bell's palsy; while the others are known as endogenous wind due to dysfunction of the liver. The liver governs the sinews, and so dysfunction of the liver may lead to disturbances in motion of some parts of the body, such as hemiplegia and involuntary movements of the limbs. As the *Huang Di's Inner Classic · Basic Questions* states that "All Wind [diseases characterized by] tremor and vertigo are [mostly] due to [dysfunction of] the liver."

Based on the above discussion, the underlying cultural connotations of disease names in Chinese medicine can be summarized into 2 points: one is self-feeling, and the other is relationship centering metaphorizing. That is to say, disease names in Chinese medicine suggest that disease has to be understood as a kind of self-feeling – lack of ease, and a kind of relationship centering metaphorizing. Based on this understanding, it is also possible for a cancer patient with irremovable tumors to be in a state of ease and comfort if he lives in harmony with and does not suffer from tumors.

10.3.3 How to Translate Disease Names in Chinese Medicine

The methods for translating disease names in Chinese medicine can be summed up into the following four:

10.3.3.1 Adopting Natural Equivalents

It is advisable to adopt natural equivalents to translate those diseases named after the chief symptoms. For example, vomiting, cough, insomnia, somnolence, headache, lumbago, constipation, diarrhea, jaundice, sterility, abscess, hemorrhoid are used to express the diseases named as "呕（吐）", "咳（嗽）", "不眠", "嗜卧", "头痛", "腰痛", "便闭"（或"不更衣"）, "泄泻", "黄疸", "不孕", "痈", and "痔" respectively.

Notes:

1. The words "cholera", "malaria", "leprosy", "epilepsy", "dysentery" are regarded as natural equivalents for "霍乱", "疟疾", "疠癞", "癫痫", "痢疾" respectively in Chinese medicine for these disease names in the Western

culture emerged long and far before the evolution of modern Western medicine.

An interesting issue to be addressed here is that some disease names in the *Basic Questions (Su Wen)* may be of foreign origin. Here are some examples:

Li lai 癘癩: 癘, whose ancient pronunciation is *ljadh* or *rjats*, and 癩, whose ancient pronunciation is *ladh* or *rats,* the initial consonants come closer to those of the three most popular ancient European terms for *leprosy*, one might speculate about an association of *li* and *lai* with *leuke, lepra, and e-lephantiasis*;

Huo luan 霍亂, the compound *huo luan* does not correspond to the graphic structure of the vast majority of ancient Chinese disease terms, while its ancient pronunciation **hwak* luan* was formed to reflect in ancient Chinese the sound of the term *cholera* used along the travel routes from regions where the Greek term was in use to the Far East to designate a particularly violent type of diarrhea;

Fei xiao 肺消, whose ancient pronunciation is **phjats*sjaw,* literally "lung wasting", could be a rendering into Chinese of the ancient Greek term *phtisis* or lung *phtisis,* which has exactly the same meaning;

Xiao ke 消渴, wasting/melting and thirst, a label used to this day for diabetes, is a compound ideally suited to signify two obvious symptoms of the disease. An identical meaning was expressed in European antiquity by Aretaios of Cappadochia.[217]

Is it purely coincidental? Or there existed medical cultural exchange between the East and the West around the Zhou Dynasty (C.1100-256B.C.)? Anyway, these terms all came out far before the modern Western medicine and should be regarded as the terms of the natural equivalents. The above understanding further provides etymological evidence when translating 癘癩, 霍亂, 肺消, 消渴 into leprosy, cholera, lung wasting, wasting and thirst respectively.

2. *Longman Dictionary of Contemporary English* explains "abscess" as "a swelling on or in the body where PUS has gathered", "hemorrhoid" as "a swollen BLOOD VESSEL at the ANUS"[218], which accords well with the

217 Unschuld, Paul U. 2003: 203-204.

218 *Longman Dictionary of Contemporary English* [Z]. 1998: 5, 715.

explanations of the two sinograms “痈” and “痔” in the *Shuo Wen Jie Zi* or *The Origin of Chinese Characters*: “痈，肿也,” “痔，后病也.” Therefore, translating “痈” and “痔” into “abscess” and “hemorrhoid” respectively is also the use of the method of adopting natural equivalents.

10.3.3.2 Literal Translation

I advocate that disease names specific in Chinese medicine should be rendered into English in literal translation approach so as to keep the imaging thinking implied in these names and to preserve the systematicness, independence, and integrity of Chinese medicine as well. As regards to literal translation, Peter Newmark comments that

“However, in communicative as in semantic translation, provided that equivalent effect is secured, the literal word-for-word translation is not only the best, it is the only valid method of translation. There is no excuse for unnecessary ‘synonyms’, let alone paraphrases, in any type of translation.”[219]

For example, I advise to translate “伤寒”, “中风”, “热病”, “温病”, “风病”, “寒病”, “燥病”, “心风”, and “肾风” into cold-induced disease, wind stroke, febrile disease, warm disease, wind disease, cold disease, dry disease, heart wind, kidney wind respectively; and to translate “梅核气” into “plum-pit qi” not “globus hystericus”, “奔豚” into “running piglet” not “gastroenteroneurosis”, “历节风” into “joint-running wind” not “arthritis”, “风火眼” into “wind-fire eye” not “acute conjunctivitis”, although these diseases can be diagnosed as the latter ones in Western medicine in most of the cases.

Actually, English disease names in Chinese medicine formed through literal translation approach bears the following merits:

1. Accuracy in content, form, and logic, i.e. the translation gives the ideas, words, and logic of the original;

2. Conciseness and pithiness in style, i.e. the translation reproduces the conciseness and pithiness of the original compared to the lengthy paraphrase for the original is usually concise in form but profound in meaning;

3. Systematicness, i.e. the literal translation approach makes the English Chinese medical terminology being systematic, and thus faithfully reflecting

---

219 Newmark, Peter. 2001: 39.

the integrity and inter-relationship in its concept system for Chinese medical terminology forms in the way of *Qu Xiang Bi Lei* or Taking Image and Analogizing on the basis of ancient Chinese daily life experiences. For example, although 風火眼 in Chinese medicine and "acute conjunctivitis" in Western medicine actually refer to the same disease, it is ill-advised to translate 風火眼 into "acute conjunctivitis" for such a translation must confuse cultural differences between the two medical systems, and fail to produce such association of the cause (pathogenic wind-fire) and therapeutic method (coursing wind and clearing fire) with the translation "acute conjunctivitis", which, on the contrary, gives the readers the association that an "-itis" or inflammation is caused by a certain kind of bacteria or virus and should be relieved by "antibiotics".

4. Back-translation, i.e. literal translation improves or realizes translation of English Chinese medical terminology back into Chinese, thus keeping distinguishing features of Chinese medical culture and being beneficial for the double direction information interchange. In real fact, "伤寒" is usually translated into "exogenous febrile disease", which, if translated back into Chinese, should be "外感热病" not "伤寒" any more; "温病" is frequently translated into "seasonal epidemic disease" or "seasonal febrile disease", which, if translated back into Chinese, should be "季节性流行病" or "季节性热病" but not "温病". It is thus clear that English disease names formed through literal translation approach can be easily translated back to their original Chinese, and thus improving or realizing the double direction information interchange.

10.3.3.3 Paraphrase

It is advisable to paraphrase some original Chinese disease names by referring to interpretations from the Shuo Wen Jie Zi or The Origin of Chinese Characters, Yu Pian or Jade Writings, and Zhu Bing Yuan Hou Lun or Treatise on Origins and Symptoms of Diseases, etc. For example, the Shuo Wen Jie Zi or The Origin of Chinese Characters includes and explains 102 sinograms with "Chuang 疒" - denoting disease as the signific[220].

220 Originally by [Han] Xu Shen, Annotated by [Qing] Duan Yucai. 1988: 348-353.

For example, *Huang Di's Inner Classic. Basic Questions. Discourse on Strange Diseases* reads that "人有重身，九月而瘖." *The Disease Part* of *The Origin of Chinese Characters*《说文解字 · 疒部》explains that "瘖，不能言也," which can be translated into "*Yin* 瘖 means loss of voice." Accordingly, this quotation can be translated into "A pregnant woman, in her ninth month of gestation, loses her voice."

10.3.3.4 A Combination of Pinyin Transliteration and Paraphrase

In certain contexts, a combination of Pinyin transliteration and paraphrase can be used to translate some disease names by referring to some reference books. For example,

Original:《黄帝内经灵枢 · 热病》："*痱*之为病也，身无痛者，四肢不收，知乱不甚，其言微知，可治."

Translation: *Huang Di's Inner Classic. Miraculous Pivot. Discourse on Febrile Diseases*: When *fei-disease, a kind of wind disease*, is the disease, there is no pain in the body, the four limbs cannot contract, the patient's thoughts are not seriously disordered, his/her speech still bears a little sense, the disease can be treated.

Note: *Shuo Wen Jie Zi* or *The Origin of Chinese Characters* explains that "*痱*，风病也," i.e., "*Fei* 痱, a kind of wind disease." Therefore, this disease is also called "*Feng Fei* 风痱", see Volume 1 of *Zhu Bing Yuan Hou Lun* or *Treatise on Origins and Symptoms of Diseases* for "Manifestations of *Feng Fei* 风痱." In this context, "*Fei* 痱"can be rendered into English by combining Pinyin transliteration and paraphrase: *fei*, a kind of wind disease.

It is worth to note that the same disease name in different contexts may have different meanings. Or in other words, the meanings of some disease names are decided by their contexts. In such cases, the above mentioned methods should be used flexibly to translate these disease names according to their concrete conditions by consulting related reference books. Here I present 2 examples.

1. One example is *Dan* 瘅:

a) *Huang Di's Inner Classic. Basic Questions. Discourse on the Essentials of Pulse:* "*瘅*成为消中." Wang Bing 王冰 (710-804) annotated that "'*Dan* 瘅', is dampness-heat. The heat accumulates internally, and hence it changes to 'wasting center'. The signs of 'wasting center' are desire to eat and emaciation." Based on this annotation, *Dan* 瘅 can be translated into "pathogenic damp-heat". "*Xiao Zhong* 消中" can be translated by the method of combining "Pinyin transliteration and paraphrase" into "*xiao zhong*", manifesting in polyphagia and polyuria. Therefore, this quotation can be translated into "Pathogenic damp-heat may cause *xiao zhong* disease, manifesting in polyphagia and polyuria."

b) *Huang Di's Inner Classic. Basic Questions. Discourse on the True Qi of the Viscera:* "肝传之脾，名曰脾风，发*瘅*，腹中热，烦心，出黄." "'*Dan* 瘅' is interchangeable with '*Dan* 疸', and refers to 'jaundice'."[221] Zhang Zhicong 张志聪 (1616-1674) annotated that "Downward flowing of [pathogenic] fire-heat causes yellow urine." Based on the above annotations, "*Dan* 瘅" here can be translated into "jaundice", and "脾风" can be literally translated into "spleen-wind"; This quotation can be translated into "When the pathogen transmits from the liver to the spleen, spleen-wind will occur, manifesting in jaundice, a hot sensation in the abdomen, vexation, and yellow urine."

2. The other example is "*Fu Liang* 伏梁", which can be translated by the method of combining "Pinyin transliteration and paraphrase" into "*fu liang* or hidden-beam". While in concrete contexts, the disease "*Fu Liang* 伏梁" can be identified by clinical manifestations expounded in its concrete contexts.

a) *Huang Di's Inner Classic. Basic Questions. Discourse on Strange Diseases* reads that "帝曰：人有身体髀股　皆肿，环齐而痛，是为何病？岐伯曰：病名曰*伏梁*," which can be translated into

Huang Di asked, "There is a condition manifesting in swelling in the hip and legs and pain around umbilicus. What is the disease?"

Qi Bo answered, "The disease is called *fu liang* or hidden-beam."

b) 《难经 · 五十六难》："心之积，名曰伏梁，起齐上，大如臂，上至心下，久不愈，...," which can be translated into

The accumulation in the heart is called *fu liang* or hidden-beam, originating above the umbilicus, as large as an arm, extending upward to the area below the heart, lingering there for a long time, ...

George Steiner (1929–), a world-famous influential translator, educator and philosopher, discussed "Understanding as Translation" in the first chapter of his masterpiece *After Babel---Aspects of Language and Translation* in

221 Guo Aichun. 1999: 121.

1975.[222] That is to say, how to translate into the target is decided by how to understand the original. This is also true with translation of the disease names in Chinese medicine - Translation should be based on a proper relationship between the part and the whole, that is to say, translation should be based on the correct understanding of not only a specific disease name, but also the Chinese medical system as a whole. Chinese medicine and Western medicine both study the life processes and aim to prevent and treat diseases, but their philosophical foundations, cultural backgrounds, methodologies and perspectives, etc. are entirely different from each other. For example, the disease "wind-fire eye" caused by pathogenic wind-fire should be relieved by the therapeutic method of coursing wind and clearing fire. But rendering 風火眼 in Chinese medicine into "acute conjunctivitis" wipes out the association of the disease with its cause and therapeutic method. That is to say, translating disease names in Chinese medicine should have an overall point of view, which, then, makes English Chinese medical terminology embody the same relationships between the original Chinese terms and makes them be in a harmonious state.

Upon ending this part, I have to point out that translation texts here are translations redone based on the author's understanding in order to illustrate points of view, and so they are not necessarily to be the best for they are not in their original contexts.

10.4 Disease, Symptoms and Pattern: The Foundations for Individualized Treatment in Chinese Medicine

Ancient Chinese understanding of disease reflects the medical level of that time in a certain sense. Diseases involved in Chinese medicine actually include the concepts of disease, disorder, illness (ailment), and sickness in English. Besides, a "symptom", the English equivalent for "*Zheng* 症", "change in the way the body works or change in the body's appearance, which shows a disease or disorder is present and is noticed by the patient himself," such as vomiting, coughing, and headache, is also a concept of disease in Chinese medicine if it happens to be the chief complaint or the major suffering of the patient.

222 Steiner, George. 2001.

As *10.2.2* gives a detailed analysis of *Chuang* 疒, *Ji* 疾, and *Bing* 病, Chinese understanding of disease originates from a kind of direct feeling in the remote antiquity, and "*Ji Bing* 疾病" in Chinese medicine, in most of cases, should be *illness or disease in its original meaning – lack of ease*, not disease in the sense of modern Western medicine which can be determined by physical, chemical and/or other specific examinations. Here we can see a good example of pictorial thinking in understanding diseases in the Chinese way. The pictorial thinking has the advantage over the Western conceptual thinking that it is to make diseases more imaginable. This is also one condition for the individualized treatment because it makes the speaking between the patient and the physician more intimate. According to the modern textbooks on Chinese medicine, after the disease is diagnosed, the *Zheng* or Pattern should be identified before instituting the treatment to an individual patient, i.e. individualized treatment based on pattern identification.

10.4.1 What Zhang Zhongjing Proposed: Pattern Identification or Else?

Individualized treatment based on pattern identification is known as *Bian Zheng Lun Zhi* in academic words. Besides of *Zheng Ti Guan Nian* 整体观念 or holist conception, *Bian Zheng Lun Zhi* 辨证论治 or Pattern Identification and Treatment has been regarded as the other basic characteristics of Chinese medicine for quite some time. Today, the scholars, practitioners and students in the circle of Chinese medicine have been informed by the textbooks that Zhang Zhongjing 张仲景 (150-219) developed or established the principle of *Bian Zheng Lun Zhi* or Pattern Identification and Treatment in his monumental work *Shang Han Za Bing Lun* or *On Cold-induced and Miscellaneous Diseases.*

Just take *Ci Hai* or *The Sea of Words* (2002), the largest encyclopedic dictionary in China, and the world-famous *Encyclopedia Britannica* (2010) as

223 *Bian Zheng Lun Zhi* 辨证论治 can be literally translated into "identifying pattern and determining treatment".

224 *Shang Han Za Bing Lun* or *On Cold-induced and Miscellaneous Diseases* was later on systematized into two books by Wang Shuhe 王叔和 (201-280): *Shang Han Lun* or *On Cold-induced Diseases* and *Jin Gui Yao Lue* or *Synopsis of the Golden Chamber*.

examples. Zhang Zhongjing's academic achievements recorded in these two books are almost the same, which can be summarized as: initiating the principles of "six-meridian pattern identification" and "pattern identification and treatment", authoring *Shanghan Zabing Lun*, and thus making major contributions to the development of Chinese medicine. Undoubtedly, Zhang Zhongjing made great contributions to Chinese medicine, but as regards to "pattern identification and treatment", it is actually far from the truth.

A textbook entitled *Bian Zheng Shi Zhi* or *Symptom Identification and Treatment* 辨症施治 compiled by Shanghai College of Traditional Chinese Medicine (known as Shanghai University of TCM since 1993) and published in 1972 reads in its preface that

"The viewpoint of *Bian Zheng Shi Zhi* or Symptom Identification and Treatment 辨症施治 was set up in *Nei Jing* or *The Inner Classic*, the earliest classic on medicine extant in China. Based on the summarization of experiences of his forefathers, Zhang Zhongjing proposed more clearly that the principle of *Bian Zheng Shi Zhi* or Symptom Identification and Treatment 辨症施治 should be performed when treating diseases."[225]

In an academic paper by Gan Zuwang 甘祖望 (1911–) published in 2003, the author said that "We, this group of veteran physicians of Chinese medicine, did not know what was '*Bian Zheng Lun Zhi* 辨证论治' or '*Bian Zheng Shi Zhi* 辨证施治' at all before the liberation [in 1949]."[226]

In the real fact, the sinogram "证"（"証", pattern） in the "辨证论治" (pattern identification and treatment) does not even show up in any of the early classics on Chinese medicine including *Nei Jing (The Inner Classic), Nan Jing (The Classic of Difficult Issues), Shanghan Lun (On Cold-induced Diseases), Jingui Yaolue (Synopsis of the Golden Chamber)*, and *Shennong Bencao Jing (Shennong's Classic of Materia Medica)*. What appears in the early Chinese medical classics is "Zheng 證" – "the evidence (manifestations/symptoms) of a disease", which is interchangeable with "症"(symptom) in the medical contexts. And what Zhang Zhongjing discussed in each chapter of *Shanghan Lun* and *Jingui Yaolue* is "病脉*證*并治" – "disease, pulse, *symptoms* and treatment".

225 Shanghai College of TCM (ed.). 1972: 1.
226 Gan Zuwang. 2003(8): 672.

It is gratifying that Luo Xiwen 罗希文 has given proper English translations for "Zheng 證" in these two books: "symptom complex".[227] Therefore, the fact is what Zhang Zhongjing developed and established is not the principle of *Bian Zheng Lun Zhi* 辨证论治 or "Pattern Identification and Treatment" but *Bing Mai Zheng Bing Zhi* 病脉證并治 or "Identifying Disease First and Determining Treatment in Accordance with Specific Pulse and Accompanied Symptoms." But how could this fundamental misinterpretation happen?

Actually, individualized treatment in Chinese medicine should be based on Chinese understanding of disease in the following three aspects: disease, symptoms, and pattern. In different to Western thinking, Classical Chinese thinking is based on circular reasoning. We can see it also in the logical relations between disease, pattern and symptoms. In order to understand disease from symptoms and patterns, we must be aware that they are logical conditions for each other.

Hereafter is my argumentation developed based on investigation of etymologies of related Chinese characters (or sinograms), Chinese medical classics, and related modern literature as well as our understanding of Chinese medicine. Let's start from distinguishing four confusing key concepts in Chinese medicine: "證", "証", "症", and "征".

10.4.2 Four Key Concepts in Chinese Medicine: "證", "証", "症", and "征"

These four key concepts in Chinese medicine, "證", "証", "症", and "征", are very confusing even for TCM majors. Therefore, *Chinese Science and Technology Terms Journal* 科技术语研究, known as *China Terminology* 中国科技术语 since 2007, published a group of papers from some experts in the fields of Chinese medicine and Western medicine with the aim of clarifying these concepts in 2003 (See Issue 4 for details). The modern use of these sinograms are therefore clarified in the right way: "症" for "symptom or manifestation" 症状, "disease" 病症, "indication" 适应症, "contraindica-

227 Originally by Zhang Zhongjing; Translated by Luo Xiwen. *Synopsis of Prescriptions from the Golden Chamber (Jingui Yaolue)*. Beijing: New World Press; 2007. Originally by Zhang Zhongjing; Translated by Luo Xiwen. *Treatise on Febrile Caused by Cold (Shanghan Lun)*. Beijing: New World Press; 2007.

tion" 禁忌症, and "complication" 并发症; "证" for "pattern" in Chinese medicine such as "Pattern Identification and Treatment" 辨证论治 and "Pattern of Hyperactivity of Liver Yang" 肝阳上亢证, for Chinese translation of "evidence" such as "Evidence-Based Medicine" 循证医学;[228] and "征" for "syndrome" 综合征, "sign" 征象, etc.[229]

But as regards to the origin of "证"（"証", pattern） in the "辨证论治" (pattern identification and treatment), they took a firm stand to support that Zhang Zhongjing initiated this concept of "证" (pattern) and this principle of "辨证论治" (pattern identification and treatment) by quoting "观其脉*證*, 知犯何逆, 随*證*治之", in which the first "證" was interpreted as "症"(symptom), whereas the second "證" was interpreted as "证" (pattern).[230] This interpretation sounds ridiculous after investigating their etymologies for the etymologies of "证"（"証", pattern） and 证 ("證", symptom) are completely different. The sinogram "Zheng 证" happens to be the simplified writing form of both "Zheng 證" and "Zheng 証", and the simplified Chinese characters came out officially in between 1952 and 1986. It is a big pity that the Chinese texts in simplified Chinese characters write off the distinctions between "Zheng 證" and "Zheng 証". Then what are the differences between these three homonymous sinograms: "證", "証", and "症"? First, let's investigate their etymologies.

10.4.2.1 "*Zheng* 證": From "Inform Against", "Demonstrate" to "the Evidence (Manifestations/Symptoms) of a Disease"

According to the *Shuo Wen Jie Zi* or *The Origin of Chinese Characters*, "*Zheng* 證" originally means "to inform against 告也", and as we all know that, a patient has to "inform" the physician "against" (complain) his chief suffering and other symptoms in all ages when he/she sees a physician; moreover, the sinogram "*Zheng* 證" is then extended to mean "to prove", "to demonstrate", then to mean "proof or demonstration or evidence of a disea-

228 Here "Zheng 证" for pattern is the simplified writing form of "Zheng 証", while "Zheng 证" for evidence is the simplified writing form of "Zheng 證".

229 Chen Keji, et al. 2003(4): 10-11.

230 Zhu Jianping. 2003(4): 14-17; Zhu WF. 2003(4): 20-21.

se"; and therefore, this sinogram "*Zheng* 症" was created and specialized for medical contexts to mean "symptom".

Investigation of ancient Chinese medical texts shows that the sinogram "*Zheng* 症" does not show up in the medical texts until the Song Dynasty (960-1279).[231] As regards to the relationship between "*Zheng* 證" and "*Zheng* 症", the former is one of the earliest sinograms and the one in common use, while the later was created in the Song Dynasty to be used specially in the field of medicine.

10.4.2.2 *Zheng* 証: From "To Remonstrate with One's Superior to Make Him Behave '*Zheng* 正 or Upright'" to "the Central Essence of a Disease"

The sinogram "*Zheng* 证" is the simplified writing form of both "*Zheng* 證" and "*Zheng* 証", and so the distinctions between "*Zheng* 證" and "*Zheng* 証" have been written off in the Chinese texts in simplified Chinese characters. As we have discussed in the last paragraph, "proof or demonstration or manifestation or evidence of a disease", one of the extended meanings of the former one – "*Zheng* 證", results in the creating of the sinogram "*Zheng* 症" for "symptom". As regards to "*Zheng* 证" in the sense of Pattern in Chinese medicine, its original writing form is "*Zheng* 証", which follows "*Yan* 言" (word) and "*Zheng* 正".

While, "*Zheng* 正", an indicative, is a key concept in Chinese culture. Its oracle writing form follows "口 (city)" and "  (foot)", indicating "heading straightly for the city (the target)"; later on, the "口 (city)" transformed into a solid spot in its bronze writing form, and then into a horizontal since the lesser seal script. The *Shuo Wen Jie Zi* or *The Origin of Chinese Characters* explains "*Zheng* 正" with "*Shi* 是". "*Shi* 是", an associative compound, written as  in the bronze script and  in the seal script, follows "*Ri* 日(sun)" and "*Zheng* 正", indicating the sun being in the middle. Thus the original meaning of "*Zheng* 正" is straight, even, central, upright.

---

231 Xiao Mincai. 1984 (4):2.

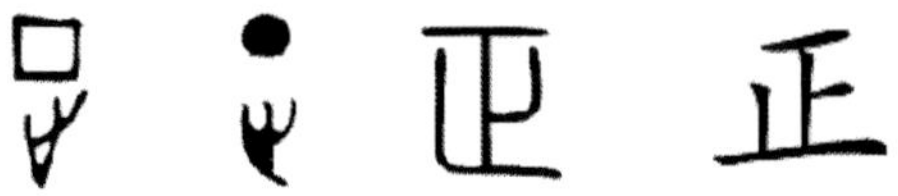

Illus. 20. "Zheng 正" From Oracle, Bronze, Lesser Seal to Regular Script

The sinogram "*Zheng* 证" with the original writing form "*Zheng* 証", originally means "to remonstrate with one's superior to make him behave '*Zheng* 正 or upright' 諫也" according to the *Shuo Wen Jie Zi* or *The Origin of Chinese Characters*.

In Chinese medicine, "*Zheng* 证/証" is a unique concept to reveal the central essence of a disease, which reflects a further and deeper understanding of a disease but is distinct from the concept of disease (as a specific kind of morbid condition), e.g. a disease may take the form of different patterns.

Briefly speaking, "*Zheng* 证" is a pathological generalization of a disease in its certain developing stage. "*Zheng* 证" indicates the location, origin, nature, and relation between the healthy *qi* of the being and the pathogenic *qi* of a disease, and reflects the essence of the pathological changes of a disease in its certain stage, and therefore, it reveals the essence of the disease much more comprehensively, deep-going, and correctly than any symptoms.[232]

Then how to translate "Zheng 证/証"? In China, it is usually translated into "syndrome" – "a medical condition that is characterized by a particular group of signs and symptoms"; and "Different syndromes are often called by the name of the person who first discovered or described them."[233] Syndrome is a word which seems to be more acceptable to the Western ears. While, in the West, the most common translation for this unique Chinese concept is "pattern". Besides, some other translators prefer "configuration", "conformation" for "Zheng 证/証", etc. You may be confused by so many different translations for "Zheng 证/証" – which should be the proper one?

Since "Syndrome" for "Zheng 证/証" and "syndrome differentiation" for "*Bian Zheng* 辨证/証" have been proposed by Prof. Lu Weibai 吕维柏 (1928-), such translations have been widely accepted by the academic circle in China but are rarely seen in English works on Chinese medicine published

232 Yin Huihe. 1st ed., 1984; fifth printing, 1988: 8.
233 *Cobuild English-Chinese Dictionary* [Z]. Harper Collins Publishers, 2006.

abroad. Just suppose – how can we differentiate "Climacteric Syndrome" again into "Syndrome of Liver Kidney Yin Deficiency" and "Syndrome of Yin Deficiency and Fire Exuberance"?

Kaptchuk commented that "From a modern Western perspective, it is tempting to translate the Chinese words as 'differentiating syndromes', but that rendering would distort the uniqueness and potential validity of the Chinese idea. 'Syndrome' is a purely descriptive term, suggesting an arbitrary grouping of signs and symptoms that is meaningless without an underlying cause. 'Syndrome' implies that something is missing."[234]

Although we know the original meaning of "*Zheng* 証/证" and its interpretation in the contexts of Chinese medicine – "the central essence of a disease", the word "pattern", the most popular translation for this concept, which implies a picture or an image of a disease in a certain specific stage, can still be regarded as a proper English interpretation for "Zheng 証/证".

10.4.2.3 The Origin of "*Zheng* 证/証" and "*Bian Zheng* 辨证/証" in Chinese Medicine: "Dialectics" since 1955

Zhang Xugu 章虚谷 proposed "*Bian Zheng Lui Zhi* 辨證论治" in 1825,[(12)] in which "證" should be interpreted as "症 symptom" for "证" as the simplified writing form of both "証" and "證" came out no earlier than 1952. Therefore, "*Bian Zheng Lui Zhi* 辨證论治" proposed by Zhang Xugu bears the same meaning as "*Bian Zheng Shi Zhi* 辨證施治" advocated before by Zhou Zhigan 周之干 (1508?-1586) in the 16th century, i.e. "symptom identification and treatment."

Actually, *Bian Zheng Lun Zhi* 辨证(証)论治 with today's significance and interpretation: "Pattern Identification and Treatment", or "Identifying Pattern and Determining Treatment", or "Treatment Determined according to Identified Pattern", is a quite new invention by Ren Yingqiu 任应秋 (1914-1984) since he published two papers successively on *Zhong Yi Za Zhi* 中医杂志 or *Journal of Traditional Chinese Medicine* in 1955.[235] In one paper published in No.2 Issue - "*Great Homeland Medical Achievements*", it reads that

234 Kaptchuk T.J. 2000: 216.
235 Ren Yingqiu. 1955 (2): 1; Ren Yingqiu. 1955 (4): 19.

“Homeland medicine (i.e. Chinese medicine) has solved problems in the clinical practice for thousands of years mainly because of the establishment of the treating system of ‘*Bian Zheng Lun Zhi* 辨证论治’, which functions to understand a disease as a kind of damage to the normal inter-relations between the organism and its environments. – The disease is not only decided by dysfunctions of the organism, but also influenced by the restoration of the damaged inter-relations and the recovery-promoting phenomena.

“Therefore, regard a disease as a unity of opposites, use yin and yang, exterior and interior, cold and heat, deficiency and excess etc. to stand for the two poles of contradictions, distinguish and identify the contradiction relations between the pathological and physiological mechanisms with both opposite and supplementary perspectives, and then determine the treatment ...

“The method ‘*Bian Zheng Lun Zhi* 辨证论治’ of yin and yang, exterior and interior, cold and heat, deficiency and excess is the most important key to treatments in homeland medicine, which relates to each other, restricts each other, develops at any time, and always moves and changes in an extremely complicated manner. Therefore, under no circumstances, it can be handled in an isolated, obstinate and mechanically anatomy-orientated way. If you do not follow this method, you are not able to distinguish and identify the mechanisms of a disease, and will not get the desired therapeutic effects.”[236]

What can we see from the above quoted part from this paper?

If you are familiar with the paper entitled “*On Contradictions*” by Mao Zedong 毛泽东 (1893-1976) published in 1937, you will see that “*Bian Zheng Lun Zhi* 辨证论治” is an direct outcome of political influences from Mao Zedong Thought. “*On Contradictions*” reads that

“The world view of materialist dialectics advocates studying the development of everything from its inside, from its relations to the others, i.e. regarding the development of a thing as a kind of inexorable movement inside itself, and movement of everything inter-relating to and inter-influencing the other things around it.”

236 Ren Yingqiu. 1955 (2): 1.

Mao Zedong Thought was written into the *Party's Constitution* where it was stipulated as the guideline for all the work of the communist party of China in 1945. Since then it has been regarded as the guideline to direct the revolution and construction of the socialist China. And it is well known that "*Shi Shi Qiu Shi* 实事求是", i.e. Seeking Truth from Facts, is its quintessence. As we have discussed in 10.4.2.2, "*Shi* 是" and "*Zheng* 正" are a pair of synonymous sinograms, which are mutually interpreted with each other.

Mao Zedong Thought is greatly influenced by dialectical materialism, or in other words, the Chinanized dialectical materialism, the central idea of which is from Hegel (1770-1831) and advocates that all the historical emergences, changes, and developments result from the struggle between the two opposites inside them. The word "dialectics" is of Greek origin, and originally means "arguing for truth". The *Oxford Advanced Learner's English-Chinese Dictionary* (the 7th edition, Oxford University Press, 2009) explains it as bearing two meanings: "(philosophy) a method of discovering the truth of ideas by discussion and logical argument and by considering ideas that are opposed to each other;" and "(formal) the way in which two aspects of a situation affect each other."

Here, we have to acknowledge that translating "dialectics" into "*Bian Zheng* 辩证" is really a great creation. "*Bian Zheng* 辩证", the Chinese translation for "dialectics", literally means "arguing for truth", and this compound bears the exact same pronunciation as the "*Bian Zheng* 辨证" in Chinese medicine, which literally means "distinguishing and identifying truth" and is usually translated into "Identifying Pattern" or "Pattern Identification", in which "Zheng 证" or Pattern indicates the true essence of a disease.

Therefore, we can draw this conclusion that "*Bian Zheng* 辨证 or Pattern Identification" in Chinese medicine is an outcome of political influences from Mao Zedong Thought, and originates directly from "dialectics" in the philosophy of dialectical materialism.

Actually materialist dialectics has exerted enormous and profound influences on TCM, the Chinese medicine evolved in China from classical Chinese medicine (CCM) since 1949. TCM is an outcome of systematizing the knowledge contained in classical Chinese medical texts from perspectives of materialist dialectics. For example, in the *Basic Theories of Chinese Medicine*, the 5th edition textbook on basic theories for TCM higher education in China, it quotes that

> "Engels (1820-1895) pointed out in the *Dialectics of Nature* that 'No matter what kinds of attitude natural scientists would take, they have always been under the control of philosophy.' Medicine, just like the other branches of natural science, has always been under the control and influence of a certain world outlook. Chinese medicine formed and developed on the basis of long term medical practice, and has been deeply influenced by ideas of the ancient materialism and dialectics in the course of its formation, and therefore, viewpoints of materialism and dialectics have run through its theoretical system."

And in this textbook, the yin-yang and five phases are regarded as "materialism and dialectics in ancient China."

10.4.3 Methodology of Treatment in Chinese Medicine: A Historical Outline

10.4.3.1 *Wu Shi Er Bing Fang or Prescriptions for Fifty Two Diseases*: Treatment Determined Based on Disease Diagnosis and Tailored According to Accompanied Symptoms

In the early stage of the history of Chinese medicine, treatments were mainly determined according to disease diagnosis. The *Wu Shi Er Bing Fang* or *Prescriptions for Fifty Two Diseases*, identified as a piece of work in the 3rd century B.C., a silk scroll unearthed at No. 3 Mawangdui Han Tomb in Changsha, Hunan province in 1973, and the earliest medical document extant in China, demonstrates that treatments were primarily determined based on disease diagnosis and sometimes tailored according to accompanied symptoms at that time.

For example, "*Ju* or deep-rooted ulcers are treated with seven medicinal substances: Radix Ampelopsis, Radix Astragali, Peony, Cinnamon, Ginger, Pepper, and Dogwood. Double Radix Ampelopsis for Bone *Ju*, double Radix Astragali for Flesh *Ju*, double Peony for Kidney *Ju*, and each dosage for each of the other six. Then put a pinch [of the prescription] into a cup of wine, and then drink it five to six times a day. ..." That is to say, Deep-Rooted Ulcers were generally treated with the seven medicinals, but dosages differed according to different accompanied symptoms. Such records have shown the high level back then of the treatment methodology in Chinese medicine.

10.4.3.2 Huang Di Nei Jing or Huang Di's Inner Classic: Treatment Determined Based on Disease Diagnosis and Origin Examination

The *Huang Di Nei Jing* or *Huang Di's Inner Classic*, the earliest systematic, complete and greatest medical classic extant in China, also stresses the importance of disease diagnosis, which is taken as the major foundation for the treatments. It mentions more than 100 disease names, and expounds the viewpoint that a clear and definite diagnosis is a prerequisite to a proper treatment. Treatment based on disease identification is its major treating methodology, and a specialized formula is designated for a specific disease. "*Ji Shi Li* 鸡矢醴" or Chicken Droppings Wine for distension, "*Sheng Tie Luo Yin* 生铁落饮" or Fresh Iron Flakes Beverage for anger and mania, and "*Ze Xie Yin* 泽泻饮" or Alisma Beverage for Wine Wind[237] are all examples of medication determined according to disease diagnosis.

More important, the famous nineteen items on pathogenesis stated in the chapter 74 of *Huang Di Nei Jing Su Wen* have been functioned as concise principles and examples to dominate complicated medical happenings in the clinical practice, which contains the seed of the idea of "Pattern identification and Treatment". Among the 19 items on pathogenesis, some show that the same clinical manifestation(s) may have different pathogenesis, for example, "All spasm and neck rigidity are ascribed to dampness," "All fever with impaired consciousness and convulsion is ascribed to fire," and "All sudden muscular spasm and rigidity is ascribed to wind," which indicates that spasm and convulsion may result from different pathogenic factors: dampness, fire, and wind; while some others demonstrate that different clinical manifestations may share the same pathogenesis, for example, "All cramps, rigidity, and turbid urine are ascribed to heat," "All abdominal distension and fullness is ascribed to heat," and "All acid eructation and spouting diarrhea with urgency for evacuation are ascribed to heat," which indicates that different clinical manifestations such as cramps, turbid urine, ab-

---

237 What kind of disease is Wine Wind? In the chapter 46 of *Huang Di Nei Jing Su Wen* it is stated that
"Huang Di said, 'Someone suffers from the body being hot and sluggish, sweating as if he is taking a bath, aversion to wind and shortness of breath. Which disease is that?'
Qi Bo answered, 'The disease is called wine wind'."

dominal distension, vomiting, diarrhea, etc. may result from the same pathogenic factor: heat.

That *Huang Di Nei Jing* contains the seed of the idea of "Pattern identification and Treatment" also implies in its many other chapters. For example, the chapter 43 entitled "*On Blockage*" of *Huang Di Nei Jing Su Wen* shows that the blockage disease[238] is diagnosed first, and different kinds of blockage disease are further identified according to different pathogenic factors – wind, cold and dampness, different seasons, and different viscera. It reads that

> Huang Di asked, "How does a blockage disease emerge?"
> Qi Bo answered, "When the three pathogenic factors, i.e., wind, cold, and dampness, arrive together, they may interact and cause a blockage disease.
> In case the pathogenic wind predominates, this may cause 'migratory blockage'.
> In case the pathogenic cold predominates, this may cause 'painful blockage'.
> In case the pathogenic dampness predominates, this may cause 'fixed blockage'.
> [Huang] Di asked, "There are five [types] of this [disease]. Why is that?"
> Qi Bo answered, "Encountering these [pathogenic factors] in winter may cause bone blockage.
> Encountering these [pathogenic factors] in spring may cause sinew blockage.
> Encountering these [pathogenic factors] in summer may cause vessel blockage.
> Encountering these [pathogenic factors] in the late summer may cause muscle blockage.
> Encountering these [pathogenic factors] in autumn may cause skin blockage."

Later on Huang Di and Qi Bo discussed how the blockage diseases of the five *zang* organs develop and manifest clinically respectively when these five types of blockage proceed into and lodge in their correlating organs.

238 Blockage disease refers to a diseased state characterized by invasion of the pathogenic factors that cause stagnation of qi and blood and blockage of the meridian vessels.

To sum up, the *Huang Di Nei Jing* or *Huang Di's Inner Classic* stresses the importance of disease diagnosis, which is taken as the major foundation for the treatments, and tailored according to different pathogenic factors.

10.4.3.3 Shang Han Za Bing Lun or On Cold-induced and Miscellaneous Diseases: Treatment Determined Based on Disease Diagnosis and Tailored According to Accompanied Symptoms

The information that Zhang Zhongjing 张仲景 (150-219) developed or established the principle of *Bian Zheng Lun Zhi* 辨证(証)论治 or "Pattern Identification and Treatment" is well known for the circle of Chinese medicine no matter in China or the other parts of the world. But obviously, this is totally wrong for the sinogram "Zheng 証" does not even show up in Zhang Zhongjing's monumental work *Shang Han Za Bing Lun* or *On Cold-induced and Miscellaneous Diseases.*

A comprehensive survey of Zhang Zhongjing's works shows that *Shang Han Lun* or *On Cold-induced Diseases* and *Jin Gui Yao Lue* or *Synopsis of the Golden Chamber* are both chaptered according to *Disease Names* not anything else, e.g. Tai Yang Disease, Yang Ming Disease, Shao Yang Disease, Tai Yin Disease, Shao Yin Disease, Jue Yin Disease, and Cholera in *Shang Han Lun*, Malaria, Apoplexy, Arthralgia, Pulmonary Abscess, Cough, Inspiratory Dyspnea, Dysuria, Edema, Jaundice, etc. and Gynecological Diseases in *Jin Gui Yao Lue*; and that a disease presents clinically with similar chief symptoms; and that a treatment, in most cases, a formula, is prescribed for a disease and is tailored for the same disease but with different accompanied symptoms.

For example, Cinnamon Twig Decoction (Guizhi Decoction) is formulated for a disease named *Tai Yang Zhong Feng* 太阳中风 or Greater Yang Disease·Wind Attack, as the 13th clause reads that "The greater yang disease with manifestations including headache, fever, sweating and aversion to wind is an indication of Cinnamon Twig Decoction," which implies that this is the primary disease of the decoction calling for the original formula; the 14th clause reads that "The greater yang disease with manifestations including stiff and taut neck and back but with sweating and aversion to wind in the meanwhile is an indication of Cinnamon Twig Decoction Plus Pueraria;" the 21st clause reads that "The greater yang disease after purgation with manifestations of skipping pulse and fullness in the chest is an indication of Cinnamon Twig Decoction Minus Peony;" the 22nd clause reads that "(The greater yang disease) with slight chill is an indication of Cinnamon Twig Decoction Minus Peony Plus Aconite." In the above-mentioned clauses except the 13th, the primary manifestations that Cinnamon Twig Decoction aims to relieve remain almost the same, and so does the primary formula. Therefore, therapeutic effects are guaranteed by slightly changing the original formula according to slightly changed manifestations, i.e. tailoring the primary formula by adding pueraria, ephedra or removing peony or removing peony and meanwhile adding aconite.

Practitioners of later generations have elaborated a lot on "treatment determined on the basis of disease diagnosis and tailored according to accompanied symptoms" proposed by Zhang Zhongjin.

Zhu Gong 朱肱 (1150?-1125?) said in his *Lei Zheng* (證) *Huo Ren Shu* or *Book on Systematized Symptoms for Saving Life* that "There are totally 113 formulas in Zhongjing's *On Cold-induced Diseases*. If a disease corresponds to its formula, just use the formula as it is; if differences occur, just modify the formula according to different accompanied symptoms."

Ke Yunbo 柯韵伯 (1662-1735) commented in his *Shang Han Lai Su Ji* or *Collection of Renewal of Cold-induced Diseases* that "Zhongjing's formulas are set for diseases not for meridians. It is his flexible way to apply a formula according to its accompanied symptoms." This comment also indicates that the so-called "Six-Meridian Pattern Identification" is also a later invention not Zhang Zhongjing's original intention.

Xu Dachun 徐大椿 (1693-1771) said in his *Yi Xue Yuan Liu Lun* or *The Origin and Development of Medicine* that "If patients' major sufferings are generally the same but probably with different signs and symptoms, there is no need to construct another formula and the formula formulated for the major symptoms (sufferings) can just be modified according to different accompanied symptoms."

As the part of the titles of all these chapters "病脉證并治" suggests, Zhang Zhongjing's real intention is to diagnose the Disease first, then to institute the treatment according to the specific pulse and the symptom complex of the diagnosing time for a specific individual. The symptom complex or "Zheng 證" means the proof, demonstration, or evidence of a disease, i.e. the manifestations or symptoms of a disease.

10.4.3.4 *Bian Zheng Lun Zhi* or Pattern Identification and Treatment: An Overall Development of the Former Methodologies of Treatment in Chinese Medicine

Before Western medicine transmitted to China, ancient Chinese medical experts tried to summarize the methodology of the treatments in Chinese medicine by using refined words. For example, Zhang Zhongjing 张仲景 (150-219) named it "*Bing Mai Zheng Bing Zhi* 病脉證并治", i.e. "treatment determined based on disease diagnosis and tailored according to pulse and accompanied symptoms"; Zhu Danxi 朱丹溪 (1281-1358) called it "*Mai Yin Zheng Zhi* 脉因證治", i.e. "treatment determined according to pulse, origin, and symptoms"; Zhou Zhigan 周之干 (1508?-1586) summarized it as "*Bian Zheng Shi Zhi* 辨證施治", i.e. "instituting treatment based on symptom identification"; Zhang Jiebin 张介宾 (1563-1640) named it "*Zhen Bing Shi Zhi* 诊病施治", i.e. "instituting treatment based on disease diagnosis"; Qin Jingming 秦景明 (1568-1644) authored an monograph entitled "*Zheng Yin Mai Zhi* 症因脉治", i.e. "treatment determined according to symptoms, origin, and pulse"; Xu Dachun 徐大椿 (1693-1771) named it "*Jian Zheng Shi Zhi* 见症施治", i.e. "instituting treatment based on manifested symptoms"; Zhang Xugu 章虚谷 proposed "*Bian Zheng Lun Zhi* 辨證论治" in 1825, i.e. "instituting treatment based on symptom identification", which actually bears the same meaning as "*Bian Zheng Shi Zhi* 辨證施治" advocted by Zhou Zhigan 周之干 in the 16th century; etc. But obviously, they did not come to an agreement on this point.

The principle of *Bian Zheng Lun Zhi* 辨证(証)论治 or "Pattern Identification and Treatment" advanced by Ren Yingqiu results not only from political influences of Mao Zedong Thought and "dialectics" in philosophy, but also an overall development of the former methodologies of treatment in

239 The sinogram "Zheng 证" is the simplified writing form of the two original complex sinograms: 證 and 証, whose original and extended meanings are different from each other.

Chinese medicine. In other words, *Bian Zheng Lun Zhi* 辨证(証)论治 or "Pattern Identification and Treatment" not only meets the political needs of a specific historical period, but also promotes the all-round development of Chinese medicine in general. Since then, an agreement on how to summarize the methodology of the treatments in Chinese medicine by using refined words has been gradually reached, first nationwide and then worldwide, i.e., *Bian Zheng Lun Zhi* 辨证(証)论治 or "Pattern Identification and Treatment".

Here it is worth to note that history of Western science shows that the development of Western science is also influenced by political and social situations of a specific historical period. For example, *The Structure of Scientific Revolutions* by Thomas S. Kuhn (1922-1996)[240] refutes by referring to the history of physics that scientific development goes in a direct line but goes by jumps, and these jumps are guided by paradigms. For paradigms political and social situations have been influential but not the only reasons. Therefore it is wrong to contend Nicolaus Copernicus (1473-1543) had refuted Claudius Ptolemaeus (100?-170?): The system of Copernicus is based on another paradigm than the system of Ptolemaeus.

10.4.4 Disease, Symptoms and Pattern: The Foundations for Individualized Treatment in Chinese Medicine

The real clinical practice of Chinese medicine in China usually goes along the following procedure:

First, clarifying the chief complaint of the patient, and gathering his/her data by both examination methods of Western medicine and Chinese medicine;

Second, diagnosing the disease in Western medicine and Chinese medicine respectively;

Third, identifying the pattern for the patient and formulating treating principles;

Fourth, determining a basic formula, which may need to be tailored according to accompanied symptoms. Under certain conditions where the

240 Kuhn, Thomas S. *The Structure of Scientific Revolutions* [M]. 2nd Revised edition. Chicago: University of Chicago Press, 1970.

chief complaint of the patient is too serious or too emergent, the chief complaint should be relieved first. That is to say, the prescription for the patient should embody the principle of "In emergency cases treat the acute symptoms, and in non-acute cases treat the root of the disease."

It is worth to note that leading experts in Chinese medicine and/or integrative medicine have advocated and expounded for years from different perspectives that treatment should be determined based on disease diagnosis in Western (or Chinese) medicine and pattern identification in Chinese medicine.[241]

Based on the linguistic conceptual analysis and textual research of "*Zheng* 证（證; 証）" and "*Bian Zheng* 辨证", What Zhang Zhongjing really proposed is clarified, i.e. treatment determined based on disease diagnosis and tailored according to accompanied symptoms, which has functioned as the guideline for clinical practice in the last thousands of years. Ren Yingqiu invented the concept "*Zheng* 证" and the principle "*Bian Zheng Lun Zhi* 辨证论治" by distorting Zhang Zhongjing's academic ideas, which came out from the political influences and directly from "dialectics" in philosophy. This conceptual enlargement of "*Bian Zheng* 辨证" came out for the purpose of emphasizing the differences between Chinese medicine and Western medicine: Chinese medicine relieves diseases from their roots while Western medicine relieves just symptoms.

To sum up, Individualized treatment is one of the greatest advantages of Chinese medicine. If it is can be understood and explained on the theoretical level – not only demonstrated by practices, a problem in basic theory must be solved: this basic characteristics of Chinese medicine as individualized treatment needs that disease diagnosing, pattern identifying, and symptom considering function together. In the other case there would be a conceptual gap which makes the individualized treatment just an outcome of the doctor's intuition.

241 Liu Ping, Ji Guang, et al. 2010 (6): 565-570; Chen Keji. 2011(8): 1016-1017; Wang TW. 2011(8): 1025-1026.

Chinese medicine needs to be developed and modernized in the way it was formed rather than to be westernized in accordance with Western scientific methods and criteria.

- The Author

11 Metaphorizing: A Vital Way to Develop and Modernize Chinese Medicine

As we know now that the theories of *qi*, yin-yang, five phases, visceral manifestation (*zang xiang*), vessels (*jing luo*) and Chinese herbal medicine, the fundamental theories of Chinese medicine, were mainly formed by means of metaphorizing or *Qu Xiang Bi Lei*, and Chinese medicine has been mainly developed also in this way, and thus sharing the same unique Chinese cultural and philosophical background. They are not discovered or detected by the modern Western scientific technology or methods, so their origin and essence cannot be revealed by Western scientific way, either. They can be only understood by means of interpreting metaphors.

In the recent years, a famous research on acupuncture was done in Germany. Assurance companies in Germany wanted to know if acupuncture is really effective in treating some diseases, such as the low back pain, migraine, and headache in the sense of science, of course, the Western science, and so they sponsored a series of studies on the effect of acupuncture. This was a huge research project which had lasted some years and used many millions of Euros.[242, 243, 244, 245] They grouped patients into 3. The first group was treated by conventional therapy, pills of Western Medicine or put into the waiting list control; the second group was treated by real acupuncture given by German acupuncture experts; and the third group was treated by sham acupuncture, superficial needling at non-acupuncture points. The results were in every aspect funny. Firstly, Western medicine or conventional therapy or waiting list control was worse than acupuncture treatment group

242 Klaus Linde, Andrea Streng, Susanne Jurgens, et al. 2005, 293: 2118-2125.

243 Dieter Melchart, Andrea Streng, Andrea Hoppe, et al. 2005, 331 (8): 376-382.

244 Michael Haake, Hans-Helge Muller, Carmen Schade-Brittinger, et al. 2007, 167 (17):1892-1898.

245 Klaus Linde, Claudia M. Witt, Andrea Streng, et al. 2007, 128 (3): 264-271.

for the low back pain, tension-type headache and migraine; secondly, the sham acupuncture group had almost the same effect as the real acupuncture.

Can we draw a conclusion that acupuncture theories are all nonsense? Can acupuncture and Chinese herbal medicine be treated and researched in the same way as Western drugs? Of course not. The pure objective therapeutic effects have never been possible in the acupuncture treatment because mind-regulating has been attached great significance for both the patient and practitioner from the very beginning of acupuncture treatment.

Modernization of Chinese medicine has been a hot issue for dozens of years. The problem now is how to modernize but not westernize Chinese medicine. Therefore first it is essential to regard the differences between Chinese medicine and Western medicine, and the advantages of Chinese medicine as well. I advocate that there are no ranking but just different cultures, and that all cultures and sciences should be treated on an equal footing.

In Chinese medicine, *Qu Xiang Bi Lei* or Taking Image and Analogizing, the metaphorizing process, not only states, constructs its theoretical system, guides its clinical practice, but is also a vital way to develop the system. Chinese medical experts are good at taking image and analogizing, and applying metaphorizing to make new explorations so as to develop Chinese medicine. See *2.2.3.3 Making New Explorations* for details.

Metaphorizing is also a vital approach to modernize Chinese medicine – to develop and modernize in the way how it was formed and has developed in the past thousands of years. Here I give you some examples.

11.1 Metaphorizing: Pattern Identification based on Microcosmic Findings

Identifying pattern and instituting treatment is a major feature of Chinese clinical medicine. "Pattern Identification based on Microcosmic Findings" refers to a method of identifying pattern by using microcosmic findings gained through modern science and technology such as gastroscopy and ultrasound techniques but guided by Chinese medical theories.[246] For example, the color and state of the gastric mucusa can be seen through gastroscopy, so the light color usually indicates deficiency of *Qi* and blood; congestion and

246 See Xue Feifei. The Emergence and Development of Pattern Identification based on Microcosmic Findings [D]. Beijing University of Chinese Medicine, 2006.

edema indicate the pattern being heat; the gastric mucusa in red and white check with submucous blood vessels visible indicates *qi* deficiency and blood stasis.

11.2 Metaphorizing: Discovery and Application of Effects of Tripterygium Wilfrodis

Li Leishi[247] discovered for the first time the therapeutic effect of Tripterygium Wilfrodis (*Lei Gong Ten,* 雷公藤) in treating various chronic nephritis, lupus nephritis, and purpuric nephritis, and spread it to the whole country through metaphorizing its immunosuppressive action in taking effect in treating nephritis and allergic dermatological diseases.

11.3 Metaphorizing: A Vital Way to Reveal Essence of Patterns

Zheng 证 or Pattern is a specific and significant concept in Chinese medicine. Actually, both acupuncture and herbal treatments are based on pattern understanding and identifying. That is to say, prescriptions of both acupoints and medicinal agents should be formulated according to the same procedure: *Li* or Theory – *Fa* or Method – *Fang* or Prescription – *Yao* or Agents (acupoints or herbs), a thinking way of the comprehensive application of Chinese medical theories, diagnosing and treating methods in the clinical practice. Therefore revealing the essence of the common patterns of acupuncture and herbal treatments bears both theoretical and practical significance.

Studies on essence of patterns of Chinese medicine are usually performed by the reductionist and analytic approach with Western scientific methods, i.e. interpreting patterns of Chinese medicine with modern science. This approach has been very fruitful in these years, and is also very important. For example, the pattern of Yin Deficiency can be interpreted by lab indexes of endocrine system, blood system, energy metabolism, cyclic nucleotide, trace elements, blood lipid, etc., and the research outcome can provide a foundation for further studies on its possible causes and pathogenesis as well as prevention and treatment of related diseases in Western medicine.

247 Li Leishi. 1998, 18 (12):707.

But how do we deal with these data and go one step further? My answer is to trace back to the source of a pattern, to investigate how this pattern was formed in Chinese medicine, and analyze the data in the way of metaphorizing, and then try to take metaphorizing as the philosophical approach to do the research. For example, inflammation is a pathological condition in Western medicine, manifesting in local redness, swelling, pain, ulcer and dysfunction as well as fever of different degrees, leukocytosis, fatigue, poor appetite, and so on, which is usually treated by antibiotics; While inflammation in Chinese medicine can be generally identified as fire - excessive fire which connects with heat, damp, phlegm, *qi* stagnation, or blood stasis, and deficient fire which connects with yin deficiency, and thus accordingly the fire can be relieved or reduced by different methods – clearing heat, eliminating dampness, resolving phlegm, freeing *qi*, promoting the flow of blood, or supplementing yin, which can be achieved with acupuncture or herbal prescriptions. In this case fire is the key metaphor, which runs through the aspects from the theoretical understanding of inflammation to its clinical treatment. The modern research can also take this point of view into consideration – fire as the central metaphor, and try to reveal the essence of fire of different kinds and their relationship to different inflammations in Western medicine. To sum up, metaphorizing is a vital way to reveal essence of patterns of Chinese medicine.

11.4 Metaphorizing: Philosophical Examinations of Treatments of Cancer

Of all major diseases that afflict us today, perhaps the most feared, and in many ways the most mysterious, is cancer. Cancer has become an increasingly prominent and feared cause of death. In modern Western medicine, the treatments of cancer can be generally classified into three forms, surgery, radiotherapy, and chemotherapy. Surgery is effective when the primary tumor has not begun to invade the tissue around it; Radiotherapy and chemotherapy are supposed to inhibit, kill the malignant cells, and/or increase the body resistance to the tumor cells. Such approaches achieve success in some cases, but at the same time produce serious side effects. Some patients did not die of cancer but died of radiotherapy or/and chemotherapy.

Based on the principle of comprehensive treatments and the care of the well-being of the cancer patient, Chinese medicine cannot be ignored when concerning the treatment of cancer, esp. for patients who have just undergone a surgical operation, or whose cancer is in the late stage or where metastasis happens. A lot of successful cases reported in China have shown that Chinese medicine can make the active malignant cells rest, thus making a tumor patient live with the tumor, or we could say, live in harmony with the tumor. Chinese medicine takes the being as a whole, cares the relationship among the phonomena and events that happen to the being at the same time, and activates the self-healing and self-organizing power of the being.

Here I propose this topic - How to Deal with Tumor: Killing, Inhibiting, or Living in Harmony with it? Killing and inhibiting are approaches of allopathic medicine, i.e. Western medicine. Then how can a human being live in harmony with tumor? Chinese herbal medicine and acupuncture can work as coordinators to coordinate, harmonize the relationship between the normal cells and the malignant cells. Whether coordinators are efficient or not hinges on the qualification of the practitioner, the patient's condition, and the relationship between the doctor and the patient, etc. The therapeutic effects reflect in several aspects, such as the life quality of tumor patients being improved, the survival rate being raised, and the survival time being lengthened, etc.

Please don't misunderstand me! I do not let you give up the Western approaches to tumor treatments; I just propose to combine (or integrate if possible) the available treating methods, such as surgical operation, radiotherapy, chemotherapy, acupuncture, moxibustion, and Chinese herbal medicine, in a proper way so as to benefit tumor patients as much as possible.

Besides, there are some other examples to show the importance of metaphor thinking in developing and modernizing Chinese medicine, such as:

"Healthy Qi", "Immunity", and pharmacological effects of "Qi-Tonifying" agents: Huang Di's Inner Classic states that "If the Healthy *Qi* resides inside the body, then the pathogenic factors cannot find a way to invade it." Modern research results read that *Qi*-Tonifying agents such as Huangqi or Radix Astragalus can improve both the humoral and cellular immunity, strengthen leukocyte's phagocytic power, and increase the ratio of T cell and lymphocyte's transformation rate.

"The lungs stand interior-exterior relationship with the large intestine": This is clearly stated in the *Huang Di's Inner Classic*. In the clinical practice, patients with serious dysfunction of the intestinal tract are always accompanied by acute respiratory failure or adult respiratory distress syndrome (RDS); Pathological anatomical studies on dead bodies with lung diseases

show that the large intestine and the small intestine are both seriously aerated, the mucous layer of the small intestine is necrotic with ulceration; Experimental studies with rabbits or rats as the objects demonstrate that ischemic dysfunction of intestinal tract is the underlying cause for damage of the lungs and that relieving constipation relates to transformation of the lung tissue from the abnormal pathological changes to the normal.

Multi-disciplinary approaches to "the kidneys opening into the ears": "The kidneys open into the ears" is also stated in the *Huang Di's Inner Classic*. In the clinical practice, Kidney-Supplementing method can achieve satisfactory therapeutic effect in treating tinnitus and deafness; A series of studies have proved the relationship between the kidneys and the ears from the aspects of adrenocortical hormone (ACH), thyroid hormone and the effects of Kidney-Supplementing medicinal agents in treating tinnitus and deafness by applying modern physiological, morphological, histochemical, and pharmacological methods; Research results also suggest that applying Kidney-Supplementing method to treat toxic deafness caused by ototoxic diuretics, gentamicin, and kanamycin is a quite satisfactory method, which also provides new theoretical and clinical evidence for treating deafness with this method.

I would like to finish this book with this quotation from the Chapter 25 of *Lao Tzu*:

> "Therefore, Dao is great.
> Heaven is great.
> Earth is great.
> Man is great.
> In the world, there are four great things, and man is one of them.
> Man abides by the earth.
> Earth abides by the heaven.
> Heaven abides by Dao.
> Dao abides by the nature."

Metaphorizing bridges Dao (The Way) of the Nature and Medicine. "Heaven", "Earth", and "Man" compose a whole system; In *Lao Tzu*, Dao abides by the nature; In the *Huang Di's Inner Classic*, medicine abides by the Dao; In essence, medicine abides by the nature. That is the way of seeing, thinking and working of Chinese medicine.

Transmitting Chinese medicine in the West began in the 17th century, originating from the real therapeutic effects of Chinese medical therapies, namely the transmission of "Skills", such as pulse taking & reading skills, moxibustion treatment for gout, acupuncture treatment for arthritis, translation of Chinese herbal medicine (such as *Ben Cao Gang Mu* or *The Compendium of Materia Medica* 《本草纲目》) and forensic medicine (such as *Xi Yuan Lu* or *Records for Washing Away Injustice* 《洗冤录》), etc. In the 20th century "the craze for acupuncture" and "the craze for Chinese medicine" in the West are also closely related to the success of acupuncture anesthesia in the Mainland China. Chinese medicine is now spreading at an unprecedented speed, scale and depth in the West after several rises and falls in the last more than 300 years. Transmission of "Way" or its philosophical foundations, in addition to "Skills", is also a need and choice of the era when reflecting on the advantages and disadvantages of modern science and Western Medicine.

- The Author

Epilogue

Transmitting Trend of Chinese Medicine in the West: From Skills to Way

The exchange and transmission of Chinese medicine in the West started in the 17th century (Ming dynasty, 1368-1644). The earliest introductions of Chinese medicine to the West come from missionaries, who introduced their own experiences with Chinese medicine in China to the West with curiosity. Matteo Ricci (1552-1610), a celebrated Italian missionary, arrived in Macau in 1582, and then opened the prologue to the first large scaled cultural exchange between China and Europe in the world's history. One of the earliest introductions of Chinese medicine to the West is from *Matteo Ricci's Reading Notes:*

Medical skills and methods in China were very different from those we were accustomed to. The pulse-taking methods were the same as ours, and practitioners were quite successful in treating diseases. Generally speaking, the medicinal substances they used were very simple such as grasses, roots, stalks and the like. In fact, the Chinese art of healing was all contained in the laws and rules they observed when using the herbal substances. There were no public medical schools here in China. Everyone who wanted to be a practitioner should be taught by another one who was proficient in the way of healing. It was possible to get a degree in medicine by passing a test held by Imperial Hospitals in Nanjing and Beijing, the two capitals of the Ming Dynasty. But it was just a form, could not bring any benefit to those with it. A practitioner with a medical degree was not more authoritative nor more respected than one without the degree because anyone was allowed to practice medicine no matter he/she was good at the art of healing or not. [248]

Michel-Pierre Boym (1612-1659), a Polish missionary from Jesuit to China in the 17th century, is another pioneer who made outstanding contributions to the transmission of Chinese medicine in the West following Matteo Ricci.

1 Materia Medica, Pulse Lore, Acupuncture and Moxibustion (1656-1849)

1.1 Michel-Pierre Boym's Contributions to Transmission of Chinese Materia Medica and Pulse Lore in Europe

Michel-Pierre Boym served as the chief physician of Polish king Sigismond. He paid attention to Chinese materia medica during his mission in China and wrote "*Flora Sinensis*" in Latin, which is actually an abridged Latin translation of "*Ben Cao Gang Mu* or *The Compendium of Materia Medica* 《本草纲目》". It is the earliest literature on Chinese herbal medicine which was introduced to the West and was published in Vienna in 1656; in 1664 the book was translated into French and got published as well. He also compiled *Clavis Medica ad Chinarum Doctrinam de Pulsibus*, a truly comprehensive presentation of Chinese medicine, including six parts: Latin translation of "*Mai Jing* or *The Pulse Classic*" by Wang Shuhe (王叔和, 201-280) , diagnosis by observing the tongue and complexion, names of 289 Chinese medicinal items, 143 pieces of wood layout and 30 pieces of copper layout of medicinal substances. The book was published in 1680 in Frankfurt, Germany (Latin).

The book was renamed *Specimen Medicinae Sinicae* and was published in 1682 in Frankfurt in the name of Cleyer de Cassel with 68 illustrations of meridians and viscera as the appendix at the end of the book since there were enmities between the Jesuit and the Dutch East India Company (Vereenig

248 Translated from Chinese. Originally by Ricci Matteo. Translated by He Gaoji, Wang Zunzhong, Li Shen. 1983: 34.

de Oostindische Compagnie, abbreviated as VOC). Michel-Pierre Boym's name was resumed until 1686 when the original version was published. Medicus Sinensis, one of the Michel-Pierre Boym's unpublished manuscripts, may be lost. It is worth mentioning that Michel-Pierre Boym's works of introducing Chinese medicine had a far-reaching influence in Europe, parts of which were translated into French, Italian, English, etc. For example, in 1707, John Floyer (1649-1734), a British doctor, compiled and published *The Physician's Pulse-watch* by combining the English version of Michel-Pierre Boym's manuscripts of Chinese pulse lore with his own papers, which is the earliest English work on pulse lore.[249] All in all, the works of Michel-Pierre Boym attracted the attention of western scholars and inspired them to study Chinese medicine.

1.2 Early Introduction of Acupuncture and Moxibustion to Europe by Rhyne and Busschof

Chinese acupuncture and moxibustion are time-honoured therapies. Acupuncture originated from needling with healing stones while moxibustion came from cauterization or fire/heat burning. In the middle of the 17th century, acupuncture and moxibustion were introduced into Europe through Japan. Moxibustion was transmitted into Europe earlier than acupuncture. According to the authors' study, Treatise of the Gout authored by Herman Busschof (dates unknown) and published in 1676 in London is the first English work on Chinese medicine. Busschof, a staff of the Dutch East India Company, had suffered from gout with the symptom of pain in feet for 14 years in Indonesia, was cured by moxibustion. Therefore he compiled a book in Dutch (1675, Amsterdam) to introduce how to treat gout with moxibustion. The book was translated into English in 1676 from Dutch (See Illus. 21)250. Busschof created the word "moxibustion" to express "ai jiu 艾灸" by combing "mugusa", from Japanese "*moe kusa*", meaning "burning herbs", and "-bustion", the contracted form of the Latin word "combustio", "combustion" in English.

---

249 Ma Boying, Gao Xi, Hong Zhongli, 1993: 605; Li Xisuo, Chen Shangsheng, 2002: 425-426.
250 Wong, Chinmin K. & Fu Weikang, 1963: 28.

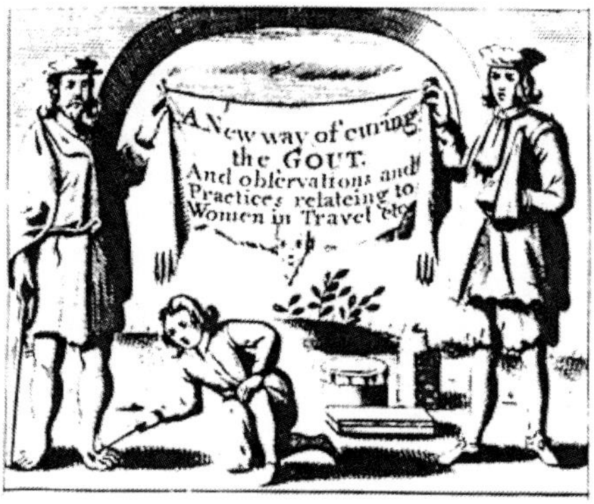

Illus. 21. Frontispiece of *Treatise of the Gout* by Herman Busschof (1676)

In 1683, Willem Ten Rhyne (1647-1700), another staff of Dutch East India Company, who graduated from the Medical School of Leiden University in Holland, published *Dissertatio de Arthritide: Mantissa Schematica:De Acupunctura*. It is the first literature of systematically introducing acupuncture to Europe although it is not the first literature of mentioning acupuncture in a Western language. Willem Ten Rhyne thus became the first person to transmit acupuncture to the West. The English word "acupuncture" used today is from the Latin word "acupunctura (acu + punctura)" he created in the book. In the book there are four charts of acupuncture points he got from Japan, of which two are the originals of China and the other two were drawn by Japanese. Rhyne introduced the names, meanings and distributions of the fourteen meridians in details. The Illus. 22 – a chart of acupuncture points is from Willem ten Rhyne's *Dissertatio de Arthritide* (London: Impensis R. Chiswell, 1683; Picture source: Wellcome Library, London).

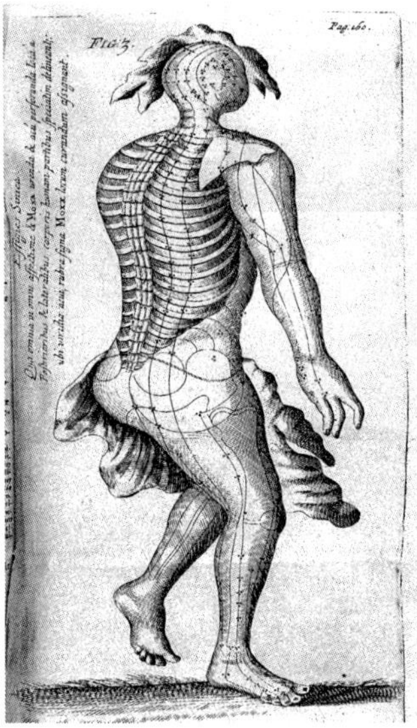

Illus. 22. Chart of Acupuncture Points from
Willem Ten Rhigne's *Dissertatio de Arthritide*

"Acupuncture and Moxibustion" have been in use ever since they were created in the 17th century, which are a pair of truly standardized translation in English Chinese medical terminology and are also a pair of medical subject headings of MEDLARS (Medical Literature Analysis and Retrieval System).

1.3 Early Translations of Chinese Medical Classics in *The General History of China*

In 1735, France published a big book on China -*Description de l' Empire de la Chine,* which is based on reports of missionaries to China in the 17th century, known as one of the "three masterpieces"[251] of European Sinology in the 18th century, the important literature and book for Europeans to understand China and its medicine. Wong, Chinmin K. in a paper entitled *Investigations of Western-Language Translations of Chinese Medical Classics* men-

251 The other two are *Jesuit Communications Set* and *Chinese Miscellaneous Essays.* All published in France.

tioned this book by referring that "*A Geographical, Historical, Chronological, Political, and Physical Description of the Empire of China* written by a Frenchman named Jean-Baptiste Du Halde was published in Paris in 1735."[252]

Jean-Baptiste Du Halde (1674-1743) was a missionary of Jesuit in Paris. The book attracted the attention of British publishers immediately after it was published in France and the English version was published in the following year 1736, namely Watts J. Edition. After the first printing, it was successively reprinted in 1739 and 1740 in four volumes. The Illus. 23 is the front cover of the fourth volume of its second English Watts J. Edition. From the cover we can see how lengthy its English title is: *The General History of China: Containing a Geographical, Historical, Chronological, Political, and Physical Description of the Empire of China, Chinese-Tartar, Korea and Tibet.* Two volumes of a complete translation were published successively in 1738 and 1742, namely Cave E. edition.

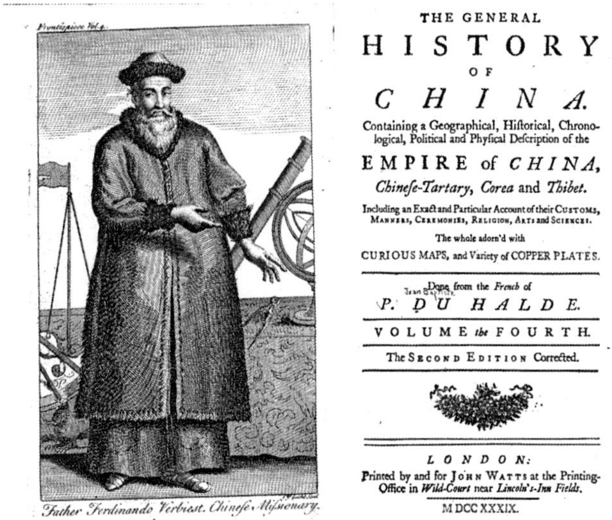

Illus. 23. Front Cover of the Fourth Volume
of the Second English Watts J. Edition of *The General History of China*

252 Wong, Chinmin K., 1928: 103-105.

Concerning the part of Chinese medicine in *The General History of China,* Huang Qichen 黄启臣 proposed according to his studies that its third volume was about Chinese medicine, which introduced unique Chinese medical skills, including translation of *Mai Jing* or *The Pulse Classic* 《脉经》, *Mai Jue* or *The Pulse Lore in Rhyme* 《脉诀》, *Bencao Gangmu* or *The Compendium of Materia Medica* 《本草纲目》, *Shennong Bencao Jing* or *Shennong's Classic of Materia Medica* 《神农本草经》, *Mingyi Bielu* or *Records of Famous Physicians* 《名医必录》(《名医别录》), *Yiyao Huilu* or *Collection and Records of Medicine* 《医药汇录》 and many Chinese medical prescriptions.[253]

On the basis of studies on contents related to Chinese medicine in the English Cave E. edition of The General History of China, Wong, Chinmin K. held that the book contains pulse theory, medicinal substances and prescriptions, and health protection, among which *Mai Jue* or *The Pulse Lore in Rhyme* 《脉诀》 by Gao Yangsheng (高阳生, dates unkown), the earliest complete English translation of Chinese medical classic in the West, is on the pulse theory; medicinal substances and prescriptions refer to translation of some volumes of *Bencao Gangmu* or *The Compendium of Materia Medica* 《本草纲目》 by Li Shizhen (李时珍, 1518-1593), its first English abridged version; as for health protection, the transliteration of the book title resembles *Changsheng or Longevity* 《长生》or *Zunsheng or Respecting Life* 《遵生》 or the like, but the contents are different from each other.[254]

From the above we can draw a conclusion that the earliest English translation of Chinese medical classics originates from the part of Chinese medicine of the English edition of *The General History of China.* Since then there was a great upsurge in learning and studying Chinese medicine among Europeans, exerting a profound impact on modern medicine, zoology, botany and doctrine of evolution in the Western Europe.

253 Huang Qichen, 1992: 54-62.

254 Qiu Le, 2011: 459-464.

1.4 Influences of *Bencao Gangmu* in Europe

In 1812, Jean-Pierre Abel-Rémusat (1788-1832), a French scholar, published his M.D. (Doctorate in Medicine) dissertation on *Bencao Gangmu* or *The Compendium of Materia Medica* 《本草纲目》; later on, both of his books *Dissertaio de Glosso-semeiotice, rive de signis morborum quae e lingua sumuntur, praesertim apud Sinenses* (1813) and *Recherches historiques sui la medicine des Chinois, etc* (1813) did further studies and gave further introductions to *Bencao Gangmu*, and thus promoting its spread in Europe.

Missionaries felt incredible that Chinese herbal medicine can cure many diseases, but its effectiveness is after all a fact. So they studied Chinese herbal medicine and associated them with botany, thus promoting the further development of botany in Europe.

Charles Robert Darwin (1809-1882), a great British biologist, quoted some information about the formation of colors of goldfishes from *Bencao Gangmu* to illustrate that animals have artificial selection problems in his book *The Descent of Man*. Besides, he repeatedly referred to *Bencao Gangmu* in the second chapter *Artificial Selection* of his another book *The Variation of Animals and Plants under Domestication.* According to the statistics, there are as much as 104 places mentioning herbal medicine and Chinese medicine in the works by Darwin.[255] This shows that Chinese medicine and Chinese herbal medicine also have a considerable impact on Darwin's doctrine of evolution.

1.5 Contributions from Other Missionaries to China

In addition, Dominicus Parrenin (1665-1741), a French Jesuit, had also made outstanding contributions to transmitting Chinese medicine to Europe. He made a scientific appraisal about Chinese medicine that Chinese medicine is significantly effective in treating some diseases, but is not as good as Western medicine in theory, esp. the lagging behind of anatomy. This conclusion was later accepted by Voltaire (1694-1778). In his work *Essai Sur Les Moeurs*, he discussed Chinese medicine, "In China, medical theories still remain igno-

255 Pan Jixing, 1954; 1959: 521-525.

rant and wrong, but Chinese practitioners are quite successful in their practices."[256]

Dominicus Parrenin also sent materials about how to treat tuberculosis with Donkey-hide gelatin (Ejiao, 阿胶) to the French Academy of Science from Macau. In the *Report from Beijing Missionaries* he picked up *Xi Yuan Lu* or *Records for Washing Away Injustice* 《洗冤录》 as the world's first work on forensic medicine. In the fourth volume of *Report from Beijing Missionaries*, Pierre Martial Cibot (1727-1780) also introduced Chinese understanding of the pathology of smallpox and methods of how to treat it in China. Since then, Chinese medicine esp. medical skills became popular in Europe.

1.6 General Features of the Translations on Chinese Medicine

During this period, translators were all Europeans, among which some of them were staff of Dutch East India Company and most of them were European missionaries in China. Translation contents are mostly their own experiences in Chinese medicine, or overviews of Chinese medicine, or related to acupuncture and moxibustion, or history of Chinese medicine, or herbal medicine, or pulse lore, etc. Besides, English translations of *Mai Jue* or *The Pulse Lore in Rhyme* and *Bencao Gangmu* or *The Compendium of Materia Medica* were also published and they were included in *The General History of China.*

As for the translation form, it involves abridged, edited and full translations; as for the translation strategy, it involves foreignization and domestication, among which foreignization reflects that early compilers or translators of English translations of Chinese medicine accepted and respected the uniqueness of Chinese culture; as for translation methods, transliterations or Chinese characters (or sinograms) were used to translate most of the culturally-loaded terms in Chinese medicine, on the basis of which literal translations, free translations and paraphrases were flexibly combined with them when Latin translations were retained in the meanwhile.

256 Voltaire, 1963: 398.

2 Translation and Transmission of Chinese Medical Classics in Europe (1850-1950)

Places of publication of Chinese medical works in English were expanded from London, Britain to Beijing, Tianjin, Shanghai, Guangdong in China, and Baltimore, Philadelphia, in the United States, etc. During this stage, the initial stage of translating Chinese medical classics, *Xi Yuan Lu* or *Records for Washing Away Injustice*《洗冤录》(1855, 1875-1924), *Huangdi Neijing* or *Huangdi's Inner Classic*《黄帝内经》(1949, 1950), *Bencao Gangmu* or *The Compendium of Materia Medica* 《本草纲目》(1871-1941), *Jiuhuang Bencao* or *Materia Medica as Famine Food*《救荒本草》(1946), etc. were partly translated into English. As for the translation form, it involves abridged, selected, and edited translations, but none of them are full translations.

2.1 Translation and Transmission of *Xi Yuan Lu*

Xi Yuan Lu or *Records for Washing Away Injustice*《洗冤录》 written in 1247 by Song Ci (宋慈, 1186-1249), an official in the Southern Song Dynasty (1127-1279), is the first relatively complete monograph on forensic medicine in China and in the world as well – it has a great influence on the history of the world forensic medicine. Its contents are substantially rich, reflecting the abundant accumulation of knowledge and practical experiences in pathology, anatomy, pharmacology, surgery, orthopedics, and laboratory tests, etc., and showing an advanced level in technology and experiences. The book has a high scientific value," and "has once been translated into Dutch, English, French, German, Korean, and Japanese languages, etc."[257]

It was first transmitted to Korea, Japan, and then to Europe since its coming out: In 1779, *Chinese Journal of History, Art and Science* first published its abridged translation in Paris, France; In 1882, Ern Martin, a French doctor, published a thesis on its summary in *Far Eastern Review;* In 1908, a separate edition of its French translation was officially published; In June of 1853, "*Royal Asiatic Society Newspaper*" of Britain published Dr. W.A. Harland's thesis (M.D.) – *Collected Evidences* of *Records for Washing Away Injustice;* In 1875, the translation by Dr. H.A. Giles[258], a sinologist of Cam-

257 Xia Zhengnong, 2002: 1827.

258 Giles, H.A. (Herbert Allen Giles, 1845-1935), Chinese name: 翟理斯, British, a

bridge University, was published in instalments in *The China Review;* In 1924, *The Journal of the Royal Society of Medicine* reprinted the book and then its separate edition was published afterwards.

We can say that two English translations of *Xi Yuan Lu* 《洗冤录》 were got published during this stage: one published in Hong Kong: Harland, W. A. *Notice of a Chinese Work on Medical Jurisprudence*, entitled *Se Yuen Luh*, or "*Records of the Washing away of Injuries*". Hongkong, 1855; the other published in London: Giles, H.A. *The "His Yuan Lu"* or *"Instructions to Coroners"*. London: John Bale, Sons & Danielsson, 1924.

As for the second translation, Wong, Chinmin K. introduced it in his paper *Investigations of Western-language Translations of Chinese Medical Classics* like this: "It was translated by Dr. H.A. Giles, a famous scholar in Oriental Culture of Cambridge University. Giles previously served as a consul to China. When he was in Ningbo in 1873, he saw autopsies by administrative officers, who always carried *Xi Yuan Lu* or *Instructions to Coroners* in hand, which arouse his interests to study and translate it." In his view, "The wording is smooth and clear" and "The approach is correct and proper."[259]

In addition, a Dutch translation by Degrijs, a Dutch man, was published in Batavia in 1863; and a German version translated from a French translation by Hoffmann was published in 1908.

2.2 Translation and Transmission of *Huangdi Neijing*

Three English translations of *Huangdi Neijing* 《黄帝内经》 came out in this period.

The first one is from Dawson, Percy. M., who published a thesis to introduce *Huangdi's Inner Classic · Basic Questions* in *Annals of Medical History* in 1925;

The second is from Ms. Ilza Veith, a PhD candidate at Institute of History of Medicine of Johns Hopkins University at that time, who translated the first 34 chapters of *Huangdi Neijing· Su Wen* into English based on the manuscripts from an organic chemist J.W. Lindau with a large space to introduce Chinese medicine along with the translation: Veith, Ilza. *The Yellow Emperor's Classic of Internal Medicine*. Baltimore: The Williams & Wilkins Co., 1949;

---

famous Sinologist, the second professor in Sinology of Cambridge University.

259 Wong, Chinmin K., 1928: 103-105.

The third is from Dr. Huang Wen 黄雯, who translated an important part of *Huangdi's Inner Classic* into English along with comments and annotations and got it published as a separate edition: Wong, W. *Nei Ching, the Chinese Canon of Medicine*. Reprint from the Chinese Medical Journal – Special Medical History Number, V. 68. No.1 & 2. Shanghai, 1950.

2.3 Translation and Transmission of *Bencao Gangmu*

The translation of *Bencao Gangmu* 《本草纲目》 has always been a hot spot since its coming out. After Michel-Pierre Boym's (1612-1659) edited translation in Latin - *Flora Sinensis*, which is actually an abridged translation of *Bencao Gangmu*, there are still some other translations:

1. Smith, F. P. *Contribution towards the Materia Medica and Natural History of China*. Shanghai: American Presbyterian Mission Press, 1871. The book has thousands of herbs, mostly from *Bencao Gangmu*.

2. Stuart, G. A. *Chinese Materia Medica · Vegetable Kingdom* (Extensively revised from Dr. F. Porter Smith's Work). Shanghai: Presbyterian Mission Press, 1911. Its contents are roughly from the herbs in the volumes 12 to 37 of *Bencao Gangmu* and is arranged in Latin alphabetical order, with three indexes of Chinese, English and botanical names, which is convenient to review and check. [260]

3. Read, B. E. & Pak, C. *The Pen Ts'ao Minerals and Stones*, Peking: Peking Society Natural History Bulletin, 1928;

Read, B.E. *Chinese Materia Medica · Animal Drugs*, 1931; *Chinese Materia Medica · Avian Drugs* 1932; *Chinese Materia Medica · Dragon and Snake Drugs*, 1933; *Chinese Materia Medica · Turtle and Shellfish Drugs*, 1937; *Chinese Materia Medica ·Fish Drugs*, 1939; *Chinese Materia Medica · Insect Drugs*, 1941. Peiping: The French Book Store.

Read, B. E., with a full name of Bernard Emms Read (1887-1949) and a Chinese name of 伊博恩, a British missionary to China, was a pharmacologist and a pioneer in Chinese pharmacology research.[261] He successively translated and published the parts of *Minerals and Stones*, *Animal Drugs*, *Avian Drugs*, *Dragon and Snake Drugs*, *Turtle and Shellfish Drugs*, *Fish Drugs*,

---

260 Wong, Chinmin K., 1935: 1167-1170.
261 Zhao Jimeng, 2012.

Insect Drugs, etc. of the *Bencao Gangmu* on the basis of the translation from Mills R., an American, between 1928 to 1941, namely the volumes from 8th to 37th and the volumes from 39th to 52nd, altogether 44 volumes, accounting for 86% of the book. Among the 44 translated volumes, except the part of *Minerals and Stones* from a joint translation with Pak, C., all the other parts were translated by himself. In the process of translation, Read identified the scientific names of herbs listed in the *Bencao Gangmu* as many as possible, stated effective ingredients and gave explanations according to Chinese and foreign references with an appendix of indexes with Chinese and foreign names of medicinal items. Many scholars and many works studied his translation. A widely-accepted evaluation about it is that the translation faithfully conveys the essence of the original, has a greater influence than most of the other English versions, and is a masterpiece for a full translation and further research on *Bencao Gangmu*.

Besides, French and German translations of *Bencao Gangmu* were got published as well.

It is worth noting that besides of translating *Bencao Gangmu*, Read also translated a part of the *Jiuhuang Bencao*《救荒本草》compiled by Zhu Di 朱棣 (1360-1424), the third emperor of the Ming Dynasty (1368-1644). There are 414 species of herbal plants in the translation, which was published in 1946 in Shanghai: Read, B.E. *Famine Food listed in the Chiu Huang Pen Ts'ao*. Shanghai: Henry Lester Institute of Medical Research, 1946.

3 Overall Translation of Chinese Medicine (1951-1991)

This is a period of overall translation of Chinese medicine. The contents of translation cover almost every aspect of Chinese medicine from its theories to skills, involving acupuncture and moxibustion, Chinese herbal medicine, basic theories, clinical medicine, and Chinese medical classics, etc.

In the years from 1956 to 1960, Chinese government established 20 colleges of Chinese medicine, which showed that, in addition to maintaining the traditional methods of transmitting Chinese medicine – "secret transmission" and "individual transmission", Chinese medicine was transmitted on a large scale in China mainly through a westernized, modernized, and professionalized mode, i.e. "the standardized mode of transmission".

Then it came into the 1970s. A historical fact needs to be clarified: People of all circles in America have always thought that the public awareness of acupuncture and moxibustion was aroused because of James Reston

(1909-1995)'s reports about his experiences during his visit in China with the former U.S. President Richard Milhous Nixon (1913-1994) in 1972, during which he suffered from an acute attack of appendicitis and was cured by acupuncture anesthesia. In real fact, it was in July 1971 that James Reston, a famous journalist and columnist of the *New York Times*, accepted an invitation alone and visited China with his wife.

Henry Alfred Kissinger (1923-) had just ended his trip to Beijing (July 9th – 11th) on one day before Reston's arrival in Beijing, and announced that President Nixon would visit China before May of the next year. During Reston's visit in China, he asked for medical treatment in Beijing because of the unbearable abdominal pain and was finally diagnosed with an acute attack of appendicitis. Because of his serious condition, he was hospitalized at noon of July 17th in the Peking Anti-Imperialist Hospital (now the "Peking Union Medical College Hospital"). Five famous doctors of the hospital, including a famous surgeon Dr. Wu Weiran 吴蔚然 (1920–), et al. held a consultation and decided to give him an operation on that evening. After the operation, Reston felt unbearable abdominal distending pain, which was relieved by acupuncture given by an acupuncturist of the hospital – Dr. Li Zhanyuan 李占元. As Reston said there was "no recurrence of the problem thereafter."[262]

Thereafter, Reston visited an operation under acupuncture anesthesia in Shanghai: "It is an amazing experience for me to see you doing tumor resection under acupuncture anesthesia in Shanghai." On July 26th, the US *New York Times* published special reports on the launch of Apollo and meanwhile splashed the story on the front page: "Now, About My Operation in Peking" with the headline "Now, Let Me Tell You About My Appendectomy in Peking." James Reston's significant influence and the position of *New York Times* in the press made his reports authentic, and therefore China's acupuncture was known as the "Oriental Apollo" in the United States. Because of the reports, James Reston's visit in China caught the world's attention and started a craze for acupuncture in the United States, attracting a careful review of acupuncture therapy from a Western power for the first time. Unexpectedly, this event also encouraged Prof. Paul U. Unschuld (1943–) to research Chinese medicine, making an attempt to systematically introduce

262 Reston, 1971.

the long-standing history and current situation of Chinese medicine to the West.[263]

Soon afterwards, U.S. former President Richard Nixon watched a surgery under acupuncture anesthesia during his visit in China in February 1972. In the same year, the U.S. National Institute of Health (NIH) funded the first research project on acupuncture therapy, thus bringing acupuncture research to a climax for the first time. Therefore Chinese medicine and acupuncture got into the United States again. And then, Chinese medical theory and skills like acupuncture, moxibustion, herbal medicine, massage, *qi gong* or breathing exercise, diet therapy, ancient Chinese medical language and Chinese medical classics followed to have full access to the United States.

As a follow-up, *The American Journal of Chinese Medicine* and *American Journal of Acupuncture* started their regular publications in 1973 in the USA;

The Theoretical Foundation of Chinese Medicine: Systems of Correspondence by Manfred Porket, a German Scholar, was published by Cambridge, Mass. and. London: MIT Press in 1974;

Celestial Lancets: a History and Rationale of Acupuncture and Moxa by Dr. Lu Gwei-Djen and Dr. Joseph Needham was published first by Cambridge University Press in 1980 and then reprinted in 2002 by Routledge Curzon in London;

Dr. Henry C. Lu, a Chinese Canadian, translated and published *A Complete Translation of The Yellow Emperor's Classics of Internal Medicine and the Difficult Classic* (1978; 2004);

Prof. Ted J. Kaptchuk, a scholar from Harvard Medical School, authored and published *The Web That Has No Weaver: Understanding Chinese Medicine*, the 1st edition, in 1982 and *Chinese Medicine: The Web That Has No Weaver*, the 2nd revised edition, in 2000, both of which have been one of the bestsellers on Chinese medicine in the West since its coming out, and successfully introduce Chinese medicine to the West and were reprinted numerous times and aroused immerse repercussions in the West;

Giovanni Maciocia started to publish his series of textbooks on Chinese medicine in 1989 – *The Foundations of Chinese Medicine*, which has been one of the major series of textbooks for training practitioners of Chinese medicine in the West;

---

263 Zheng Jinsheng, 2013: 3.

Dr. Nigel Wiseman's translation *Fundamentals of Chinese Medicine* (co-translated with Andrew Ellis, 1985) and his *Glossary of Chinese Medical Terms and Acupuncture Points* (1990) were published successively by Paradigm Publications;

During this stage, Prof. Paul U. Unschuld published a series of books on Chinese medicine at University of California Press, including *Medicine in China: A History of Pharmaceutics* (1986), *Nan-Ching: The Classic of Difficult Issues* (1986), *Medicine in China: A History of Ideas* (1988), *Forgotten Traditions of Ancient Chinese Medicine: The I-hsueh Yuan Liu Lun of 1757 by Hsu Ta-ch'un* (1990);

WHO (World Health Organization) issued the standardization of the English terms of acupuncture: *A Proposed Standard International Acupuncture Nomenclature* (Geneva, 1989) and *Standard Acupuncture Nomenclature* (Revised ed., Manila, 1991) as the outcome of the international cooperation since 1982.

During this stage, English translations of Chinese medicine in China are as follows:

In China, several International Acupuncture Training Centers were set up in Shanghai, Beijing, Nanjing, etc. by the aid of WHO. Ministry of Public Health and State Administration of TCM of China organized experts to compile and translate textbooks for beginners and advanced learners, i.e. *Essentials of Chinese Acupuncture* (1975, 1980) and *Chinese Acupuncture and Moxibustion* (1987), which have been used to train international acupuncturists up till now;

Dr. Luo Xiwen (罗西文, 1945-2012), a research fellow of China Academy of Social Sciences, translated and published *Shanghan Lun* 《伤寒论》: *Treatise on Febrile Diseases Caused by Cold* (Shanghan Lun, Beijing: New World Press, 1986), prefaced by Dr. Joseph Needham (1900-1995);

English-Chinese Edition of Practical Book Library on Chinese Medicine 《英汉对照实用中医文库》 (Zhang Enqin 张恩勤, 1990), and *English-Chinese Edition of A Practical Complete Collection of Chinese Medicine and Pharmacology* 《英汉实用中医药大全》 (Xu Xiangcai 徐象才, 1990-92) were published in China, which thus laid foundation for translation of different subjects of Chinese medicine;

Ou Ming (歐明, 1924–), Xie Zhufan (謝竹藩, 1924–), Shuai Xuezhong (帥學忠), et al. compiled and published different editions of "Chinese-English Dictionary of Chinese Medicine".

4 Translation and Studies on Chinese Medicine: From Standardization of Its English Terminology, English Translation & Research of Its Classics, to Interpretation of Its Way (1992–)

4.1 Standardization of English Translation of Chinese Medical Terminology

A great number of English works on Chinese medicine have got published at both home and abroad since 1992, covering foundations of Chinese medicine and acupuncture, all clinical subjects, and Chinese medical classics, including English translations and English writings. Among them, the domestic presses and academic journal editorial departments on Chinese medicine have not yet appointed a standard English terminology for their English publications on Chinese medicine; While in the United States, Paradigm Publications and Blue Poppy Press, two of the three major Chinese medical literature publishing houses, have appointed English Chinese medical terminology formulated by Dr. Nigel Wiseman as the standard terminology for their publications.

Dr. Nigel Wiseman's *English-Chinese and Chinese-English Dictionary of Chinese Medicine* (Changsha: Hunan Science & Technology Press, 1995), and *A Practical Dictionary of Chinese Medicine* (Brookline, Massachusetts: Paradigm Publications, 1998; Beijing: People's Medical Publishing House, 2002) were successively published and the free online dictionary *Paradigm Online TCM Dictionary* (an updated version in 2011) is available at the website of Paradigm Publications - http://www.paradigm-pubs.com/TermList to promote this terminology, which contains more than 35,000 entries and convenient two-way access – Chinese-English, English-Chinese.

The research project "Standard English Translation of TCM Nomenclature" chaired by Prof. Xie Zhufan (谢竹藩, 1924–) and sponsored by the State Administration of TCM results in the publications of *Classified Dictionary of Traditional Chinese Medicine* (New Edition) in 2002 and *On the Standard Nomenclature of Traditional Chinese Medicine* in 2003 by Foreign Language Press in Beijing to promote this terminology at home and abroad respectively.

Chinese Terms in Traditional Chinese Medicine and Pharmacy 《中医药学名词》, the research outcome of a project "*Research on Standardization of Basic Terms in Traditional Chinese Medicine and Pharmacy* (Chinese-English)", which was sponsored by Ministry of Science and Technology of China and chaired by Academician Wang Yongyan (王永炎, 1938–), Prof.

Liang Jusheng 梁菊生, Prof. Zhu Jianping 朱建平 of China Academy of Chinese Medical Sciences, was examined and approved by the China National Committee for Terms in Sciences and Technologies and published by Science Press (Beijing) in 2005. But its standard English terminology set off controversies among the academic circle in China. For example, Prof. Xie Zhufan 谢竹藩 et al. found various mistakes among the English equivalents in the book *Chinese Terms in Traditional Chinese Medicine and Pharmacy*, which were classified into eight categories: grammatical errors, violation of English idioms, total ignorance of the original implications, partial reflection of the Chinese original, erroneous use of general medical terms, erroneous use of specific medical terms, violation of medical principles, and wrong interpretation of pharmaceutical concepts. For each category, three examples were given. The mistakes found in the book counted up to ten times the number of examples. In addition, much more English equivalents were found in want of standardization. However, since the book was published as a formal document with compulsory application approved and promulgated by China National Committee for Terms in Sciences and Technologies, it has given wrong directions domestically and made an unfavorable impact abroad.[264]

In 2004, World Health Organization（WHO）launched the work of "*International Standardization of Terminology on Traditional Medicine*" and announced *WHO International Standard Terminologies on Traditional Medicine in the Western Pacific Region* on October 16th, 2007, and thus laying a foundation for standardization of traditional medicine in the future. Actually there are also some mistakes in this proposal, such as "terminologies" in the title, triple "energizers" for 三焦, and so and so forth.

4.2 English Translation and Research of Chinese Medical Classics

Translations of many Chinese medical classics were got published at home and abroad up till this period. *Huang Di Nei Jing* 《黄帝内经》or *Huangdi's Inner Classic* (including *Su Wen* 《素问》or *Basic Questions* and *Ling Shu* 《灵枢》or *Miraculous Pivot*), *Shennong Bencao Jing*《神农本草经》 or *Shennong's Classic of Materia Medica*, *Shang Han Lun* 《伤寒论》or *On Cold-induced*

264 Xie Zhufan, et al. 2006: 169-172.

Diseases and *Jingui Yaolüe* 《金匮要略》or *Synopsis of the Golden Chamber* by Zhang Zhongjing (张仲景, 150-219), *Mai Jing* 《脉经》 or *The Pulse Classic* by Wang Shuhe (王叔和, 201-280), *Zhenjiu Jiayi Jing* 《黄帝针灸甲乙经》 or *The Systematic Classic of Acupuncture and Moxibustion* by Huangfu Mi (皇甫谧, 215-282), *Zhong Zang Jing* 《中藏经》 or *The Classic of the Central Viscera*, whose authorship is attributed to Hua Tuo in legends (华佗, ?-203), *Beiji Qianjin Yaofang·Furen Fang* 《备急千金要方 · 妇人方》or *Prescriptions Worth a Thousand in Gold for Every Emergency* (*Invaluable Prescriptions for Emergencies*) · *3 Volumes of Gynecology* by Sun Simiao (孙思邈, 581-682), *Yin Hai Jing Wei* 《银海精微》 or *Essential Subtleties on the Silver Sea*, whose authorship is attributed to Sun Simiao in legends, *Xi Yuan Lu* 《洗冤录》 or *Records for Washing Away Injustice* by Song Ci (宋慈，1186-1249), *Pi Wei Lun* 《脾胃论》 or *The Treatise on Spleen and Stomach* by Li Gao (李杲, 1180-1251), *Heart Approach to Gynecology* 《妇科心法要决》, the part of gynecology of *Yi Zong Jin Jian* 《医宗金鉴》 or *Golden Mirror of Medicine*, the official textbook of Chinese medicine of the Qing Dynasty (1644-1911), *Bencao Gangmu* 《本草纲目》 or *The Compendium of Materia Medica* and *Binhu Mai Xue* 《濒湖脉学》 or *Lakeside Master's Study of the Pulse* by Li Shizhen（李时珍, 1518-1593）, *Ge Zhi Yu Lun* 《格致余论》or *Extra Treatises Based on Investigation and Inquiry* and *Dan-Xi Zhi Fa Xin Yao* 《丹溪治法心要》 or *The Heart & Essence of Dan-Xi's Methods of Treatment* by Zhu Zhenheng (朱震亨,1281-1358), *Wen Bing Xue* 《温病学》 or *Warm Disease Theory*, *Fu Qing-zhu Nu Ke* 《傅青主女科》 or *Fu Qing-Zhu's Gynecology* by Fu Qing-zhu (傅青主, 1607-1684), *Yixue Yuan Liu Lun* 《医学源流论》 or *The Origin and Development of Medicine* by Xu Dachun（徐大椿, 1693-1771), *Yi Lin Gai Cuo* or *Correcting the Errors in the Forest of Medicine* 《医林改错》 by Wang Qingren (王清任, 1768-1831), etc., have been fully translated into English, but the translation versions are confused with good or bad qualities.

And some classics have two or more translations, e.g. *Huang Di Nei Jing Su Wen* 《黄帝内经素问》 has around 10 translations, and other classics like *Huang Di Nei Jing Ling Shu* 《黄帝内经灵枢》, *Nan Jing* 《难经》, *Shang Han Lun* 《伤寒论》, *Jingui Yaolue* 《金匮要略》, *Mai Jing* 《脉经》, and *Binhu Mai Xue* 《濒湖脉学》 etc. have at least two translated versions. Besides, translations of medical manuscripts from Mawangdui Han tomb (No. 3) unearthed in 1973[265] and Dunhuang[266] discovered in 1900 have also got published: *Early Chinese Medical Literature: the Mawangdui Medical Manuscripts* (Donald John Harper, 1998) and *Medieval Chinese Medicine: The Dunhuang Medical Manuscripts* (Needham Research Institute Series, Vivienne Lo & Christopher Cullen, 2005). [267]

Among the translations of classical Chinese medical texts, *Huang Di Nei Jing Su Wen Project* and *Bencao Gangmu Project* chaired by Prof. Paul U. Unschuld (1943–) are the two largest, most time-consuming, most costly projects on the research and translation of Chinese medical classics involving the most extensive international cooperation and with most research outcomes ever. On May 25th. 2011, *Huang Di Nei Jing Su Wen* and *Bencao Gangmu* were both included into the Memory of the World Register by UNESCO (United Nations Educational，Scientific and Cultural Organization)，which shows that Prof. Unschuld's selection of research topics just hit the mark.

Huang Di Nei Jing Su Wen Project sponsored by Volkswagen Foundation and German Research Foundation (DFG) was accomplished through 22 years (1989-2011) of international cooperation with Hermann Tessenow, a philologist of Institute of History of Medicine of Munich University, and Zheng Jinsheng 郑金生, a research fellow of China Academy of Chinese Medical Sciences. The University of California Press successively published

265 "The Mawangdui Medical Manuscripts" represent the richest cache of ancient medical manuscripts ever found in China, which was identified as the medical knowledge in third and early second century B.C. China, including discussions of meridians, physiological theories and pathology, prescriptions & recipes for the treatment of ailments and for the practice of macrobiotic hygiene, sexual treatises, and illustrations of hygienic exercises.

266 In 1900, a Chinese Daoist Priest Wang Yuanlu (王圆箓, 1850?-1931) uncovered a cache of thousands of paintings and manuscripts in the Silk Road town of Dunhuang 敦煌 in the northwest China. Formerly walled up in a man-made cave in about 1035, these materials now constitute one of the most valuable sources on China and central Asia during the first millennium CE. Its medical parts are known together as *Dunhuang Medical Manuscripts* 敦煌医书.

267 You may know the available translations of classical Chinese medical texts in details at http://www.redwingbooks.com.

their research outcomes: *Huang Di Nei Jing Su Wen: Nature, Knowledge, Imagery in An Ancient Chinese Medical Text* (2003), a research monograph to comprehensively introduce *Huang Di Nei Jing Su Wen*; *Dictionary of Huang Di Nei Jing Su Wen* (2008), a research tool and index of *Huang Di Nei Jing Su Wen* with 1,886 Chinese characters as the key link; *Huang Di Nei Jing Su Wen: An Annotated Translation of Huang Di's Inner Classic – Basic Questions* (2 Volumes, 2011), a full translation of the 79 chapters of the Wang Bing (王冰, 710-804) annotated *Su Wen* based on methods of linguistic anthropology.

The *Bencao Gangmu* Project first approved in 1988, re-started in 2008 in international cooperation with experts of different fields of study. This project, another time-consuming research project, is currently in smooth progress. *Historical Chinese Illness Terminology*, which analyzes around 4,500 terms of diseases, the first volume of the first research outcome *A Dictionary of the Bencao Gangmu* (4 Volumes), will be published in 2014.

4.3 Understanding the "Way" of Chinese Medicine

It is worth noting that Chinese medicine has gradually gained a legal identity and status as well as understanding and acceptance by the American government during this period. On March 7th, 2000, William Jefferson Bill Clinton (1946–), a former U.S. President, issued No. 13147 Executive Order and approved the establishment of White House Commission on Complementary and Alternative Medicine, C.A.M for short. After about two years of investigation and research by C.A.M., the FINAL REPORT of the *White House Commission on Complementary and Alternative Medicine Policy* was announced at the end of March, 2002. In the report clearly safe and effective CAM medical practices and products are required to incorporate into the routine health care in the United States and increasing funding for the study of these treatments is also proposed.[268] As the report is from the American government, it has undoubtedly a significant and far-reaching impact on the existing health care system and the development of integrative medicine. So far, Chinese medicine, acupuncture and moxibustion in America have gained a "legal identity and status".

268 See http://whccamp.hhs.gov//finalreport.html in details.

4.3.1 Chinese Medicine: A Complete Medical System Rooted in Chinese Culture

Science depends on culture. This point of view has been developed through

1. Thomas Samuel Kuhn (1922-1996), one of the most influential philosophers of science of the twentieth century, see *The Structure of Scientific Revolutions*, Chicago: University Of Chicago Press, 1996;
2. Paul Feyerabend (1924-1994), a critic of Karl Popper's "critical rationalism" and one of the twentieth century's most famous philosophers of science, see *Against Method*, London: New Left Books, 1975; and *Realism, Rationalism and Scientific Methods: Philosophical Papers,* Volume 1, Cambridge: Cambridge University Press, 1981;
3. Friedrich G. Wallner (1945-), the founding father of Constructive Realism, an intercultural and interdisciplinary philosophy of science with the aim of making the manifold scientific approaches depending on different cultures understandable, see *Constructive Realism: Aspects of A New Epistemological Movement*, Wien: W. Braumueller, 1994.

In December 2006, Food and Drug Administration (FDA) mentioned that traditional Chinese medicine is a complete medical system with its own theory and practice, derived from classical Chinese culture and evolved simultaneously and independently with Western medicine in the *Guidance for Industry on Complementary and Alternative Medicine Products and Their Regulation* by the Food and Drug Administration (DRAFT GUIDANCE). Of course Traditional Indian medicine is no exception (FDA, 2006). The original is as follows:

"The term 'complementary and alternative medicine' (CAM) encompasses a wide array of health care practices, products, and therapies that are distinct from practices, products, and therapies used in 'conventional' or 'allopathic' medicine. Some forms of CAM, such as traditional Chinese medicine and Ayurvedic medicine, have been practiced for centuries, whereas others, such as electrotherapy, are more recent in origin.", and that "NCCAM describes whole medical systems as involving 'complete systems of theory and practice that have evolved independently from or parallel to allopathic (conventional) medicine.' These may reflect individual cultural systems, such as traditional Chinese medicine and Ayurvedic medicine."

This statement from FDA in 2006 shows the general official acknowledgement of cultural dependency of medical systems. As for Chinese medicine, it is a culturally dependent medical system deeply rooted in the culture and philosophy of the country it originated from: China. That is to say, Chinese medicine is not simply an old healing art indigenous to China with a basic understanding of the human body and diseases and mainly composed of effective herbal formulas and acupuncture techniques nor a healing system that can be gauged according to Western scientific criteria, but is a systematic, independent and complete medical system in and of itself, rooted in Chinese culture, that cannot be adapted to suit the Western conventional medical approach.

4.3.2 The Way of Chinese Medicine: *Qu Xiang Bi Lei* or Metaphorizing

Chinese medicine as we know it today is the product of a systematic organization of the knowledge contained in the ancient Chinese medical classics. Up until now, Chinese medicine has still claimed that it follows the system founded in classical texts such as *Huang Di Nei Jing* or *Huang Di's Inner Classic*, *Nan Jing* or *The Classic of Difficult Issues*, *Shang Han Lun* or *On Cold-induced Diseases*, *Jin Gui Yao Lue* or *Essential Prescriptions of the Golden Cabinet*, *Shen Nong Ben Cao Jing* or *Shennong's Classic of Materia Medica*, essentially. As all the ancient Chinese medical classics bear historical, cultural, and medical values, the study of their English translation cannot be confined to the field of History and Literature of Chinese medicine, it is rather the key and difficult point of cross-cultural transmission and exchanges of Chinese medicine.[269]

Based on the research outcome of the author's cooperation with Prof. Dr. Friedrich G. Wallner (1945-) on the projects "Cultural Dependency of Medical Knowledge: A Comparison between Chinese Medicine and Western Medicine from the Perspectives of Philosophy of Science"(2007-2010), "Theory, Methodology and Structure of TCM" (2008-2011; 2012–), One Branch Project of Joint Research Project of the TCM Research Cluster Austria together with the Sino-Austrian Collaborating Centre for Chinese Medicine Research: TCM and Age Related Diseases, sponsored by Austria, and "A Corpus-based Translation Study on Classical Chinese Medical Texts" (2009-2013) sponsored by China, the way of Chinese medicine is interpreted as: Chinese medicine takes *Tian Ren He Yi* 天人合一 or The

269 Lan Fengli, 2012: 253-258.

Unity of Heaven and Humankind, as its ontological presupposition and *Qu Xiang Bi Lei* 取象比类 or Taking Image and Analogizing, as its core methodology; *Qu Xiang Bi Lei* is the process and the way of forming metaphors in Chinese medicine. Chinese medicine, from the writing form it is recorded in and carried on, to the formation of its concepts, to its terminology, its way of formulation, its logic, and even to the system in its entirety, it is essentially metaphorical. Interpreting metaphors is, therefore, the key to understand Chinese medicine, thus enabling it being carried forward and developed.[270]

4.3.3 How to Keep the Way in Translations of Classical Chinese Medical Texts

Based on the interpretation of Chinese medicine in the sense of philosophy of science and a C-E comparable corpus of ancient Chinese medical classics (Chinese Corpus composed of 13 ancient Chinese medical classics with 1.485 millions of sinograms; English Corpus composed of 22 translations of the above mentioned classics with 2.62 millions of words), the research project "A Corpus-based Translation Study on Classical Chinese Medical Texts" sponsored by National Social Sciences and Philosophy Foundation of China studies the English translation of these ancient Chinese medical classics. Through this process, the following conclusions were reached:

1. In view of preserving the unique features of each of the two languages of Chinese medicine and Western medicine, as well as their complementarity and the differing philosophical foundations of both medical systems, the necessity of applying certain translating principles so as to preserve the metaphors, the systematic quality, wholeness and independence of the Chinese medical concepts, should be strictly observed. In this regard, "foreignization" or a source-target translation approach should be adopted, and the excessive use of Western medical terms to translate Chinese medical concepts should be avoided. Consequently, literal translation based on metaphor cognition and etymology investigation should be taken as the chief method in translating Chinese medical terminology.

270 Lan Fengli & Wallner, Friedrich. 2014: 87-93.

2. In view of the fact that all ancient Chinese medical classics bear historical, medical and cultural values, the classics require an extremely close *translation*, not an 'interpretation' of the original, as the translation itself should be able to support as many different interpretations as the original does. For this purpose, the original Chinese text (including terms, structure of the sentences and discourses as well as the figures of speech contained in it) should be given a literal translation wherever/whenever possible. Meanwhile, reliable commentaries from both the experts of the past and the translator should be added in the notes in order to provide the English readers with the opportunity to experience the process of studying Chinese medical classics in a way similar to that of the Chinese readers.[271]

To sum up, transmission of Chinese medicine in the West started in the 17th century, originating from the real therapeutic effect of Chinese therapies, i.e. the transmission of "Skills" such as pulse-taking & reading skills, moxibustion treatment for gout, acupuncture treatment for arthritis, translation and introduction of Chinese herbal medicine (e.g. *Bencao Gangmu* 《本草纲目》 or *The Compendium of Materia Medica*) and forensic medicine (e.g. *Xi Yuan Lu* 《洗冤录》 or *Records for Washing Away Injustice*), and so and so forth. In the 20th century "the craze for acupuncture" and "the craze for Chinese medicine" in the West are also closely related to the success of acupuncture anesthesia in the Mainland China. After more than 300 years of rises and falls, Chinese medicine is now spreading at an unprecedented speed, scale and depth in the West. Transmission of "*Dao* or Way", in addition to transmission of "Skills", is also a need and choice of the era when reflecting on the advantages and disadvantages of modern science and Western Medicine. As Prof. Paul U. Unschuld repeatedly emphasizes that "People like a medicine not because it is effective, but because they like the ideas it is based on (or they think it is based on)."[272]

271 Lan Fengli. 2014: Abstract.

272 Quoted as a secondary source from Dr. Nigel Wiseman's Lectures in Shanghai: Wiseman, N. *Chinese Medical English in the Wider Context of International Communication* (Lecture 1). Series of Lectures at Shanghai University of TCM. June 3, 2013.

Chief References

1 Addison Wesley Longman Limited. *Longman Dictionary of Contemporary English* [Z]. Beijing: The Commercial Press, 1998.

2 Andrews M.M., Boyle J.S. (eds). *Transcultural Concepts in Nursing Care*[C]. 4th ed. Philadelphia: Lippincott Williams and Wilkins, 2003.

3 *Britannica Concise Encyclopedia* (Chinese Version), 2010.

4 Cassirer, Ernst. *An Essay on Man: An Introduction to a Philosophy of Human Culture* [M]. New Heaven: Yale University Press, 1944.

5 Chalfant, H. P. *Medical Sociology* [M]. Shanghai: Shanghai People's Publishing House, 1987.

6 Chen Biliu. *Nan Jing* with Modern Chinese Interpretation [M]. Beijing: People's Medical Publishing House, 1963.

7 Chen Hongwei. *Foundation of Chinese-English Translation* 汉英翻译基础 [M]. Shanghai: Shanghai: Shanghai Foreign Language Education Press, 1998.

8 Chen Keji, et al. Suggestions for Standard Usage of "证", "症", "征" and Related Medical Terms [J]. *China Scientific and Technical Terms Journal*. 2003 (4): 10-11.

9 Chen Keji. Treatment Concept of Combining Disease Diagnosis with Pattern Identification and Its Application in Clinical Practice [J]. *Chinese Journal of Integrated Traditional and Western Medicine*. 2011(8): 1016-1017.

10 Collin, P.H. *Dictionary of Medicine* [Z]. Beijing: Foreign Language Teaching and Research Press, 2001.

11 Department of History of Sciences of Shanghai Jiao Tong University, Translator; Needham, Joseph, Author. *Science and Civilisation in China Series* [M]. Shanghai: Shanghai People's Publishing House, 2001: 149.

12 *Dictionary of Commonly Used Sinograms in Archaic Chinese* [Z]. Beijing: Commercial Press, 1998.

13 Dieter Melchart, Andrea Streng, Andrea Hoppe, et al. Acupuncture in patients with tension-type headache: randomised controlled trial [J]. *British Medical Journal*. 2005, 331 (8): 376-382.

14 Dong Hongle. *Metaphorization in Scientific Discourse* [M]. Shanghai: Fudan University Press, 2005.

15 Fung Yu-Lan. *A Short History of Chinese Philosophy* [M]. English Version. London and New York: The MacMillan Co., 1948; English-Chinese Version. Tianjin: Tianjin Academy of Social Science Press, 2007; 2010 Third Print.

16 Gan Yang, Translator; Author: Cassirer Ernest. *An Essay on Man* [M]. Shanghai: Shanghai Translation Publishing House, 2004.

17 Gan Zuwang. On the Word Item "*Bian Zheng Lun (Shi) Zhi* 辨证论(施)治" [J]. *Liaoning Journal of Traditional Chinese Medicine*. 2003(8): 672.

18 GuYankui. *Dictionary of Etymologies of Chinese Characters* [Z]. Beijing: Yu Wen Press, 2008; 2010.
19 Guo Aichun. *Huang Di Nei Jing Su Wen* with Collations, Annotations and Modern Chinese Interpretation [M]. Tianjin: Tianjin Science and Technology Press, 1st ed. 1981; 2nd ed. 1999.
20 Guo Guichun. *Metaphor, Rhetoric, and Scientific Interpretation* [M]. Beijing: Science Press, 2007.
21 He Jiuying, Hu Shuangbao, Zhang Meng. *A Grand Exposition of Culture of Chinese Characters* [M]. Peking University Press, 1995: 195-196.
22 He Yumin. *Differences, Perplexity and Choice: A Comparative Study of Chinese Medicine and Western Medicine* [M]. Shenyang: Shenyang Press, 1990.
23 Hou Weirui. *English Styles of Writing* [M]. Shanghai: Shanghai Foreign Language Education Press, 1988.
24 Hsu, Elisabeth. *The Transmission of Chinese Medicine* [M]. Cambridge: Cambridge University Press, 1999.
25 Huang Qichen. Transmission and Influences of Chinese Culture in Europe from 16th to 18th Century[J] . *Journal of Sun Yatsen University* (Social Science Edition), 1992, 4: 54-62.
26 Jaspers, Karl. *The Origin and Goal of History* [M]. Translated by Michael Bullock. New Haven, CT: Yale University Press, 1953; Reprint. Westport, Connecticut: Greenwood Press, 1977.
27 Kaptchuk, Ted J. *Chinese Medicine: The Web That Has No Weaver* [M]. Revised ed. London, Sydney, Aukland, Johannesburg: Rider, 2000.
28 Klaus Linde, Andrea Streng, Susanne Jurgens, et al. Acupuncture for Patients With Migraine: A Randomized Controlled Trial [J]. *The Journal of the Amerian Medical Association (JAMA)*. 2005, 293: 2118-2125.
29 Klaus Linde, Claudia M. Witt, Andrea Streng, et al. The impact of patient expectations on outcomes in four randomized controlled trials of acupuncture in patients with chronic pain [J]. *Journal of the International Association for the Study of Pain*. 2007, 128 (3): 264-271.
30 Kuhn, Thomas S. *The Structure of Scientific Revolutions* [M]. 2nd Revised edition. Chicago: University of Chicago Press, 1970.
31 Lakoff, George; Johnson, Mark. *Metaphors We Live By* [M]. Chicago: The University of Chicago Press, 1980.
32 Lan Fengli. Use the Translating Experiences of Other Countries for Reference to Bring about An Advance in Translation of Chinese Medicine in China [J]. *Chinese Journal of Integrated Traditional and Western Medicine*. 2003, 23(8): 627-28.
33 Lan Fengli. Cultural Connotations and English Translation of Ancient Chinese Medical Classics: Study on English Translation of *Huang Di Nei Jing Su Wen* [D]. PhD. Dissertation. Shanghai University of Traditional Chinese Medicine, July 2005.

34 Lan Fengli. Influence of *Huang Di's Inner Classic* on *The Origin of Chinese Characters* [J]. *Chinese Journal of Medical History*. 2006, 36(4): 201-205.
35 Lan Fengli. The Origin of Yin-Yang as Chinese Medical Terms and Their Translation [J]. *Chinese Translators Journal*. 2007, 28(4): 69-72.
36 Lan Fengli. *A Corpus-Based Study on Cultural Connotations and Translation of Fundamental Concepts in Classical Chinese Texts* [D]. Shanghai: Shanghai Jiao Tong University, 2008.
37 Lan Fengli. Philosophical Reflections on Standard English Terminology of Chinese Medicine [J]. *Medicine and Philosophy*, 2010, 31 (7): 72-73.
38 Lan Fengli, Wallner Friedrich G., and Wobovnik Claudia (eds.). *Shen, Psychotherapy and Acupuncture: Theory, Methodology and Structure of Chinese Medicine*[C]. 2011.
39 LanFengli. *Culture, Philosophy, and Chinese Medicine: Viennese Lectures* [M]. Frankfurt am Main: Peter Lang, 2012.
40 Lan Fengli. Taking Image and Analogizing: The Metaphorizing Process and the Way of Forming Metaphors in Chinese Medicine [J]. *Journal of Dialectics of Nature*, 2014, 36(2): 97-93.
41 Lan Fengli. *A Corpus-based Translation Study on Classical Chinese Medical Texts*[M]. Forthcoming.
42 Li Ding. *Interpretation of Difficult Issues on Acupuncture* [M]. Shanghai: Shanghai University of Traditional Chinese Medicine Press. 1998: 99-191.
43 Li Jingwei, Ou Yongxin, Yu Ying'ao, et al. *A Concise Dictionary of Chinese Medicine* [Z]. Beijing: China Press of Traditional Chinese Medicine, 2001.
44 Li Lei (editor). New Century TCM English Course. Shanghai: Shanghai Foreign Language Education Press, 2006.
45 Li Leishi. Personal Experiences in Integrating Chinese Medicine with Western Medicine [J]. *Chinese Journal of Integrated Traditional and Western Medicine*, 1998, 18 (12):707.
46 Li Xisuo, Chen Shangsheng. *5,000 Years of Sino-Foreign Cultural Exchange*[M]. Beijing: World Knowledge Press, 2002.
47 Li Xisuo, Lin Yanqing, Li Mengzhi, et al. *5,000 Years of History of Sino-Foreign Cultural Exchange* (Vol. 2) [M]. Beijing: World Knowledge Press, 2001.
48 Narrated by Li Yangbo, Systematized by Liu Lihong, et al. *Opening the Door of Chinese Medicine: Introduction to Doctrine of Periods and Qi*. Beijing: China Press of TCM, 2004.
49 Liang Donghan. *Sinograms* [M]. Shanghai: Shanghai Education Press, 1984.
50 Liang Fanrong. *Acupuncture and Moxibustion* [M]. Beijing: China Press of Traditional Chinese Medicine, 2005.
51 *Ling Shu Jing*. Taiyuan: Shanxi Science and Technology Press, 1992.
52 Ling Yikui. Textbook for Medical Higher Education (5th Edition): *Chinese Herbal Medicine* [M]. Shanghai: Shanghai Scientific and Technical Publishers, 1984: 1.

53 Liu Ping, Ji Guang, et al. Combination of disease diagnosis with pattern identification and Construction of Theoretical System of Integrative Medicine [J]. Chinese Journal of Integreted Traditional and Western Medicine. 2010 (6): 565-570.
54 Luckman J. *Transcultural Communication in Nursing* [M]. Albany, NY: Delmar Publishers, 1999.
55 Ma Boying, Gao Xi, Hong Zhongli. *History of Sino-Foreign Medical Cultural Exchange: Sino-Foreign Cross Cultural Communications*[M]. Shanghai: Wenhui Press, 1993.
56 Ma Boying. *A History of Medicine in Chinese Culture* [M]. Shanghai: Shanghai People's Press, 1994.
57 Originally by Matteo, Ricci. Translated by He Gaoji, Wang Zunzhong, Li Shen. *Matteo Ricci's Reading Notes on China* [M]. Beijing: Zhonghua Book Company, 1983.
58 Michael Haake, Hans-Helge Muller, Carmen Schade-Brittinger, et al. German Acupuncture Trials (GERAC) for Chronic Low Back Pain: Randomized, Multicenter, Blinded, Parallel-Group Trial With 3 Groups [J]. *Archive of Internal Medicine*. 2007, 167(17):1892-1898.
59 Michel Foucault. *The Birth of the Clinic* [M]. New York: Vintage Books, 1973.
60 Needham, Joseph. *Science and Civilization in China* [M] (Volume 1). Translation. Beijing: Science Press & Shanghai: Shanghai Ancient Books Press, 1990.
61 Newmark, Peter. *Approaches to Translation* [M]. Shanghai: Shanghai Foreign Language Education Press, 2001.
62 Ni, Maoshing. Trans. *The Yellow Emperor's Classic of Medicine* [M]. Boston, Massachusetts: Shambhala, 1995.
63 Nida, Eugene A. *Language, Culture and Translating* [M]. Shanghai: Shanghai Foreign Language Education Press, 1993.
64 Ong Bendick. M.A. Thesis: *A Study of Pre-Qin "Daoist" Thoughts: From Guodian to Jixia* [D]. National University of Singapore, 2004.
65 *Oxford Dictionary of English*, 2nd Edition, Oxford University Press, 1998, 1999, 2001, 2003, 2005.
66 Pan Jixing. Transmission of Chinese Culture in the West and Its Influences on Darwin[J], *Science*, 1954 (10).
67 Pan Jixing. Transmission of Chinese Biological Works in Europe before the Time of Darwin [J]. *Bulletin on Biology*, 1959 (10): 521-525.
68 Pan Wenguo. *Sinogram as the Basic Unit and Chinese Language Study* [M]. Shanghai: East China Normal University Press, 2002.
69 Pang Pu. *A Corpus of Meditation* [M]. Shanghai: Shanghai People's Publishing House. 1982.
70 Pang Pu. *Observing One in Three: Textual Criticisms and Explanations of Chinese Traditional Thoughts* [M]. Shenzhen: Haitian Press, 1995.

71 Qiu, Jane. China Plans to Modernize Traditional Medicine [J]. *Nature*, April 2007: 590-591.
72 Qiu, Jane. 'Back to the future' for Chinese herbal medicines [J]. *Nature*, 2007 (6): 506-507.
73 Qiu Le. A General Review of Research on Historical Facts of English Translation of Ancient Traditional Chinese Medicine Books [J]. *Journal of Chinese Integrative Medicine*, 2011; 9(4): 459-464.
74 Ren Jiyu. *History of Buddhism in China* (Volume1) [M]. Beijing: China Social Sciences Press, 1985.
75 Ren Yingqiu. Great Homeland Medical Achievements [J]. *Journal of Traditional Chinese Medicine*. 1955 (2): 1.
76 Ren Yingqiu. The System of Pattern Identification and Treatment in Chinese Medicine [J]. *Journal of Traditional Chinese Medicine*. 1955 (4): 19.
77 Reston, James. Now, Let Me Tell You About My Appendectomy in Peking [N]. *New York Times*, Monday July 26, 1971.
78 Shanghai College of TCM (ed.). *Bian Zheng Shi Zhi* 辨症施治. Shanghai: Shanghai Renmin Chubanshe, 1972.
79 Shen Qingsong (known as Vincent Shen in the West). *Shen Qingsong's Self Selections* [M]. Jinan: Shandong Education Press, 1995.
80 Spector, R.E. *Cultural Diversity in Health and Illness* [M]. 6th ed. Upper Saddle River NJ.: Pearson/Prentice Hall, 2004.
81 Steiner, George. *After Babel---Aspects of Language and Translation* [M]. Shanghai: Shanghai Foreign Language Education Press, 2001.
82 Sun Baozhi. *Introduction to Clinical Medicine* [M]. 2nd Ed. Beijing: Higher Education Press, 2003.
83 Teaching and Research Section of History of Foreign Philosophy, Department of Philosophy, Peking University. *Philosophy of Ancient Greece and Rome* [M]. Beijing: SDX Joint Publishing Company. 1957: 73-91.
84 Unschuld, Paul U. *HUANG DI NEI JING SU WEN: Nature, Knowledge, Imagery in An Ancient Chinese Medical Text* [M]. Berkeley, Los Angeles and London: University of California Press, 2003.
85 Unschuld Paul U., Tessenow Hermann. Trans. *Huang Di Nei Jing Su Wen* (Vol.1). Berkeley and Los Angeles: University of California Press, 2011: 42-44.
86 Veith, Ilza. Trans. *The Yellow Emperor's Classic of Internal Medicine*. 1st Ed., Baltimore: The Williams & Wilkins Co., 1949; 2nd Ed., Berkeley, Los Angeles, London: University of California Press, 1966, 1972.
87 Voltaire. *Essai Sur Les Moeurs* (Vol.2) [M]. Paris: Gamier, 1963.
88 Wallner, Fritz G. *How to Deal with Science If You Care for Other Cultures: Constructive Realism in the Intercultural World* [M]. Wien: Wilhelm Braumuller, 1997.
89 Wallner, F. G. *Five Lectures on the Foundations of Chinese Medicine* [M]. Frankurt am Main: Peter Lang, 2009.

90 Wallner F.G., Kubiena G., Jandl M.J. (eds). *Understanding Traditional Chinese Medicine* [C]. Frankfurt Am Mein: Peter Lang, 2009.
91 Wallner F.G., Schmidsberger F., Wimmer F.M. (eds.). *Intercultural Philosophy: New Aspects and Methods* [C]. Frankfurt am Main: Peter Lang, 2010.
92 Wallner F.G., Lan FL, Jandl M.J. (eds.). *The Way of Thinking: Theory, Methodology and Structure of Chinese Medicine* [C]. Frankfurt Am Main: Peter Lang, 2010.
93 Wallner F.G., Lan FL, Jandl M.J.(eds.). *Chinese Medicine and Intercultural Philosophy: Theory, Methodology and Structure of Chinese Medicine* [C]. Frankfurt Am Main: Peter Lang, 2011.
94 Wang Hongtu. Great Compendium of Studies on *Huang Di Nei Jing* [M]. Beijing: Beijing Press, 1997.
95 Wang Lan, Zhou Guangbiao, Liu Ping, et al. Dissection of Mechanisms of Chinese Medicinal Formula Realgar-Indigo Naturalis as an Effective Treatment for Promyelocytic Leukemia [J]. *PNAS (Proceedings of the National Academy of Sciences of the United States of America)*, 2008, Vol. 125 (12): 4826-4831.
96 Wang Rongpei, Wang Hong (eds.). *English Translation of Chinese Classics* [M]. Shanghai: Shanghai Foreign Language Education Press, 2009.
97 Wang Xiaolong. *A Practical Dictionary for Sinograms in Chinese Medicine* 实用中医字典 [Z]. Beijing: Academy Press 学苑出版社, 2001.
98 Wang TW. Establishment of Diagnostic Standards of Combination of Disease Diagnosis with Pattern Identification [J]. *Chinese Journal of Integreted Traditional and Western Medicine*. 2011 (8): 1025-1026.
99 Wang Yuxiong. *Investigation into Origins of Image* [M]. Hefei: Anhui Education Press, 1996.
100 *Webster's Encyclopedic Unabridged Dictionary of the English Language* (New Revised Edition) [Z]. New York: Gramercy Books, 1994.
101 Wei Zhengtong. *A History of Chinese Thoughts* [M]. Shanghai: Shanghai Bookstore Publishing House, 2003.
102 Wilhelm, Baynes. Bollingen Series. *The I Ching*. Princeton: Princeton University Press, 3rd ed., 1967; 27th printing in 1997.
103 Wiseman Nigel, Ellis Andrew. *Fundamentals of Chinese Medicine* [M]. Revised ed. Brookline Massachusetts: Paradigm Publications, 1996.
104 Wiseman, Nigel. *English-Chinese & Chinese-English Dictionary of Chinese Medicine* [Z]. Changsha: Hunan Science and Technology Press, 1996.
105 Wiseman, Nigel. Translation and Transmission of Chinese Medicine in the West [J]. *Medicine and Philosophy*. 2001, 22(7): 51-54.
106 Wiseman Nigel, Zhang Yuhuan. *Chinese Medical Characters Volume One: Basic Vocabulary* [M]. Brookline, Massachusetts and Daos, Mexico, 2003.
107 Wiseman, Nigel. *Chinese Medical English in the Wider Context of International Communication* (Lecture 1). A Series of Lectures at Shanghai University of TCM. June 3, 2013.

108 Wong, Chinmin K. Investigations of Western-Language Translations of Chinese Medical Classics [J]. *National Medical Journal of China*, 1928, 14(2): 103-105.
109 Wong, Chinmin K. Investigations of English Translations of *Bencao Gangmu* [J]. *National Medical Journal of China*, 1935, 21(10) : 1167-1170.
110 Wong, Chinmin K. & Fu Weikang. *Title Catalogue of Writings on Chinese Medicine in Foreign Languages* (1656-1962) [M]. Shanghai: Museum of History of Medicine of Shanghai College of Traditional Chinese Medicine, 1963.
111 World Health Organization. *WHO International Standard Terminologies on Traditional Medicine in the Western Pacific Region*. 2007.
112 Wu Guanghua. *The Chinese-English Dictionary* [Z]. 3rd Edition. Shanghai: Shanghai Translation Publishing House, 2010.
113 www.zdic.net
114 Xia Zhengnong. *Ci Hai* or *An Unabridged Comprehensive Dictionary* or *Sea of Words* [Z]. Shanghai: Shanghai Lexicographical Publishing House, 2002.
115 Xiao Jiansheng. *Chinese History Revisited* [M]. Hong Kong: New Century Press, 2009.
116 Xiao Mincai. Connotations of and Sinograms Related to "*Bian Zheng* or Pattern Identification" [J]. *Journal of Beijing College of Chinese Medicine*, 1984 (4):2.
117 Xie Zhufan. *On the Standard Nomenclature of Traditional Chinese Medicine* [M]. Beijing: Foreign Languages Press, 2003.
118 Xie Zhufan, Liao Jiazhen, Liu Ganzhong, et al. Comments on the English Equivalents of Chinese Terms in Traditional Chinese Medicine and Pharmacy [J]. *Chinese Journal of Integrated Traditional and Western Medicine*, 2006, 26 (2): 169-172.
119 Xing Yurui. The Theories and Methodology in the *Huang Di's Inner Classic* [M]. Xi'an: Shaanxi Science and Technology Press, 2004.
120 Composed by Xu Shen (Han Dynasty), Annotated by Duan Yucai (Qing Dynasty). *Shuo Wen Jie Zi* or *The Origin of Chinese Characters* [Z]. Shanghai: Shanghai Ancient Books Press, 1987.
121 Xu Youyu. *"Copernican" Revolution: Linguistic Transfer in Philosophy* [M]. Shanghai: Joint Publishing House, 1994.
122 Xue Feifei. The Emergence and Development of Pattern Identification based on Microcosmic Findings [D]. Beijing University of Chinese Medicine, 2006.
123 Yang Bojun, Xu Ti. *Dictionary of Zuo's Spring Autumn Annals* [Z]. Beijing: Zhonghua Book Company. 1985: 559.
124 Yang Bojun, Xu Ti. *Zuo's Spring Autumn Annals in Modern Chinese* [M]. Changsha: Yuelu Book Company, 1993.
125 Ye Shuxian, Tian Daxian. *The Mysterious Numbers in Ancient China* [M]. Beijing: Social Sciences Academic Press, 1998.
126 Yin Huihe. National Textbook for TCM Higher Education· *The Basic Theories of Chinese Medicine*. Shanghai: Shanghai Scientific and Technical Publishers. 1st ed., 1984; fifth printing, 1988.

127 Zhang Boyu. *Chinese Internal Medicine* [M]. Shanghai: Shanghai Scientific and Technical Publishers. 1989.
128 Zhang Daqing, Translator; Porter, Roy, Author. *The Cambridge Illustrated History of Medicine* [M]. Changchun: Jilin People's Publishing House, 2000.
129 Originally by Zhang Zhongjing; Translated by Luo Xiwen. *Synopsis of Prescriptions from the Golden Chamber (Jingui Yaolue)* . Beijing: New World Press. 2007.
130 Originally by Zhang Zhongjing; Translated by Luo Xiwen. *Treatise on Febrile Caused by Cold (Shanghan Lun)*. Beijing: New World Press. 2007.
131 Zhao Jimeng. *A Brief History of Modern Pharmacology of Chinese Herbal Medicine in China* [D]. Master Dissertation of China Academy of Chinese Medical Sciences, 2012.
132 Zheng Jinsheng. Prof . Unschuld's Path of Researching the History of Medicine in China [J]. *The Chinese Journal for the History of Science and Technology*, 2013, 34(1): 1-17.
133 Zhu Anyi. Interpreting Yin and Yang [J]. *Journal of Sichuan College of Education*, 2005, 21（3）: 47-48.
134 Zhu Jianping. On Standard Usage of Medical Sinograms "证", "症", and "征". *China Scientific and Technical Terms Journal*. 2003(4): 14-17.
135 Zhu WF. Concepts and Evolutions of Terms "证", "症", and "征". *China Scientific and Technical Terms Journal*. 2003(4): 20-21.
136 Zuo Min'an. *Detailed Interpretation of Chinese Characters: Origin and Evolution of 1,000 Sinograms* [M]. Beijing: Jiuzhou Press, 2005.

Historical Bibliography

(Before 1911)

Historical bibliography quoted in the book is listed here. The titles are arranged in chronological order by dynasty. Each entry includes the original Chinese, Pinyin transliteration, and an English translation or rendering of the Chinese title, as well as a brief introduction.

Pre-Qin Days (Before 221 B.C.)

论语
Lun Yu, or *The Analects of Confucius:* the first Confucian classic in book form appearing in the early Warring States Period (475-221 B.C.), comprising 20 chapters. It is a record of the words and deeds of Confucius (551-479 B.C.) and his disciples. The core idea of *The Analects* is *Ren* or Benevolence, which means "to love people". According to *The Analects*, to realize benevolence one has to use "*Li* or Rite or Propriety" as a norm for "To Restrain One's Selfishness and Restore Propriety is Benevolence". Besides, *The Analects* still embodies Confucius's political advocation of rule with virtue and opposition to harsh government, and his educational thought of "making no social distinctions in teaching" and of "teaching disciples in accordance with their aptitude".

詩經
Shi Jing, or *The Classic of Poetry:* translated variously as *The Book of Songs* and *The Book of Odes*, the earliest existing collection of Chinese poems and songs. It comprises 305 poems and songs, with the earliest range from the 10th to the 7th centuries B.C. The collection is classified into three parts according to their genre, namely *feng* 风, *ya* 雅 and *song* 颂: *Feng* 风, 160 folk songs of different localities; *Ya* 雅, 105 festal songs or odes; and *Song* 颂, 40 hymns and eulogies. *The Analects of Confucius* reads that "In *The Classic of Poetry* there are [around] 300 poems. But the essence of them can be covered in one sentence: 'Have no depraved thoughts'."

書經, 尚書
Shu Jing, or *The Classic of Documents; Shang Shu*, literally *Esteemed Documents:* translated variously as "*The Classic of History*", "*The Classic of Documents*", "*The Book of History*", "*The Book of Documents*". It is the earliest compilation of documentary records related to events from the Yu Shun through Xia, Shang to Zhou Dynasties until the reign of Duke Mu of Qin (Qin Mu Gong), i.e. from ca. 22th Century to 621 B.C., in ancient history of China.

禮記

Li Ji, or *The Classic of Rites*: also known as *The Book of Rites, The Book of Customs, The Record of Rites*, described the social forms, governmental system, and ancient ceremonial rites of the Zhou Dynasty (ca. 1050 – 256 B.C.). The work is not to be confused with the two other classical texts on rites: *Zhou Li* or *The Rites of Zhou [Dynasty]* 周禮, which is a collection of bureaucratic establishment with characteristics of archives; and *Yi Li* or *The Book of Etiquette and Ceremonies* 儀禮, which records complicated ceremonial procedures of Zhou rulers, something like a schedule of a professional master of ceremonies.

易经

Yi Jing, or *The I Ching*, or *The Classic of Changes:* also commonly known as *The Book of Changes* and *Zhou Yi*. It is one of the oldest classical Chinese texts, which "was completed by three sages, namely Fu Xi 伏羲, Wen Wang 文王 and Confucius, through three eras". Fu Xi made the Eight Trigrams by observing the Heaven and the Earth; King Wen of Zhou Dynasty (Zhou Wen Wang) doubled the Eight Trigrams into Sixty-Four Hexagrams and gave text comments on them; Confucius composed *Shi Yi* or *Ten Wings* 十翼 to interpret the sixty-four hexagrams, and thus transforming *The I Ching* from a divination book to a philosophical masterpiece, and finally to a classic of Confucianism. Actually, being composed of symbols (trigrams & hexagrams) and interpreting words, it is also a remarkable piece of writing on metaphor, and occupies an immeasurable place in the metaphor studies of China.

春秋

Chun Qiu, or *The Spring and Autumn Annals*: the official chronicle of the State of Lu covering the period from 722 to 481 B.C.. It is the earliest surviving Chinese historical text to be arranged on annalistic principles. Its contents involve various aspects such as politics, military affairs, economics, culture, astronomy, meteorological phenomena, material production, and social life, which are original records with correct time, place and figure of that time. The text is extremely concise and, if all the commentaries are excluded, about 16,000 sinograms long. Because of this its meaning can only be appreciated with the aid of ancient commentaries, especially the traditional *Zuo Zhuan* or *Commentary of Zuo [Qiuming]*.

左传，左氏春秋

Zuo Zhuan, *Zuo Shi Chun Qiu*, or *Zuo's Spring Autumn Annals:* a historical record from 722 to 453 B.C. which forms the three records or elucidations relative to events coverd in *Confucius's Spring and Autumn Annals*, and an important Confucian classic. Its authorship is generally attributed to Zuo Qiuming 左丘明 (502? – 422? B.C.) of the Spring and Autumn Period.

老子，道德经

Lao Zi, or *Lao Tzu; Dao De Jing,* or *Dao Te Ching:* the most important Daoist text, also known as *Dao Te Ching,* as the Chapter 51 reads that "All things respect Dao and value Te". Its authorship is attributed to Lao Tzu 老子 (580? – 500 B.C.). Dating back to the 3rd century B.C., it has 81 short chapters, contains altogether 5,635 sinograms, which is composed by 815 different ones. It contains many paradoxes and profound teachings on living in harmony with the nature.

荀子

Xun Zi, or *Xun Tzu*, or *The Book of Xun Tzu:* an important Confucian classic involving such aspects as philosophy, politics, ways of conducting oneself in society and doing scholarly research as well as academic augumentation. It is a collection of essays chiefly by Xun Tzu 荀子 (300? – 230? B.C.), who spread Confucianism throughout China and developed it as the realistic wing of Confucianism. Unlike the aphoristic style of *The Analects of Confucius* and *Mencius*, Xun Tzu was a more rigorous thinker and wrote elaborately argued essays with well-knit syntax, plenty of metaphors and parallel constructions in form.

庄子

Zhuang Zi, or *Chuang Tzu:* a famous Daoist book named after its purported author Chuang Tzu 庄子 (369? – 286? B.C.), also known as *Nan Hua Zhen Jing* or T*rue Classic of Southern Florescence* since 742 A.D. alluding to the tradition that Chuang Tzu came from South China. According to *Han Shu Yi Wen Zhi* or *Treatise on Literature* of *History of the Former Han Dynasty*, it had 52 chapters, but only 33 has transmitted down until today, among which 7 are inner chapters, 15 outer chapters, and 11 miscellaneous chapters. The authorship of the inner chapters is generally attributed to Chuang Tzu himself, and the others to his followers and other Daoists afterwards. The popular version of *Chuang Tzu* with 33 chapters nowadays was compiled by Guo Xiang 郭象 (252-312) of the Western Jin Dynasty (265-316).

Chuang Tzu bears very high values in both literature and philosophy. Its achievements in the literature are mainly embodied in the aspects of romantic writing, realistic description, fables in different poses and with different expressions as well as forceful, boundless, free and natural language. Prose in *Chuang Tzu* can be regarded as the beginning of the romantic writings in China.

周礼

Zhou Li, or *The Rites of Zhou [Dynasty]*: a collection of bureaucratic establishment of the Zhou Dynasty (ca. 1050 – 256 B.C.) with characteristics of archives. It has six essays on respectively Heaven, Earth, Spring, Summer, Autumn, and Winter Officials. *Zhou Li* has become one of the Confucian classics, and one of the "Three Rites" with the other two *Li Ji* or *The Classic of Rites* and *Yi Li* or *The Book of Etiquette and Ceremonies* since the Tang Dynasty (618-907).

国语

Guo Yu, or *Records of States:* the earliest monograph of the history of different states from around 990 to 453 B.C. extant in China.

韩非子

Han Fei Zi, or Han Fei Tzu: a collection of essays by Han Fei 韩非 (281? – 233 B.C.), a famous philosopher, thinker, and political commentator, who epitomized the thought of the Legalist School. His essays are well-knit with strict precise reasoning, penetrating, incisive analysis, and a trenchant humurous pen.

吕氏春秋

Lyu Shi Chun Qiu, or *Lyu's Spring and Autumn Annals*: an encyclopedic classical Chinese text compiled around 239 B.C. under the patronage of the Chancellor of Qin Dynasty Lyu Buwei 吕不韦 (?-235 B.C.), and a typical representative work of the Eclectics. Several chapters of it such as *Shang Nong* or *Valuing Farming*, *Bian Tu* or *Differentiating Soils*, *Shen Shi* or *Observing Seasons*, etc. are regarded as important materials to study the thought of the School of Agriculturalists.

管子

Guan Zi, or *Guan Tzu:* a collection of viewpoints of different thoughts of school including Schools of Legalists, Literati, Yin-Yang, Names, Militarists, and Agricultualists. The authorship is said to be Guan Zhong 管仲 (ca. 723? or 716? – 645 B.C.), a famous politician, militalist, and Prime Minsiter of the State of Qi, of the Spring and Autumn Period. The current version, originally 86 articles and 76 remaining until now, was edited and finalized by Liu Xiang 刘向 (77? – 6 B.C.) of the Western Han Dynasty.

山海经

Shan Hai Jing, or *The Classic of the Mountains and Seas*, a classical Chinese text of the Pre-Qin Days, and largely a fabled geographical and cultural account of Pre-Qin China as well as a collection of mythology.

黄帝内经，内经

Huang Di Nei Jing, or *Huang Di's Inner Classic*: also known as *The Nei Jing*, comprising *Su Wen* 素问 or *Basic Questions*, and *Ling Shu* 灵枢, or *Miracullous Pivot*, the earliest systematic, complete and greatest medical classic extant in China. The authorship was attributed to an ancient legendary ruler Huang Di or Yellow Emperor (2698? – 2589? B.C.). But actually the work was a product of various unknown authors in the Warring States Period (475-221 B.C.), and it is comparable in importance to the *Hippocratic Corpus* in Greek medicine. It is not only the breeding ground of the ontological concepts and fundamental theories of Chinese medicine, but also an important component part of excellent cultural heritage of China. It has been guiding the development of Chinese medicine for over 2,000 years. As Donald Harper said, it is "the essential reference for ancient Chinese medicine and a valuable to research on early Chinese civilization".

Qin and Han Dynasties（221 B.C. – 220 A.D.）

尔雅
Er Ya, or *Approaching to the Standard:* one of "the Thirteen Classics" on Confucianism, and the earliest dictionary to explain meanings of *Ci* or significant single or compound sinograms arranged according to meanings. It was finished in between the Warring States Period and the early Han Dynasty, and was first recorded in the *Treatise on Literature* of *The History of the Former Han Dynasty.* It is regarded as the first book on explaining words in ancient books in China, and has exerted important influences on exegetic studies, phonology, etymology, dialects, and philology.

淮南子
Huai Nan Zi, or *Huai Nan Tzu:* a collection of essays of the Western Han Dynasty (206 B.C. – A.D. 24), also known as *Huai Nan Hong Lie* or *Liu An Zi* for its compilation was directed by a royal family member, Duke of Huainan Liu An 刘安 (179-122 B.C.). Based on thoughts of Daoist School before 221 B.C., it synthesizes essence of other thoughts of school like Schools of Yin-Yang, Mohists, Legalists, and Literati, and is listed as a work of the Eclectics by *Treatise on Literature* of *History of the Former Han Dynasty*.

史记
Shi Ji, or *The Historical Records,* or *The Records of Grand Historian:* China's first dynastic history, completed ca. 86 B.C. by Sima Qian 司马迁 (145 or 135 ? – ca. 86 B.C.), who is regarded as the father of Chinese historiography because of his highly praised work. It is a general history of China covering more than two thousand years from a legendary ruler Huang Di 黄帝 (2698? – 2589? B.C.), known as the Yellow Emperor in the West, to Emperor Han Wu Di Liu Che (156-87 B.C.), and thus laying a solid foundation for later Chinese historiography.

难经，黄帝八十一难经
Nan Jing, or *The Classic of Questioning*, or *The Classic of Difficult Issues*: also known as *Huang Di's Eighty One Difficult Issues*, originally compiled during the first century A.D. by an unknown author though its authorship is often ascribed to Qin Yueren 秦越人 (407-310 B.C.). It deals with fundamental theories in the form of questions and answers. Acupoints, needling method, physiological and pathological conditions to *Jing Luo* or the vessels, and pulse-taking method are all discussed. "It marked the

apex and the conclusion of the initial development phase of a conceptual system of health care based on the doctrines of the Five Phases and yinyang. As the classic of the medicine of systematic correspondence, the *Nan-Ching* covers all aspects of theoretical and practical health care within these doctrines in an unusually systematic fashion. Most important is its innovative discussion of pulse diagnosis and needle treatment". (From the Inside Front Cover of the *Nan-Ching*, translated and annotated by Paul U. Unschuld, published by The University of California Press, 1986.)

春秋繁露

Chun Qiu Fan Lu, or *The Luxuriant Dew of the Spring and Autumn Annals:* an important Confucian classic, and one of the works that was attributed to Dong Zhongshu 董仲舒 (179-104 B.C.), a famous thinker and politician, who proposed "To proscribe all non-Confucian schools of thoughts and to espouse Confucianism as the orthodox state ideology", which was taken by Han Wu Di Liu Che 刘彻 (156-87 B.C.). And thereafter Confucianism was established as an official religion of China and the leading philosophical thought in China until 1905. The book deified Confucius by propogating the doctrine of *Tian Ren Gan Ying* or Interactions between Heaven and Man and integrating yin-yang and five phases into an ethical and political framework, which lays down rules for deciding the legitimacy of a monarch as well as providing a set of checks and balances for reigning a monarch. Such a proposal legitimated the emperors' autocratic government for thousands of years since Han Wu Di in China.

神农本草经

Shen Nong Ben Cao Jing, or *Shennong's Classic of Materia Medica:* the earliest monograph on materia medica in China and one of "The Four Great Classics" on Chinese medicine, believed to be a work of the first century B.C. with its authorship attributed to Shennong, a god in charge of agriculture and medicine. The original ancient work has been lost. Its contents have been preserved in quotations in the books on materia medica of the past ages. It records properties, flavors, actions and indications of 365 medicinals in three grades: top, medium, and lower in details. Scholars restored it by collecting quotations from the books on materia medica of its later ages.

新论 · 形神

Xin Lun · Xing Shen, or *Body and Spirit* of *New Argumentation*: the first treatise on body and spirit in the history of Chinese philosophy by Huan Tan 桓谭 (23 B.C. – 50 A.D.), which advances a famous metaphor – the relationship between body and spirit is just like that between the candle and its flame, in which candle metaphorizes the body and flame the spirit.

汉书·艺文志

Han Shu Yi Wen Zhi, or *Treatise on Literature* of *The History of the Former Han Dynasty:* the earliest literature on bibliography and the earliest systematic title catalogue extant in China, compiled by Ban Gu 班固 (A.D. 32-92), who took the *Qi Lue* 七略 by Liu Xiang 刘向 (78-8 B.C.) and his son Liu Xin 刘歆 (50 B.C.? – 23 A.D.) as the primary source. Liu Xiang and Liu Xin were the first two persons in the history of China to systematize the available books, which were presented to the Han Imperial Court from the whole country after the event of burning books (of poetics, master philosophers and their school thoughts) in 213 B.C. in Qin Shi Huang's reign. They were put in charge of writing a catalogue of the books that were stored in the imperial library in the late first century B.C. Their survey began in 26 B.C. Their catalogue, called *Qi Lue*, was later lost, but not before it was used by Ban Gu to compile the bibliographical monograph - *Treatise on Literature*, a part of *Han Shu* or *The History of the Former Han Dynasty*.

论衡

Lun Heng, or *Critical Essays:* an important work finished around 86 A.D. by Wang Chong 王充 (27-100 A.D), a famous thinker, philosopher, and educator. It contains 85 essays with one missing and over 200,000 sinograms. It has been listed in the category of the Eclectics in the bibliographies since *Sui Shu Jing Ji Zhi* or *Treatise on Classics and Documents* of *The History of Sui Dynasty* by Wei Zheng 魏征 (580-643), the second oldest historical bibliography after *Treatise on Literature* of *The History of the Former Han Dynasty*. The author discussed significant issues on philosophy, politics, religion, and culture, augued against the viewpoint of Interaction between Universe and Man proposed by Dong Zhongshu, held that all things in the universe, including man and universe, are all natural existant beings resulting from a natural process known as the movement and mutation of *qi*, and Universe is not a deified God; denied the existance of *Gui* or Ghost; and opposed the ideology of "Esteeming the Universe and Following the Old".

说文解字

Shuo Wen Jie Zi, or *The Origin of Chinese Characters: Shuo Wen Jie Zi* literally means "explaining pictographs and analyzing composite sinograms". I prefer to translate the title into *The Origin of Chinese Characters*. It is the first comprehensive systematic dictionary of sinograms arranged by sections with shared components, called radicals (*bùshǒu*, lit. "section headers") and finished in 100 A.D. by Xu Shen 许慎 (A.D. 58? – 147?) of the Eastern Han Dynasty. It is also the first dictionary which interprets the original meaning of a sinogram by analyzing its structure and gives the rationale behind it, sometimes the etymology of the sinogram as well. Actually, it is far beyond a dictionary, and moreover it can be interpreted from cultural and philosophical perspectives. It is indeed the case that no monograph on philosophy of Chinese language has ever been available up till today except this book.

伤寒杂病论
Shang Han Za Bing Lun, or *Treatise on Cold-induced and Miscellaneous Diseases:* a famous work by a world famous medical expert Zhang Zhongjing 张仲景(150-219), systematized and rearranged into "*Shang Han Lun* or *On Cold-induced Diseases*" and "*Jin Gui Yao Lue* or *Synopsis of the Prescriptions from the Golden Chamber*", which are regarded as the two of the "Four Great Classics on Chinese Medicine" (the other two are *Huang Di's Inner Classic* and *Shennong's Classic of Materia Medica*), and have been the required readings and courses for majors of Chinese medicine even up till today.

伤寒论
Shang Han Lun, or *On Cold-induced Diseases:* one of the most influential works in the history of Chinese medicine, the part on "cold-induced diseases" of *Treatise on Cold-induced and Miscellaneous Diseases,* rearranged by Wang Shuhe in 10 volumes.

金匮要略
Jin Gui Yao Lue, or *Synopsis of the Golden Chamber:* one of the most influential works in the history of Chinese medicine, the part on "miscellaneous diseases" of *Treatise on Cold-induced and Miscellaneous Diseases,* dealing with miscellaneous diseases of internal medicine, and some external and women's diseases, rearranged by Wang Shuhe in 3 volumes and 25 chapters, including 262 prescriptions.

The Three Kingdoms (220-265)

广雅
Guang Ya, or *Supplement to Er Ya:* an encyclopediac dictionary to explain meanings of *Ci* or significant single or compound sinograms in literature before Wei (220-265), one of the Three Kingdoms by Zhang Yi 张揖, Doctor of Wei Kingdom (220-265). As an supplement to *Er Ya* 尔雅, it includes 18,150 sinograms.

脉经
Mai Jing, or *The Classic of Pulse Diagnosis*: written by Wang Shuhe 王叔和 (201-280), which records 24 pulses and is generally acknowledged as the standard work and the earliest comprehensive monograph on sphygmology extant.

The Northern and Southern Dynasties (420-589)

神灭论
Shén Miè Lùn, or *On the Annihilation of the Spirit*: a famous work on annihilation of the Spirit by Fan Zhen 范缜 (ca. 450-515), a Chinese philosopher and thinker of the Southern Dynasty. It insists on the primary importance of the materials, systematically expounds the viewpoints of atheism, points out that man is the unity of body and spirit, and metaphorizes the relationship between the body and the spirit as that between the sword and its sharpness.

全元起注素问
Quan Yuaqi Zhu Su Wen, or *Quan Yuanqi's Annotated Version of Su Wen:* the earliest annotated version of *Su Wen* or *Basic Questions* in China by Quan Yuanqi 全元起 (?-?), a famous medical expert living in the Northern and Southern Dynasties. It lost in between Norther Song (960-1127) and Southern Song (1127-1279) Dynasty. A famous modern Chinese scholar Duan Yishan 段逸山 (1940–) tried to restore it based on his research, and published the outcome entitled "Su Wen Quan Yuanqi Ben Yan Jiu Yu Ji Fu" or "Research and Restoration of *Quan Yuanqi's Annotated Version of Su Wen*" 素问全元起本研究与辑复 in 2001.

玉篇
Yu Pian, or *Jade Writings*: a dictionary arranged according to forms and structures of sinograms compiled by Gu Yewang 顾野王 (519-581) in 543.

Sui-Tang Dynasties (581-907)

五行大义
Wu Xing Da Yi, or *The Great Connotations of the Five Phases:* the most important work on five phases of the middle ancient times written by Xiao Ji 萧吉 in 594 for his emperor, a comment from Joseph Needham (1900-1995), which not only epitomised the thoughts on five phases theory before its time, but is also a must for studying the entire developing course of five phases theory in China as well as the theory of Images and Numbers of *The Book of Changes*.

诸病源候论
Zhu Bing Yuan Hou Lun, or *Treatise on Origins and Symptoms of Diseases:* the earliest monograph on origins and symptoms of diseases in China compiled by Chao Yuanfang 巢元方 (?-?), et al. in 610 with 30 volumes of detailed discussions on origins and symptoms of various diseases, including diseases of internal medicine, external medicine, gynecology, pediatrics, ENT, mouth and teeth, orthopedics and traumatology, and some infectious diseases, parasitic diseases, and surgery. It summarizes

medical achievements before 610, and consists of 67 categories with 1,720 entries and many brilliant expositions frequently cited by authors of later generations.

备急千金要方
Bei Ji Qian Jin Yao Fang, or *Invaluable Prescriptions for Emergencies:* also known as *Qian Jin Yao Fang*, or *Invaluable Prescriptions* for short, a famous work compiled by Sun Simiao 孙思邈 (581-682), in 30 volumes with a general introduction, prescriptions of various clinical branches, diets, pulse-taking, acupuncture, etc. *Da Yi Jing Cheng* or *A Great Doctor Should Be Expert in Medical Skills and Sincere to His Patients* 大医精诚, an important essay on medical ethics, is from the first volume of the book.

Song Dynasty (960-1279)

太平御览
Tai Ping Yu Lan: a large-sized *Lei Shu* or reference book with materials taken from various sources and arranged according to subjects compiled by Li Fang 李昉 (925-996), et al. from 977 to 983. It has 1,000 volumes and 5 millions of sinograms. It quotes altogether 2,579 kinds of books including 1,690 historical and classical ones, most of which have lost, therefore it has preserved plenty of valuable materials for us.

经史证类备急本草
Jing Shi Zheng Lei Bei Ji Ben Cao, or *Classic of Classified Materia Medica for Emergencies*: compiled by Tang Shenwei 唐慎微 (1056-1093) in 1082, a Confucian physician, which summarizes achievements on materia medica of the former ages, includes records on materia medica from Confucian classics, historical records, philosophical writings, and miscellaneous works as well as the Buddhist and Daoist Scriptures. It includes 1,746 kinds of medicinal agents with directions for use and preparation, and many new prescriptions. It laid a solid foundation for the development of Chinese materia medica. Li Shizhen, a Confucian physician, took it as a chief source of his monumental work *Ben Cao Gang Mu*.

本草衍义
Ben Cao Yan Yi, or *Augmented Materia Medica:* compiled by Kou Zongshi 寇宗奭 (?-?), a Confucian official, in 1116, supplementing what *Jing Shi Zheng Lei Bei Ji Ben Cao* lacks such as some medicinal agents' actions and methods to differentiate similar ones. It includes 472 medicinal agents, and suggests that the dosage of a medicinal should vary according to age, constitution, and emergent or chronic condition.

Ming Dynasty (1368-1644)

难经集注
Nan Jing Ji Zhu or *A Collection of Annotations on The Classic of Difficult Issues*: a collection of annotations on *The Classic of Difficult Issues* from Lyu Guang 吕广 of the Three Kingdoms (220-265), Yang Xuancao 杨玄操 of the Tang Dynasty (618-907), Ding Deyong 丁德用, et al. of the Song Dynasty (960-1279) by Wang Jiusi 王九思 in 1505 of the Ming Dynasty (1384-1644), the extant earliest collection of annotations on *The Classic of Difficult Issues*. It has 5 volumes and 13 chapters.

本草纲目
Ben Cao Gang Mu, or *The Compendium of Materia Medica:* finished in 1578 by Li Shizhen 李时珍 (1518-1593), appraised as the "encyclopedia of China published in 1596", which not only makes great contribution to Chinese pharmacology, but also exerts far-reaching influences on pharmacology, botany, zoology, mineralogy, and chemistry of the whole world.

六科证治准绳
Liu Ke Zheng Zhi Zhun Sheng, or *Standards of Diagnosis and Treatment in Six Branches of Medicine:* a famous work with 120 volumes by Wang Kentang 王肯堂 (1549-1613), a Confucian official, which epitomized the achievements on medicine before its time and was highly appraised by medical practitioners afterwards.

类经
Lei Jing, or *Classified Inner Classic:* a famous work of comprehensive classified studies on *Huang Di Nei Jing* with 32 volumes, and one of the representative works by Zhang Jiebin 张介宾 (1563-1640), also known as Zhang Jingyue 张景岳, a famous medical expert.

景岳全书
Jingyue Quan Shu, or *Jingyue's Complete Works*: 64 volumes by Zhang Jiebin 张介宾 (1563-1640), also known as Zhang Jingyue 张景岳, a famous medical expert.

Qing Dynasty (1644-1911)

绎史
Yi Shi: a historical record by Ma Xiao 马骕 (1621-1673), including five parts – Time Immemoria, Three Dynasties (Xia, Shang, and Western Zhou), Spring and Autumn, Warring States, and External Records.

本草崇原

Ben Cao Chong Yuan, or *The Origin of Materia Medica:* a monograph on materia medica with 3 volumes, which annotates *Shennong's Classic of Materia Medica,* by Zhang Zhicong 张志聪 (1616-1674). Based on the five circuit phases, six climatic factors, and waxing and waning between yin and yang, Zhang Zhicong founded the *Yao Qi* 药气 theory to expound actions of medicinals in details, which starts from the formation of properties and flavors, attributes of yin-yang and five-phases as well as shapes and colors of medicinals, and then is related to the machanism of curing an illness. His approach deeply influenced such medical experts as Xu Dachun 徐大椿 (1693-1771) and Chen Xiuyuan 陈修园 (1753-1823).

本草备要

Ben Cao Bei Yao, or *Essentials of Materia Medica*: a clinical manual of materia medica and a door to Chinese medicine with 8 volumes and published in 1694 by Wang Ang 汪昂 (1615-1695). It mainly draws materials from *Ben Cao Gang Mu* or *The Compendium of Materia Medica* by Li Shizhen 李时珍 (1518-1593) published in 1596 and *Shen Nong Ben Cao Jing Shu* or *Commentaries on Shennong's Classic of Materia Medica* by Miu Xiyong 缪希雍 (1546-1627) published in 1625. It has exerted deep-going and far-reaching influences on Chinese medical majors of the later ages, for example, until 1963, it had been reprinted 107 times since its first publication.

画语录

Hua Yu Lu, or *Arts of Painting:* also known as *Shi Dao Hua Yu Lu* or *Ku Gua He Shang Hua Yu Lu,* a monograph on arts of painting by Shi Dao 石涛 (1630-1724), a painting wonder, whose paintings and achievements in Daoism, Buddhism, literature, and poetry exerted far-reaching and deep-going influences on the development of classical Chinese painting, and are appreciated by the people today.

医学源流论

Yi Xuen Yuan Liu Lun, or *The Origin and Development of [Chinese] Medicine:* A collection of 99 essays on Chinese medicine by Xu Dachun 徐大椿 (1693-1771) finished in 1757. It has 2 volumes: Vol. 1 one on the vessels, *zang fu* organs, pulse, illnesses, prescriptions and medicinals, and Vol. 2 on therapeutic methods, commentaries on medical books, clinical medicine and other topics. The book presents a lot of author's original creative ideas on Chinese medicine.

LIBRI NIGRI
DENKEN ÜBER GRENZEN

Herausgegeben von Hans Rainer Sepp

Die *libri nigri* treffen sich bevorzugt an Orten, an denen die Grenzen von Wirklichkeitsbereichen, Standpunkten, Fachrichtungen sowie Kultur- und Wissenstraditionen in den Blick geraten und ihre Voraussetzungen verhandelbar werden. Begründungsabsichten nachzuspüren, gilt hier mehr, als Begründungen zu suchen, das wagende Experiment mehr als die gültige Schablone, die störende Bewegung mehr als der Drang nach Absicherung. Da die Orte für entscheidende Bewegungen meist Ränder und nicht Zentren sind und da Grenzen nicht einfach nur begrenzen, sondern vor allem Potentiale des Anderen und Fremden bergen, wird sich die Reihe auch dem Terrain des Utopischen nicht verweigern.

1 Hans Rainer Sepp
Die Grenze denken
Prolegomena zu einer Philosophie des Transkulturellen
broschiert ISBN 978-3-88309-792-3
gebunden ISBN 978-3-88309-793-0

2 Yoshiko Oshima
Zen – anders denken?
Zugleich ein Versuch über Zen und Heidegger
2. Aufl.
broschiert ISBN 978-3-88309-846-3
gebunden ISBN 978-3-88309-847-0

3 Max Lorenzen
Philosophie der Nachmoderne
Die Transformation der Kultur – Virtualität und Globalisierung
Herausgegeben von Cathrin Nielsen
broschiert ISBN 978-3-88309-668-8
gebunden ISBN 978-3-88309-668-1

4 Hisaki Hashi und Friedrich G. Wallner (Hg.)
Globalisierung des Denkens in Ost und West
Resultate des Österreichisch-Japanischen Dialogs
broschiert ISBN 978-3-88309-555-4
gebunden ISBN 978-3-88309-560-8

5 Aleš Novák
Heideggers Bestimmung des Bösen
broschiert ISBN 978-3-88309-650-6
gebunden ISBN 978-3-88309-651-3

6 André Julien S. E. Faict
Philosophische Voraussetzungen des interkulturellen Dialogs
Die vergleichende Philosophie von Hajime Nakamura
im Dialog mit Anthropologie und Hermeneutik
broschiert ISBN 978-3-88309-683-4
gebunden ISBN 978-3-88309-684-1

7 Peter Schwankl
Diplomatisches Verhalten
Ein phänomenologischer Versuch über das Wesen des Diplomatischen
Herausgegeben von Georg Lechner
broschiert ISBN 978-3-88309-517-2
gebunden ISBN 978-3-88309-516-5

8 Paul Janssen
Vom zersprungenen Weltwerden
broschiert ISBN 978-3-88309-685-8
gebunden ISBN 978-3-88309-686-5

9 Constantin Noica
De dignitate Europae
Übersetzt von Georg Scherg
Herausgegeben von Mădălina Diaconu
broschiert ISBN 978-3-88309-708-4
gebunden ISBN 978-3-88309-709-1

10 Constantin Noica
Briefe zur Logik des Hermes
Übersetzt von Christian Ferencz-Flatz und Stefan Moosdorf
broschiert ISBN 978-3-88309-434-2
gebunden ISBN 978-3-88309-435-9

11 Ananta Charan Sukla (ed.)
Art and Expression
Contemporary Perspectives in the Occidental and Oriental Traditions
broschiert ISBN 978-3-88309-710-7
gebunden ISBN 978-3-88309-711-4

12 Dean Komel
Den Nihilismus verwinden
Ein slowenisches Postscript zum 20. Jahrhundert
broschiert ISBN 978-3-88309-712-1
gebunden ISBN 978-3-88309-713-8

13 Tatiana Shchyttsova (Hg.)
In statu nascendi
Geborensein und intergenerative Dimension des menschlichen Miteinanderseins
broschiert ISBN 978-3-88309-716-9
gebunden ISBN 978-3-88309-688-9

14 Chung-Chi Yu and Kwok-ying Lau (eds.)
Phenomenology and Human Experience
broschiert ISBN 978-3-88309-722-0
gebunden ISBN 978-3-88309-723-7

15 Daniel Aebli
Wie modern ist die Antike?
Studien und Skizzen zur Altertumswissenschaft
broschiert ISBN 978-3-88309-729-9
gebunden ISBN 978-3-88309-730-5

16 Hiroo Nakamura
Für den Frieden
broschiert ISBN 978-3-88309-731-2
gebunden ISBN 978-3-88309-732-9

17 Günter Fröhlich
Anthropologische Wege
Ulmer Stadthausvorträge
broschiert ISBN 978-3-88309-733-6
gebunden ISBN 978-3-88309-734-3

18 Hans-Dieter Bahr
Die Anwesenheit des Gastes
Entwurf einer Xenosophie
broschiert ISBN 978-3-88309-761-9

19 Massimo Mezzanzanica
Von Dilthey zu Levinas
Wege im Zwischenbereich von Lebensphilosophie, Neukantianismus und Phänomenologie
broschiert ISBN 978-3-88309-750-3

20 Klaus Kanzog
Mit Auge und Ohr
Studien zur komplementären Wahrnehmung
broschiert ISBN 978-3-88309-784-8
gebunden ISBN 978-3-88309-785-5

21 Silvia Stoller und Gerhard Unterthurner (Hg.)
Entgrenzungen der Phänomenologie und Hermeneutik
Festschrift für Helmuth Vetter zum 70. Geburtstag
broschiert ISBN 978-3-88309-771-8
gebunden ISBN 978-3-88309-772-5

22 Claus C. Schnorrenberger
Chinesische Medizin –
Placebo, Wissenschaft oder Wirklichkeit?
broschiert ISBN 978-3-88309-776-3
gebunden ISBN 978-3-88309-777-0

23 Detlef Thiel
Maßnahmen des Erscheinens
Friedlaender/Mynona im Gespräch mit
Schelling, Husserl, Benjamin und Derrida
broschiert ISBN 978-3-88309-782-4
gebunden ISBN 978-3-88309-783-1

24 Leonidas Donskis
Fifty Letters from the Troubled Modern World
A Philosophical-Political Diary 2009–2012
broschiert ISBN 978-3-88309-799-2
gebunden ISBN 978-3-88309-800-5

25 Hartmut Buchner
Heidegger und Japan – Japan und Heidegger
Vorläufiges zum west-östlichen Gespräch
broschiert ISBN 978-3-88309-836-4
gebunden ISBN 978-3-88309-837-1

26 Kateřina Šolcová
Comenius im Blick
Der Briefwechsel zwischen Milada Blekastad und Dmitrij Tschižewskij
Deutsch-Tschechische Ausgabe
broschiert ISBN 978-3-88309-843-2
gebunden ISBN 978-3-88309-844-9

27 Karin Knobel
Poetik des Staubes bei Goethe und Hafis
broschiert ISBN 978-3-88309-838-8
gebunden ISBN 978-3-88309-839-5

28 Ryôsuke Ohashi
Schnittpunkte
Essays zum ost-westlichen-Gespräch
Erster Band: Dimensionen des Ästhetischen
broschiert ISBN 978-3-88309-859-3
gebunden ISBN 978-3-88309-860-9

29 Ryôsuke Ohashi
Schnittpunkte
Essays zum ost-westlichen-Gespräch
Zweiter Band: Deutsch-Japanische Denkwege
broschiert ISBN 978-3-88309-885-2
gebunden ISBN 978-3-88309-886-9

30 Aleš Novák (Hg.)
Grenzen der Transzendenz
Aus dem Tschechischen übersetzt von Jana Krötzsch
broschiert ISBN 978-3-88309-854-8
gebunden ISBN 978-3-88309-855-5

31 Boško Tomašević
Hervorgang des Seins
Das ontologische Geschehen des Dichtens
broschiert ISBN 978-3-88309-952-1
gebunden ISBN 978-3-88309-953-8

32 Gerard Visser
Nichts ist geschenkt
Ein philosophischer Essay über die Seele
Aus dem Niederländischen übersetzt von Anna Sikora
broschiert ISBN 978-3-88309-871-5
gebunden ISBN 978-3-88309-872-2

33 Marcin Rebes
Der Streit um die transzendentale Wahrheit
Heidegger und Levinas
broschiert ISBN 978-3-88309-942-2
gebunden ISBN 978-3-88309-943-9

34 Jürgen Trinks
Überleben des Phänomens im Symbolischen
Studien zur sprachphänomenologischen Kulturwissenschaft
broschiert ISBN 978-3-88309-875-3
gebunden ISBN 978-3-88309-876-0

35 Martin Cajthaml
Europe and the Care of the Soul
Jan Patočka's Conception of the Spiritual Foundations of Europe
With a Preface by Peter McCormick
broschiert ISBN 978-3-88309-887-6
gebunden ISBN 978-3-88309-888-3

36 Leonidas Donskis
Das Ende von Ideologie und Utopie?
Moralität und Kulturkritik im zwanzigsten Jahrhundert
Aus dem Englischen übersetzt von Cathrin Nielsen
broschiert ISBN 978-3-88309-883-8
gebunden ISBN 978-3-88309-884-5

37 Dean Komel
Kontemplationen
Entwürfe zur phänomenologischen Hermeneutik
broschiert ISBN 978-3-88309-903-3
gebunden ISBN 978-3-88309-904-0

38 Armin Wildermuth
Findlinge
Gefundenes und Erfundenes
broschiert ISBN 978-3-88309-944-6
gebunden ISBN 978-3-88309-945-3

39 Hisaki Hashi (Hg.)
Denkdisziplinen von Ost und West
Interdisziplinäre Philosophie in einer globalen Welt

40 Markus Ophälders
Konstruktion von Erfahrung
Versuch über Walter Benjamin

41 Ivan Chvatík and Lubica Ucník (eds.)
Asubjective Phenomenology
Jan Patočka's Project in the Broader Context of his Work

42 Terri Jane Hennings
Writing Against Aesthetic Ideology
Tom Sharpe's *The Great Pursuit* and Paul Auster's *City of Glass*

43 Irina Hron (ed.)
Thinking in Unity after Postmodernism
Figures of Unity, Presence, and Transcendence at the Millennium

44 Nicole Thiemer
Zwischen Hermes und Hestia
Hermeneutische Lektüren zu Heidegger und Derrida
broschiert ISBN 978-3-88309-946-0
gebunden ISBN 978-3-88309-947-7

45 Sumalee Mahanarongchai
Health and Disease in Buddhist Minds
broschiert ISBN 978-3-88309-950-4
gebunden ISBN 978-3-88309-951-4

46 Fengli Lan and Friedrich G. Wallner (eds.)
The Concepts of Health and Disease
From the Viewpoint of four Cultures
broschiert ISBN 978-3-88309-948-4
gebunden ISBN 978-3-88309-949-1

47 Fengli Lan
Metaphor
The Weaver of Chinese Medicine
With an Introduction by Friedrich Wallner
broschiert ISBN 978-3-95948-020-8
gebunden ISBN 978-3-95948-039-0